Portal Hypertension IV

Portal Hypertension IV

Proceedings of the
Fourth Baveno International Consensus Workshop

EDITED BY
ROBERTO DE FRANCHIS MD
Professor of Gastroenterology
Department of Internal Medicine, University of Milan, and
Head, Gastroenterology and Gastrointestinal Endoscopy Service,
IRCCS Ospedale Maggiore Policlinico, Milan, Italy

Blackwell
Publishing

Blackwell Publishing, Inc., 350 Main Street, Malden, Massachusetts 02148-5020, USA
Blackwell Publishing Ltd, 9600 Garsington Road, Oxford OX4 2DQ, UK
Blackwell Publishing Asia Pty Ltd, 550 Swanston Street, Carlton, Victoria 3053, Australia

First published 2006

Library of Congress Cataloging-in-Publication Data

Baveno International Consensus Workshop (4th : 2005)
Portal hypertension IV : proceedings from the Fourth Baveno International Consensus Workshop / edited by Roberto de Franchis.
p. ; cm.
Includes bibliographical references and index.
ISBN-13: 978-1-4051-3940-3 (hardback : alk. paper)
ISBN-10: 1-4051-3940-4 (hardback : alk. paper)
1. Portal hypertension–Congresses. I. De Franchis, Roberto. II. Title. III. Title: Portal hypertension 4. IV. Title: Portal hypertension four.
[DNLM: 1. Hypertension, Portal–Congresses. 2. Gastrointestinal Hemorrhage–complications–Congresses. 3. Liver Diseases–complications–Congresses. WI 720 B353p 2006]

RC848.P6B38 2006
616.3'62–dc22

2005023981

ISBN-13: 978-1-4051-3940-3
ISBN-10: 1-4051-3940-4

A catalogue record for this title is available from the British Library

Set in 10/13 Sabon by Newgen Imaging Systems (P) Ltd, Chennai, India
Printed and bound in Haryana, India by Replika Press Pvt Ltd

Commissioning Editor: Alison Brown
Editorial Assistant: Saskia van der Linden
Development Editor: Fiona Pattison
Production Controller: Kate Charman

For further information on Blackwell Publishing, visit our website:
http://www.blackwellpublishing.com

The publisher's policy is to use permanent paper from mills that operate a sustainable forestry policy, and which has been manufactured from pulp processed using acid-free and elementary chlorine-free practices. Furthermore, the publisher ensures that the text paper and cover board used have met acceptable environmental accreditation standards.

Contents

Contributors

JUAN G. ABRALDES MD, *Research Associate, Hepatic Hemodynamic Laboratory, Hospital Clinic, IDIBAPS, Barcelona, Spain*

AGUSTIN ALBILLOS MD, *Assistant Professor of Medicine, Department of Gastroenterology, Hospital Ramon y Cajal, University of Alcalà, Madrid, Spain*

MARIO ANGELICO MD, *Professor of Gastroenterology, Department of Public Health and Cellular Biology, Tor Vergata University Medical School, Rome, Italy*

RAFAEL BAÑARES MD, *Associate Professor of Medicine, Liver Unit, Hospital General Universitario Gregorio Marañon, Madrid, Spain*

G. BAROSI MD, *Director, Laboratory of Clinical Epidemiology, IRCCS Policlinico S Matteo, Pavia, Italy*

FLEMMING BENDTSEN MD, *Dr Med.Sci., Head, Department of Gastroenterology, Hvidovre University Hospital, DK-2650 Hvidovre, Denmark*

BRIGITTE BERNARD-CHABERT MD, *Service d'Hépato-Gastro-entérologie, Centre Hôpitalier Universitaire Robert Debré, 51100 Reims, France*

ANNALISA BERZIGOTTI MD, *Department of Internal Medicine, Cardioangiology, Hepatology, University of Bologna, 40138, Bologna, Italy*

ANDRES T. BLEI MD, *Division of Hepatology, Department of Medicine, Lakeside VA Medical Center and Northwestern University Feinberg School of Medicine, Chicago, IL 60611, USA*

JAIME BOSCH MD, *Professor of Medicine, University of Barcelona, Senior Consultant Hepatologist, Liver Unit, Chief of Hepatology Section, IMD, Hospital Clinic, Barcelona, Spain*

THOMAS D. BOYER MD, *John J Lee Professor of Medicine, University of Arizona, Liver Research Institute, Tucson, AZ 85724, USA*

ANDREW K. BURROUGHS MD, *Liver Transplantation and Hepatobiliary Unit, Royal Free Hospital, London, UK*

PAUL CALÈS MD, *CHU, University of Angers, 49933 Angers Cedex 9, France*

ANDRÉS CÁRDENAS MD, MMSC, *Liver Unit, Institut de Malalties Digestives, Hospital Clinic, IDIBAPS, University of Barcelona, Barcelona, Spain*

NAGA CHALASANI MD, *Associate Professor of Medicine, Division of Gastroenterology/Hepatology, Division of Clinical Pharmacology, Indiana University School of Medicine, Indianapolis, IN, USA*

Y.C. CHAWLA MD, *Head, Department of Hepatology, PGIMER, Chandigarh, India 160012*

ERIK CHRISTENSEN MD, *Clinic of Internal Medicine I, Bispebjerg University Hospital, Bispebjerg Bakke 23, DK-2400, Copenhagen NV, Denmark*

GENNARO D'AMICO MD, *UO Gastroenterologia, Ospedale V Cervello, 90146 Palermo, Italy*

ROBERTO DE FRANCHIS MD, *Professor of Gastroenterology, Department of Internal Medicine, University of Milan. Head, Gastroenterology and Gastrointestinal Endoscopy Service, IRCCS Ospedale Maggiore Policlinico, Milan, Italy*

ELWYN ELIAS MD, *Liver Unit, Queen Elizabeth Hospital, Birmingham B15 2TH, UK*

MICHAEL B. FALLON MD, *Department of Medicine, Division of Gastroenterology/Hepatology, University of Alabama at Birmingham, Birmingham, AL, USA*

JUAN CARLOS GARCIA-PAGAN MD, PhD, *Consultant in Hepatology, Hepatic Hemodynamic Laboratory, Liver Unit, Hospital Clinic, IDIBAPS, Barcelona, Spain*

GUADALUPE GARCIA-TSAO MD, *Professor of Medicine, Yale University, VA-CT Healthcare System, New Haven, CT, USA*

PERE GINÈS MD, *Liver Unit, Institut de Malalties Digestives, Hospital Clinic, IDIBAPS, University of Barcelona, Barcelona, Spain*

CHRISTIAN GLUUD MD, *Dr Med. Sci., Head of Department, The Cochrane Hepatobiliary Group, The Copenhagen Trial Unit, Centre for Clinical Intervention Research, Department 7102 Rigshospitalet, Copenhagen University Hospital, Copenhagen, Denmark*

LISE LOTTE GLUUD MD, *Dr Med. Sci., Senior Researcher, The Cochrane Hepato-Biliary Group, The Copenhagen Trial Unit, Centre for Clinical Intervention Research, Department 7102 Rigshospitalet, Copenhagen University Hospital, Copenhagen, Denmark*

NORMAN D. GRACE MD, FACP, FACG, *Professor of Medicine, Tufts University School of Medicine, Lecturer on Medicine, Harvard Medical School, Director of Clinical Hepatology, Brigham and Womens Hospital, Boston, MA, USA*

ROBERTO J. GROSZMANN MD, FRCP, *Professor of Medicine, VA Connecticut Healthcare System, Hepatic Hemodynamic Laboratory, West Haven, CT, and Yale University School of Medicine, New Haven, CT, USA*

ANTOINE HADENGUE MD, *Professor of Medicine, University of Geneva, Head, Division of Gastroenterology and Hepatology, Geneva University Hospitals, Hopital Cantonal, CH 1211, Geneva, Switzerland*

JENNY HEATHCOTE MD, *Professor of Medicine, University of Toronto, Toronto Western Hospital, University Health Network, Toronto, Ontario M5T 2S8, Canada*

J. MICHAEL HENDERSON MD, *Department of Surgery, The Cleveland Clinic Foundation, Cleveland, OH, USA*

YASUKO IWAKIRI PhD, *Section of Digestive Diseases, Yale University School of Medicine, New Haven, CT, USA*

HARRY JANSSEN MD, *Department of Gastroenterology and Hepatology, Erasmus MC University Hospital, Rotterdam, The Netherlands*

PATRICK S. KAMATH MD, *Professor of Medicine, Mayo Clinic College of Medicine, Rochester, MN 55905, USA*

W. RAY KIM MD, *Associate Professor of Medicine, Division of Gastro enterology and Hepatology, Mayo Clinic College of Medicine, Rochester, MN 55905, USA*

SARAH LOUISE KLINGERBERG CAND. SCIENT., *Hand Search Coordinator, The Cochrane Hepato-Biliary Group, The Copenhagen Trial Unit, Centre for Clinical Intervention Research, Department 7102 Rigshospitalet, Copenhagen University Hospital, Copenhagen, Denmark*

DAVID KRAVETZ MD, *Staff Physician, Gastroenterology Division, VA San Diego Healthcare System, Professor of Clinical Medicine, University of California, San Diego, CA, USA*

LOREN LAINE MD, *Professor of Medicine, Keck School of Medicine, University of Southern California, Los Angeles, CA, USA*

DIDIER LEBREC MD, *Laboratoire d'Hémodynamique Splanchnique et de Biologie Vasculaire, INSERM U-481, and Service d'Hépatologie, Hôpital Beaujon, Clichy, France*

FA-YAU LEE MD, *Division of General Medicine, Department of Medicine, Taipei Veterans General Hospital, Taiwan*

HAN-CHIEH LIN MD, *Professor of Medicine, Division of Gastroenterology, Department of Medicine, Taipei Veterans General Hospital and National Yang-Ming University School of Medicine, Taipei, Taiwan*

GIN-HO LO MD, *Chief, Division of Gastroenterology, Department of Medicine, Kaohsiung Veterans General Hospital, Professor, National Yang-Ming University, Taiwan, Kaohshiung, Taiwan*

PIER MANNUCCIO MANNUCCI MD, *Professor of Medicine Angelo Bianchi Bonomi Hemophilia and Thrombosis Center, Department of Internal Medicine and Dermatology, IRCCS Maggiore Hospital Mangiagalli and Regina Elena Foundation and University of Milan, Italy*

NORMAN MARCON MD, *Gastroenterologist, St. Michael's Hospital, University of Toronto, Toronto, Ontario, Canada*

CARLO MERKEL MD, *Associate Professor of Medicine, Department of Clinical and Experimental Medicine, University of Padua, Padua, Italy*

MANUELA MERLI MD, *Associate Professor of Gastroenterology, II Division of Gastroenterology, Department of Clinical Medicine, University of Rome 'La Sapienza', Rome, Italy*

ALBERTO MORABITO PhD, *Professor of Medical Statistics and Biometrics, Department of Medicine, Surgery and Dentistry, University of Milan, Milano, Italy*

RICHARD MOREAU MD, *INSERM and Service D'Hèpatologie, Hôpital Beaujon, 92118 Clichy, France*

MIGUEL NAVASA MD, *Associate Professor of Medicine, Liver Unit, IMDIM, IDIBAPS, Hospital Clinic, University of Barcelona, Barcelona, Spain*

FREDERIK NEVENS MD, *Department of Liver and Pancreatic Disease, UZ Gasthuisberg KU Leuven, Leuven, Belgium*

LUIGI PAGLIARO MD, *Professor of Medicine, University of Palermo, Internal Medicine, V Cervello Hospital, Regional Referral Center for Chronic Liver Diseases, Palermo, Italy*

DAVID PATCH MD, MBBS, FRCP, *Royal Free Hospital, London, UK*

RAMÓN PLANAS MD, *Liver Unit, Gastroenterology Department, Autonomous University of Barcelona, Unidad de Hepatologia. Servicio de Digestivo, Hospital Germans Trias i Pujol, Badalona, Spain*

MASSIMO PRIMIGNANI MD, *Department of Internal Medicine, University of Milan, Gastroenterology and Gastrointestinal Endoscopy Service, IRCCS Ospedale Maggiore Policlinico, Milan, Italy*

OLIVIERO RIGGIO MD, *Associate Professor of Gastroenterology, II Division of Gastroenterology, Department of Clinical Medicine, University of Rome 'La Sapienza', Rome, Italy*

JUAN RODÉS MD, *Professor of Medicine, University of Barcelona. Chief Executive, Hospital Clinic i Provincial, Barcelona, Spain*

FRANCESCO SALERNO MD, *Professor of Medicine, Department of Internal Medicine, University of Milan, Policlinico S. Donato, Milan, Italy*

ARUN J. SANYAL MD, *Professor of Medicine and Chairman, Division of Gastroenterology, Hepatology and Nutrition, Virginia Commonwealth University Medical Center, Richmond, VA 23298-0341, USA*

SHIV K. SARIN MD, *Department of Gastroenterology, G.B. Pant Hospital, New Delhi, India*

TILMAN SAUERBRUCH MD, *Department of Internal Medicine I, University of Bonn, Bonn, Germany*

FILIPPO SCHEPIS MD, *Gastroenterology Unit, University of Modena and Reggio Emilia, Via Del Pozzo 71, 41100, Modena, Italy*

MICHAEL SCHEPKE *Department of Internal Medicine I, University of Bonn, Bonn, Germany*

VIJAY SHAH MD, *Advanced Liver Disease Study Group and Gastroenterology Research Unit, Mayo Clinic, Rochester, MN, USA*

GAMAL SHIHA MD, *Professor of Internal Medicine, Elmansoura Faculty of Medicine, Liver and Gastroenterology Unit, Elmansoura University Hospital, Egypt*

BENJAMIN L. SHNEIDER MD, *Professor of Pediatrics, Chief, Division of Pediatric Hepatology, Mount Sinai School of Medicine, New York, NY, USA*

CHRISTINE SILVAIN MD, *Service d'Hepato-Gastroenterologie, CHU La Miletrie, 86021 Poitiers Cedex, France*

THORKILD I.A. SØRENSEN MD, *Professor, Dr Med. Sci, Institute Director, Institute of Preventive Medicine, Centre for Health and Society, Copenhagen University Hospital, Copenhagen, Denmark*

JAYANT TALWALKAR MD, *Assistant Professor of Medicine, Mayo Clinic College of Medicine, Consultant, Division of Gastroenterology/Hepatology, Mayo Clinic and Foundation, Rochester, MN, USA*

DOMINIQUE THABUT MD, *Hepato-gastroenterology Unit, Hôpital Pitié-Salpetrière, Paris, France*

DOMINIQUE-CHARLES VALLA MD, *Professor of Hepatology, Service d'Hépatologie, Fédération Médico-Chirurgicale d'Hépatogastroentérologie, Hôpital Beaujon, 92118 Clichy, France*

HENK R. VAN BUUREN MD, *Department of Gastroenterology, Erasmus MC University Hospital, Rotterdam, The Netherlands*

CÀNDID VILLANUEVA MD, *Gastrointestinal Bleeding Unit, Department of Gastroenterology, Hospital de la Santa Creu i Sant Pau, Barcelona, Spain*

JEAN-PIERRE VINEL MD, *Chef du Service d'Hépato-Gastroentérologie, Fédération Digestive de Purpan, Centre Hospitalier Universitaire Purpan, Toulouse Cedex, France*

JULIO VOROBIOFF MD, *Gastroenterology Department, University of Rosario Medical School, and Fundaciòn Villavicencio, Rosario, Argentina*

IAN R. WANLESS MD, CM, FRCPC, *Professor of Pathology, University of Toronto, Staff Pathologist, Toronto General Hospital, Toronto, Ontario, Canada*

MARCO ZOLI MD, *Professor of Medicine, Department of Internal Medicine, Cardioangiology, Hepatology, University of Bologna, S Orsola-Malpighi Hospital, 40138, Bologna, Italy*

PARTICIPANTS

Argentina: J. Vorobioff
Belgium: F. Nevens
Canada: J. Heathcote, N. Marcon, I.R. Wanless
Denmark: F. Bendtsen, E. Christensen, C. Gluud, T.I.A. Sørensen
Egypt: G. Shiha
France: B. Bernard-Chabert, P. Calès, D. Lebrec, R. Moreau, C. Silvain, D. Thabut, D.C. Valla, J.P. Vinel
Germany: T. Sauerbruch, M. Schepke
India: Y.C. Chawla, S.K. Sarin
Italy: M. Angelico, G. Barosi, G. D'Amico, R. de Franchis, P.M. Mannucci, C. Merkel, M. Primignani, F. Salerno, F. Schepis, M. Zoli
Spain: J.G. Abraldes, A. Albillos, R. Bañares, J. Bosch, J.C. Garcia-Pagan, P. Ginès, M. Navasa, R. Planas, J. Rodés, C. Villanueva
Switzerland: A. Handengue
Taiwan: F.Y. Lee, H.C. Lin, G.H. Lo
The Netherlands: H. Janssen, H. van Buuren
UK: A.K. Burroughs, E. Elias, D. Patch
USA: A.T. Blei, T.D. Boyer, N. Chalasani, M.B. Fallon, G. Garcia-Tsao, N.D. Grace, R.J. Groszmann, J.M. Henderson, Y. Iwakiri, P.S. Kamath, W.R. Kim, D. Kravetz, L. Laine, A.J. Sanyal, V. Shah, B.L. Shneider, J. Talwalkar

Preface

Portal hypertension is the haemodynamic abnormality associated with the most severe complications of cirrhosis, including ascites, hepatic encephalopathy and bleeding from gastroesophageal varices. Since variceal bleeding is a medical emergency associated with significant morbidity and mortality, the evaluation of diagnostic tools and the design and conduct of good clinical trials for the treatment of this condition have always been difficult. Awareness of these difficulties has led to the organisation of a series of meetings aimed at reaching consensus on the definitions of some key events related to portal hypertension and variceal bleeding, and at producing guidelines for the conduct of trials in this field. Such meetings took place in Groningen, the Netherlands in 1986, in Baveno, Italy in 1990 (Baveno I) and in 1995 (Baveno II), in Milan, Italy in 1992, in Reston, United States, in 1996 and in Stresa, Italy in 2000 (Baveno III). All these meetings were successful and produced consensus statements on some important points, although several issues remained unsettled.

Since the Baveno III meeting, new diagnostic tools, new drugs and new treatment strategies for portal hypertension have been developed, which might lead to important changes in the management of this condition. We thus felt that the time had come to evaluate the impact of these novelties on the diagnostic and therapeutic strategies that we follow in managing patients with portal hypertension. Therefore, with the help and encouragement of a group of friends from 16 countries, many of whom had taken part in the previous three Baveno meetings, we organised a Baveno IV workshop which took place on 28–29 April 2005.

The aims of the Baveno IV workshop were the same as in Baveno I, II and III, that is to refine and extend the definitions of key events concerning the bleeding episode, in the light of the feedback we have received from studies carried out since Baveno III, and to review and put into perspective the new diagnostic tools and the new therapeutic strategies that have been proposed in the last five years. In addition, we continued the effort that was begun in Groningen and continued in the following workshops of producing updated guidelines aimed at improving the quality of our future studies. We were very fortunate in being able to bring to this workshop many of the experts responsible for most of the major achievements of the last five years in this field.

The structure of the Baveno IV workshop included eight sessions and seven lectures. The first session was devoted to verifying the appropriateness and practicality of the definitions of key events that had been given in Baveno I , II and III, and an attempt was made to develop consensus definitions on points which were not addressed – or not agreed upon – in the previous workshops. In each of sessions 2 to 6, the chairpersons and the panellists reviewed an important topic related to the diagnosis or the treatment of portal hypertension. At the end of each session, the chairpersons proposed a series of statements which were discussed within the panel and with the other experts on the floor with the aim of reaching consensus on some important diagnostic or therapeutic issues.

Session 7 focused on an emerging entity, that is non-cirrhotic portal hypertension, comparing experiences developed in the Eastern and Western world. Session 8 was devoted to assess ways of evaluating the scientific evidence above and beyond randomised controlled trials.

The seven lectures were different in scope. The first one summarised the past history of the Baveno workshops, the impact of publications derived from those workshops on the medical literature and gave a brief survey of the new diagnostic tools, new drugs and new therapeutic strategies that have been recently proposed and will have to be evaluated in the future. The second lecture analysed the value and limits of evidence-based medicine; the third, fourth, fifth and sixth lecture addressed important clinical issues, that is the relationship between coagulation defects, fibrinolysis and portal hypertensive bleeding, the hepatopulmonary syndrome and portopulmonary hypertension, hepatorenal syndrome, spontaneous bacterial peritonitis and infections. The seventh lecture analysed the quality of trials in portal hypertension and other fields of hepatology, and was an update of a lecture on the same topic that was given at Baveno III.

These proceedings follow closely the structure of the workshop. The order of lectures and sessions is the same, except for the lectures by Dr Gluud and of Professor Pagliaro, which were moved close to session 8, as they are the ideal introductions to the latter. The consensus statements that were agreed upon at the end of each session are reported at the end of the pertinent chapters. The levels of available evidence and the strength of the recommendations are graded according to the Oxford System: (http://www.cebm.net/downloads/Oxford_EBM_Levels_5.rtf).

Our deepest thanks go to all the friends who accepted to give lectures and to serve as chairpersons and panellists of the sessions, and who helped us by working hard in the preparation of the workshop and of the chapters. We also wish to thank Sandra Covre and her staff of GPA Net, who managed brilliantly the organisation of the workshop, Jorge Cubero Sotela, Alessandra Dell' Era, Federica Fabris end Emanuele Rondonotti, who skilfully operated the computer-video projector systems throughout the workshop. In addition, we are grateful to the European Association for the Study of the Liver (EASL), the Associazione Italiana per lo Studio del Fegato (AISF), the Società Italiana di Gastroenterologia (SIGE), the Società Italiana di Endoscopia Digestiva (SIED) and the Associazione Italiana dei Gastroenterologi ed endoscopisti Ospedalieri (AIGO) who endorsed the meeting, to the Companies who sponsored the workshop and especially to Ferring Pharmaceuticals, who made the publication of this book possible through a generous grant, to Tim Akroyd for his encouragement and co-operation in this project, and to Blackwell Publishing for the timely and excellent production of this volume.

Roberto de Franchis
On behalf of the Baveno IV Scientific Committee

LECTURE

What Have We Accomplished (and What Lies Ahead)

Roberto de Franchis

INTRODUCTION

The idea of holding consensus meetings on portal hypertension was born in 1986, when Andrew Burroughs organised the first such meeting in Groningen, the Netherlands [1]. After Groningen, other meetings followed, in Baveno, Italy in 1990 (Baveno I) [2] and in 1995 (Baveno II) [3,4], in Milan, Italy in 1992 [5], in Reston, United States [6] and in Stresa, Italy in 2000 (Baveno III) [7,8]. This is the seventh meeting of this kind.

In this review, I will summarise the work previously done in the Baveno workshops I to III and outline the new diagnostic and therapeutic modalities that are emerging and will have to be evaluated in the near future.

What we have done

1 Topics covered at the Baveno I, II and III meetings.
2 Publications derived from the Baveno I, II and III workshops.
3 Quantitative impact of the Baveno I, II and III consensus on the medical literature.
4 Attendance at the Baveno workshops.

What lies ahead

1 New diagnostic tools.
2 New drugs.
3 New therapeutic strategies.

WHAT WE HAVE DONE

Topics addressed at the Baveno I, II and III workshops

- Definitions of key events.
- Diagnostic evaluation of patients with portal hypertension.
- Prognostic factors for first bleeding, rebleeding and survival.
- Therapeutic strategies in patients with portal hypertension.
- Methodological requirements of future trials.

Publications derived from the Baveno I, II and III workshops

- The Baveno I workshop was reported in the *Journal of Hepatology* in 1992 [2].
- A report of the Baveno II workshop was published in the *Journal of Hepatology* in 1996 [3].
- The proceedings book of the Baveno II workshop was published by Blackwell Science in 1996 [4].
- The Baveno III workshop was reported in the *Journal of Hepatology* in 2000 [7].
- The proceedings book of the Baveno III workshop was published by Blackwell Science in 2001 [8].

Impact of the Baveno consensus on the medical literature

Figure 1 shows the number of citations of the Baveno I–III reports in the medical literature between January 1993 and January 2005. Overall, the reports had more than 200 citations.

Attendance at the Baveno workshops

Two hundred and five participants took part in the Baveno I workshop; 81% of them were from Italy, 19% from other countries. Eighteen countries were represented.

The Baveno II workshop was attended by 252 participants, of which 74% were from Italy and 26% from other countries. Eighteen countries were represented.

The attendance of the Baveno III workshop was 385, of which 49% were from Italy and 51% from other countries. Twenty-nine countries were represented.

Four hundred and eighty five participants took part in the Baveno IV workshop; 38% were from Italy, 62% from 39 other countries. Forty countries were represented: Argentina, Australia, Austria, Belgium, Bulgaria, Canada, Chile, Costa Rica, Croatia, Czech Republic, Denmark, Egypt, Finland, France, Germany, Greece, Hong Kong, Hungary, India, Israel, Italy, Jordan, Korea, Malaysia, Mexico, Pakistan, Portugal, Romania, Saudi Arabia, Serbia-Montenegro, Slovakia, Slovenia, Spain, Sweden, Switzerland, Taiwan, Thailand, The Netherlands, United Kingdom and United States.

These data are shown graphically in Figs 2 and 3.

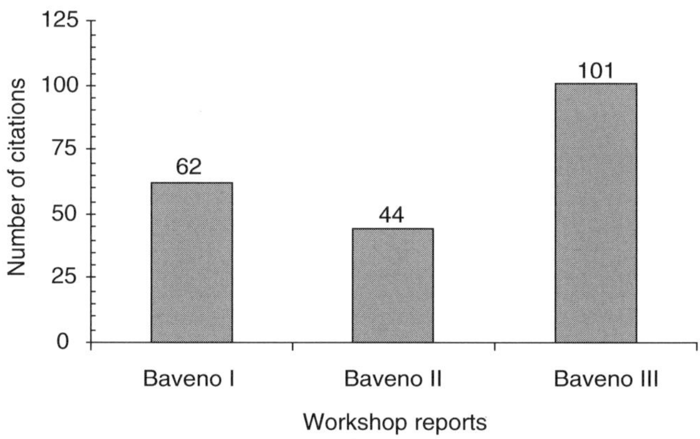

Fig. 1 Citations of the Baveno I–III reports.

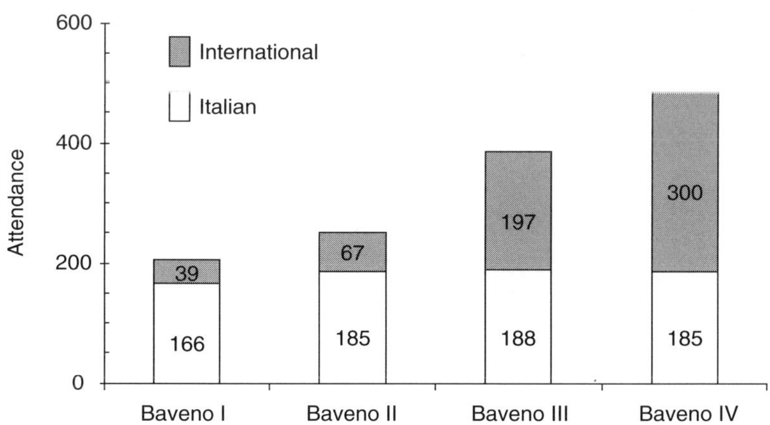

Fig. 2 Attendance at the Baveno I–IV workshops.

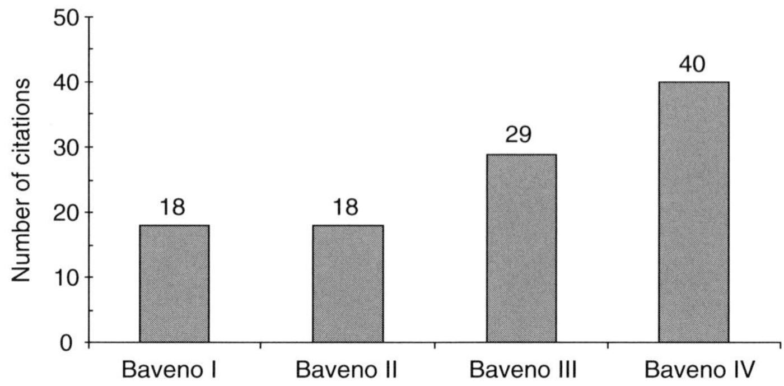

Fig. 3 Countries represented at the Baveno I–IV workshops.

WHAT LIES AHEAD

New diagnostic tools

Oesophageal endoscopic capsule (PillCam Eso)

Traditionally, upper GI endoscopy (EGD) has been the mainstay for the diagnosis of portal hypertension. Current guidelines [7] recommend that all cirrhotic patients be screened for oesophageal varices by endoscopy at the time of the diagnosis of cirrhosis: those with no varices at screening endoscopy should undergo endoscopic surveillance every 2–3 years; those with small varices at screening endoscopy should undergo endoscopic surveillance every 1–2 years.

These recommendations represent a potentially large endoscopic burden. Their application is hampered by suboptimal patient acceptance of conventional EGD. The availability of a less invasive screening test could improve patient acceptance and thus adherence to recommendations.

The recently developed oesophageal capsule endoscope (PillCam Eso®) is a new, minimally invasive tool for the study of oesophageal lesions. Plate 1 (*facing p.* 204) shows the appearance of oesophageal varices on PillCam Eso® endoscopy. In a pilot study [9], the PillCam Eso® has been compared with conventional EGD for the diagnosis and surveillance of oesophageal varices in cirrhotic patients. The study has shown a 96.9% agreement between PillCam Eso® and EGD for the diagnosis of the presence of oesophageal varices. The sensitivity, specificity, positive and negative predictive values of PillCam Eso® were 100%, 89%, 96% and 100% respectively (Fig. 4). If these data are confirmed, the PillCam Eso® could become a first-line, minimally invasive tool to screen cirrhotic patients for the presence of varices.

		Traditional Endoscopy +	Traditional Endoscopy –	
Capsule endoscopy	+	23	1	24
	–	0	8	8
		23	9	32

Overall agreement 96.9%
Positive likelihood ratio: 9.1
Negative likelihoodratio: 0.0

	Capsule endoscopy
Sensitivity	100%
Specificity	89%
PPV	96%
NPV	100%

Fig. 4 Comparison of EGD and PillCam Eso® for the diagnosis of oesophageal varices.

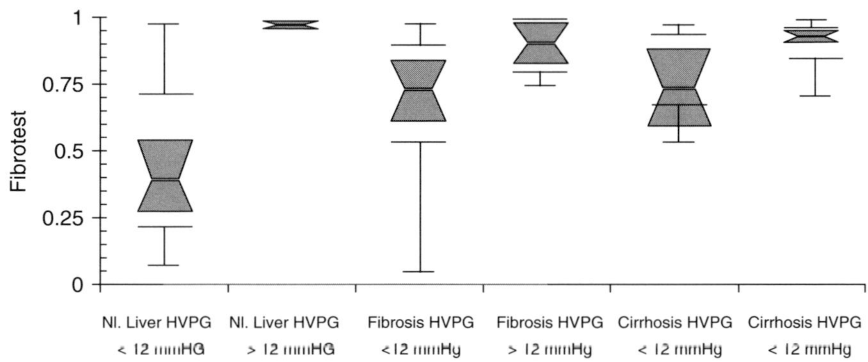

Fig. 5 Relationship between Fibrotest values and degree of portal hypertension in patients with normal liver, liver fibrosis and cirrhosis.

Fibrotest and Fibroscan

Attempts at identifying the patients with oesophageal varices by non-invasive means, in order to restrict the performance of endoscopy to the patients with a high probability of having varices have been disappointing so far [10]. It has been suggested that patients with varices could be identified non-invasively by a combination of biochemical tests [α-2-macroglobulin, haptoglobin, apolipoprotein A1, gamma-glutamyltranspeptidase and total bilirubin (Fibrotest)] and/or by transient elastography (Fibroscan). A French study [11] presented in 2004 at the AASLD meeting has shown that there is a good correlation between the values of Fibrotest and the presence of severe portal hypertension (Fig. 5). Another recent study [12] has shown a good correlation between liver stiffness measured by transient elastography and

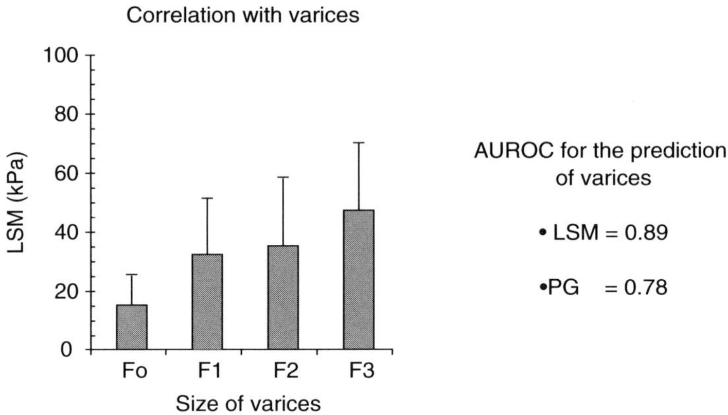

Fig. 6 Relationship between liver stiffness measured by transient elastography and presence and size of oesophageal varices (left panel). Comparison of the area under the ROC curve (AUROC) for transient elastography (LSM) and portal pressure gradient (PG) (right panel).

the presence and size of oesophageal varices (Fig. 6). Further studies with the above techniques should be carried out to define whether Fibroscan and/or Fibrotest can be used to identify non-invasively the patients with oesophageal varices.

New drugs

Interferon in the prevention of the progression of fibrosis

Attempts at preventing the development of oesophageal varices with β-blockers have given disappointing results [13,14]. The recent demonstration that interferon treatment may delay the development of varices in patients with chronic hepatitis C and hepatitis C virus (HCV)-related cirrhosis [15] (Fig. 7) suggests that interferon treatment might have a role in preventing the development of portal hypertension. this hypothesis deserves to be tested in appropriately designed studies.

Recombinant-activated factor VII (rFVIIa) in the treatment of acute variceal bleeding

It has recently been shown that the administration of recombinant-activated factor VII (rFVIIa) normalises prothrombin time in bleeding cirrhotic patients. The potential role of rFVIIa has been evaluated in a multicentre European trial [16], including 245 bleeding cirrhotic patients who were

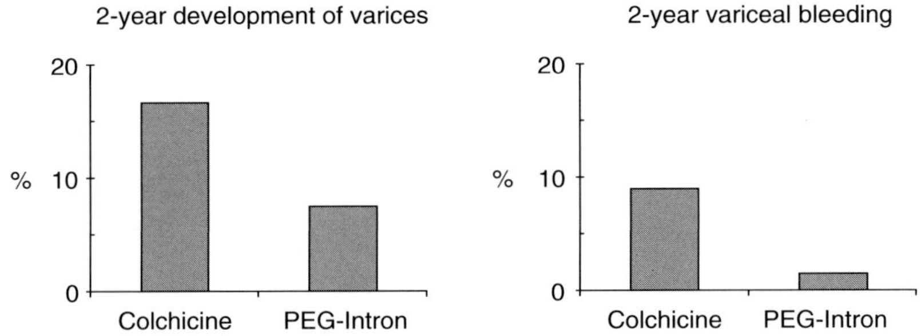

Fig. 7 Comparison between PEG-Interferon and colchicine in the prevention of the development of oesophageal varices and of variceal bleeding in patients with chronic hepatitis C and with HCV-related cirrhosis.

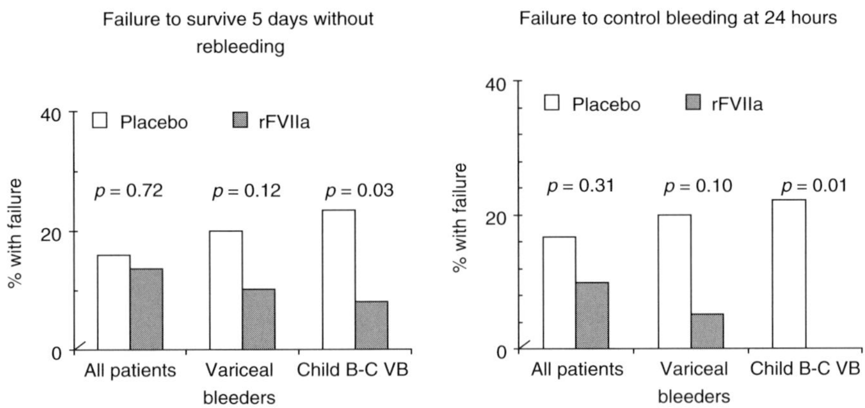

Fig. 8 Randomised controlled trial of recombinant-activated factor VII (rFVIIa) as an adjunct to endoscopic and vasoactive treatment for acute variceal bleeding.

randomised to receive eight doses of rFVIIa, 100 μg/kg or placebo in addition to combined endoscopic + pharmacological treatment. The primary end point was a composite including failure to control bleeding at 24 h, failure to prevent rebleeding between 24 h and 5 days and death within 5 days. No significant effect was found when analysing the whole patients population; however, an exploratory analysis showed that, in Child-Pugh B and C variceal bleeders, rFVIIa significantly reduced the occurrence of the primary end point (from 23% in patients receiving placebo to 8% in patients receiving rFVIIa, $p = 0.03$), and improved bleeding control at 24 h (from 88% to 100%, $p = 0.03$) (Fig. 8). These data are encouraging, but require confirmation by studies specifically targeted on the appropriate patients.

Conclusions

All these exciting new developments will have to be carefully evaluated to see whether they can be incorporated in the diagnostic/therapeutic armamentarium for portal hypertension.

REFERENCES

1 Burroughs AK ed. *Methodology and review of clinical trials in portal hypertension.* Excerpta Medical Congress Service No 763. Amsterdam, New York, Oxford, 1987.

2 de Franchis R, Pascal JP, Ancona E *et al.* Definitions, methodology and therapeutic strategies in portal hypertension. A consensus development workshop. *J Hepatol* 1992;**15**: 256–261.

3 de Franchis R. Developing consensus in portal hypertension. *J Hepatol* 1996;**25**: 390–394.

4 de Franchis R ed. *Portal hypertension II. Proceedings of the second Baveno international consensus workshop on definitions, methodology and therapeutic strategies.* Oxford, Blackwell Science, 1996.

5 Spina GP, Arcidiacono R, Bosch J *et al.* Gastric endoscopic features in portal hypertension: final report of a consensus conference. *J Hepatol* 1994;**21**: 461–467.

6 Grace ND, Groszmann RJ, Garcia-Tsao G *et al.* Portal hypertension and variceal bleeding: an AASLD single topic symposium. *Hepatology* 1998;**28**: 868–880.

7 de Franchis R. Updating consensus in portal hypertension: report of the Baveno III consensus workshop on definitions, methodology and therapeutic strategies in portal hypertension. *J Hepatol* 2000;**33**: 846–852.

8 de Franchis R (ed). *Portal hypertension III. Proceedings of the third Baveno international consensus workshop on definitions, methodology and therapeutic strategies.* Oxford, Blackwell Science, 2000.

9 Eisen G, de Franchis R, Eliakim R. Evaluation of esophageal varices by PillCam Eso as compared to upper endoscopy. In: Lewis BS, Rey JF, Seidman E (eds). *4th international conference on capsule endoscopy (ICCE) abstract book.* Yoqneam, Israel, Given Imaging, 2005; 199.

10 de Franchis R. Incidental esophageal varices. *Gastroenterology* 2004;**126**: 1860–1867.

11 Thabut D, Imbert-Bismuth F, Cazals-Hatem D *et al.* Diagnostic value of fibrosis biochemical markers (Fibrotest-Fibrosure) for the prediction of severe portal hypertension in patients with and without cirrhosis. *Hepatology* 2004;**40**(suppl. 1): 203A.

12 Kazemi F Pinto E, N'Koutchou G, Ganne-Carrié N, Trinchet JC, Beaugrand M. In Patients with cirrhosis, liver stiffness measurement (LSM) predicts the presence of oesophageal varices (OV) more accurately than portal gradient (PG). *J Hepatol* 2005;**42**(suppl. 2): 82.

13 Calés P, Oberti F, Payen JL *et al.* Lack of effect of propranolol in the prevention of large oesophageal varices in patients with cirrhosis: a randomized trial. *Eur J Gastroenterol Hepatol* 1999;**11**: 741–745.

14 Groszmann R, Garcia-Tsao G, Makuch R *et al.* Multicenter randomized trial of non-selective beta-blockers in the prevention of complications of portal hypertension: final results and identification of a predictive factor. *Hepatology* 2003;**38**(suppl. 1): 206A.
15 Curry M, Cardenas A, Afdhal NH. Effect of maintenance PEG-Intron therapy on portal hypertension and its complications: results from the copilot study. *J Hepatol* 2005;**42**(suppl. 2): 40.
16 Bosch J, Thabut D, Bendtsen F *et al.* On behalf of the European Study Group on rFVIIa in UGI haemorrhage. Recombinant factor VIIa for upper gastrointestinal bleeding in patients with cirrhosis. A randomized, double-blind trial. *Gastroenterology* 2004;**127**: 1123–1130.

ACKNOWLEDGEMENTS

The Baveno I, II, III and IV workshops were a concerted effort of the following:

Chairpersons, lecturers, panellists:

Argentina:	J. Vorobioff
Austria:	G. Krejs
Belgium:	F. Nevens
Canada:	J. Heathcote, N. Marcon, G. Pomier-Layrargues, I. Wanless
Denmark:	U. Becker, F. Bendtsen, E. Christensen, C. Gluud, S. Møller, T.I.A. Sørensen
Egypt:	G. Shiha
France:	B. Bernard-Chabert, P. Calès, D. Lebrec, R. Moreau, J.P. Pascal, C. Silvain, D. Thabut, D. Valla, J.P. Vinel
Germany:	K. Binmøller, W. Fleig, G. Richter, M. Rössle, T. Sauerbruch, M. Schepke, D. Schuppan, M. Staritz
Great Britain:	A.K. Burroughs, E. Elias, D. Patch, D. Westaby
India:	Y.C. Chawla, S.K. Sarin
Italy:	M. Angelico, G. Balducci, G. Barosi, G. Battaglia, M. Bolognesi, L. Bolondi, L. Cestari, G.C. Caletti, F. Cosentino, G. D'Amico, R. de Franchis, A. Gatta, G. Gerunda, A. Liberati, A. Maffei Faccioli, P.M. Mannucci, C. Merkel, M. Merli, G. Minoli, A. Morabito, L. Pagliaro, A. Peracchia, M. Pinzani, M. Primignani, O. Riggio, P. Rossi, C. Sabbà, D. Sacerdoti, F. Salerno, F. Schepis, P. Spina, F. Tinè, V. Ziparo, M. Zoli
Portugal:	P. Alexandrino

Spain:	J.G. Abraldes, A. Albillos, R. Bañares, J. Bosch, A. Escorsell, J.C. Garcia-Pagàn, P. Ginés, M. Navasa, J. Piqué, R. Planas, J. Rodès, C. Villanueva
Switzerland:	A. Hadengue, P. Gertsch, C. Sieber
Taiwan:	F.Y. Lee, H.C. Lin, G.H. Lo
Sweden:	C. Søderlund
The Netherlands:	H. Janssen, H. van Buuren
United States:	A. Blei, T. Boyer, Chalasani, M. Fallon, G. Garcia-Tsao, N. Grace, R. Groszmann, J.M. Henderson, Y. Iwakiri, P. Kamath, W.R. Kim, D. Kravetz, L. Laine, A. Sanyal, V. Shah, B. Shneider, J. Talwalkar, G. van Stiegmann

Organisation:

S. Covre

SESSION 1

Definition of Key Events – Last Attempt?

Andrew K. Burroughs, Paul Calès, David Kravetz, Oliviero Riggio, Dominique Thabut, Henk R. van Buuren and Patrick S. Kamath

INTRODUCTION

Following Baveno III, there has been further discussion regarding the key events in variceal bleeding, as these were still unresolved issues. In particular there has been a formal evaluation of their use based on data from a randomised clinical trial [1].

Questions related to the definition of key events were formulated by the panellists and sent out to members of other panels. In total we had 38 respondents and the results are included in the text.

EVENTS RELATED TO FAILURE TO CONTROL ACUTE VARICEAL BLEEDING

The majority of respondents ($n = 24$) felt the criteria for failure to control variceal bleeding needed changing, with only a few in disagreement ($n = 6$) and the others who did not know ($n = 8$). Time zero and death due to bleeding are not changed, but responses to the questionnaire and polls of the participating audience have resulted in new proposals for failure to control bleeding.

The issue of definition is an important one for the evaluation and understanding of all clinical studies in this setting whether randomised or not. A good example is the effect of acute sclerotherapy in various types of trials such as those comparing it combined with vasoactive drugs/balloon tamponade to the latter alone, or a direct comparison with vasoactive drugs, or compared to the combination of vasoactive drugs and sclerotherapy, or to ligation alone. In these four groupings the median efficacy of acute sclerotherapy (Fig. 9) was only 69% in trials comparing sclerotherapy to

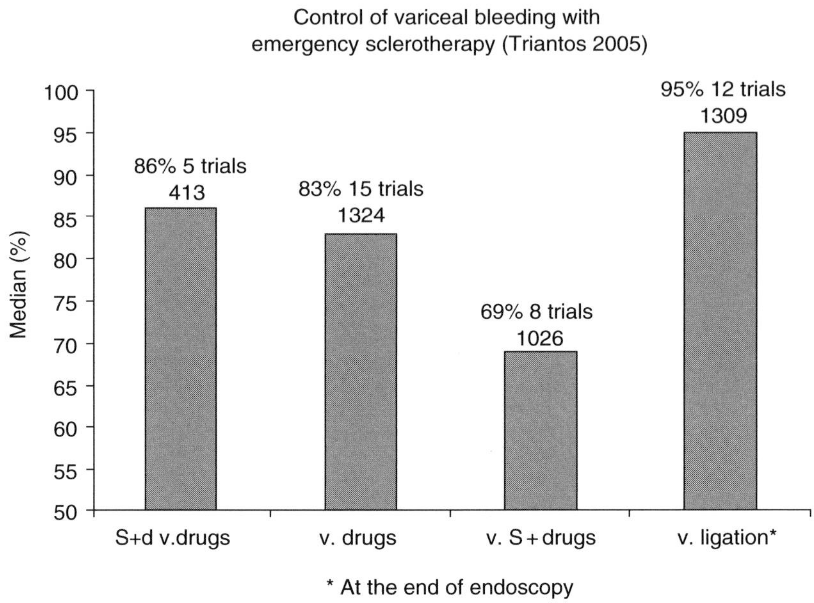

Fig. 9 The efficacy of emergency sclerotherapy alone in groups of randomised trials compared to other treatments (column 1 sclerotherapy + vasoactive drugs versus drugs; column 2 versus vasoactive drugs; column 3 versus sclerotherapy combined with vasoactive drugs and column 4 versus ligation).

combined vasoactive drugs and sclerotherapy, whereas it was 86% (together with vasoactive drugs/balloon tamponade) and 83% (direct comparison with vasoactive drugs) and 95% (versus ligation). The last high figure is explained by the assessment at the end of the endoscopic procedure, and not over subsequent time periods as in the other groups. Moreover if the issue of the assessment of the efficacy of sclerotherapy is examined further, then it can be seen that there is no systematic change over time (Fig. 10) in terms of year of publication of trials, but the discrepancy appears to be related to the assessment of trials evaluated over a 5-day period, in the group in which sclerotherapy was compared to combined vasoactive therapy and sclerotherapy (Fig. 11). This becomes even more of a problem, as it is this group of trials which suggests that the best acute therapy is a combination of vasoactive drug and sclerotherapy. This could be true, but the evaluation of the efficacy of sclerotherapy across trials means that some caution must be used in supporting this interpretation. It is unlikely that the real efficacy of sclerotherapy is very different across studies, so that these differences represent differences in definition – a problem highlighted in the past regarding trials in acute variceal bleeding [2,3].

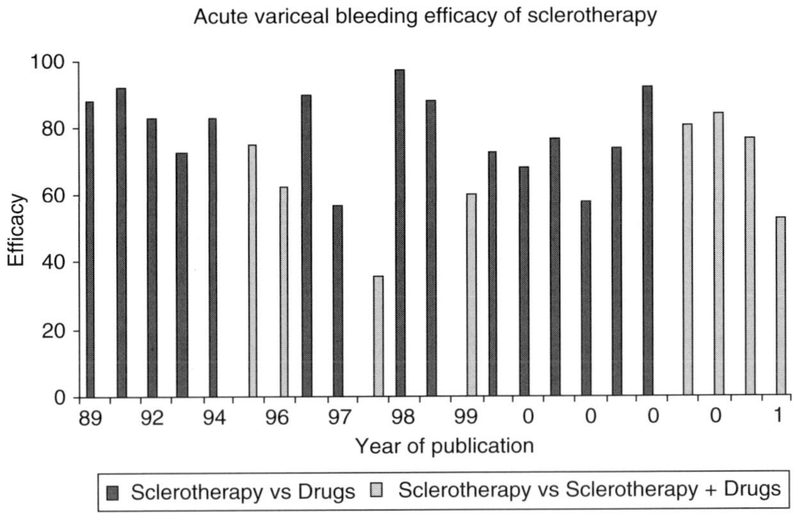

Fig. 10 The efficacy of emergency sclerotherapy alone in randomised trials comparing it to vasoactive drugs alone or the combination of sclerotherapy and vasoactive drugs with respect to the year of publication of the trial.

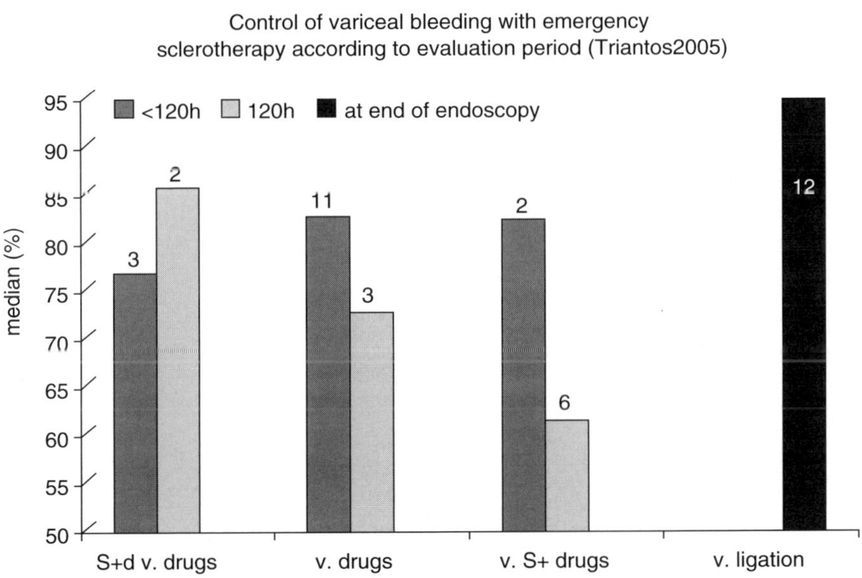

Fig. 11 The efficacy of emergency sclerotherapy alone in randomised trials comparing it to other therapies (column 1 sclerotherapy + vasoactive drugs versus drugs; column 2 versus vasoactive drugs; column 3 versus sclerotherapy combined with vasoactive drugs and column 4 versus ligation) with respect to the interval over which the efficacy was evaluated.

Table 1 Ranking of criteria used to define failure to control bleeding (including start of very early rebleeding) by 38 respondents to the Baveno IV questionnaire.

Ranking of signs of 38 responders to questionnaire	1st rank	2nd rank
Fresh haematemesis	26	8
Systolic drop > 20 mmHg	4	8
Fresh melaena	2	5
Tachycardia 120 + (on terlipressin)	1	7
Tachycardia 120 + (no terlipressin)	1	1
Haemoglobin drop? 2 g/dL	0	2

NB: Nasogastric tube aspiration was NOT asked – from Baveno 2 + 3– only 50% units use nasogastric tube aspiration

Table 2 Criteria selected by 38 respondents to the Baveno IV questionnaire in terms of blood/colloid transfusion equating with failure to control acute variceal bleeding.

Transfusion (blood)	Yes	Plasma expanders to be included	
2 units	11	yes	7
3 units	2	no	28
4 units	6	don't know	3
Units transfused corrected by baseline value	13		
None of the above	5		

Thus, the definition of failure to control acute variceal bleeding (FCB) raised the major concern for Baveno IV panellists, but resulted in some fairly consistent responses to the questionnaire. Thus, ranking of signs to define such failure showed that fresh haematemesis was either first ($n = 26$), or second rank ($n = 8$) as a criterion, with a systolic blood pressure drop of 20 mmHg or more being second as a criterion (first ranking 4, second ranking 8) (Table 1).

As regards blood or colloid requirement, the majority felt that a transfusion index taking into account the baseline value was also a criterion to define failure (Table 2). Lastly, the use of added procedures (other than first therapeutic endoscopy) was also felt to constitute failure (Table 3).

The time frame for acute variceal bleeding, which had been agreed upon at Baveno III, but not applied in many trials since 2000, was confirmed as lasting 5 days (120 h). This was despite some centres considering the end of the acute bleeding episode, in terms of the start of secondary prophylaxis, as being at admission ($n = 6$), end of 48 h ($n = 6$), end of 72 h ($n = 8$) and

Table 3 Criteria selected by 38 respondents to the Baveno IV questionnaire in terms of use of alternative procedures equating with failure to control acute variceal bleeding.

	Yes	No
2° therapeutic endoscopy? 5 days	26	12
Use a balloon tamponade	37	1
Use of Transjugular Intrahepatic Porto-systemic Shunt (TIPS) after at least One therapeutic endoscopy or as first therapy after diagnostic endoscopy	26	12

Table 4 Simplified criteria defining failure to control bleeding according to previous Baveno II/III definitions.

	Criteria	
Period	< 6 h	> 6 h
Blood units	≥ 4	≥ 2
Systolic arterial pressure	< 70 or $\nearrow < 20$	$\searrow > 20$
Heart rate	≥ 100 or $\searrow \leq 20$	$\nearrow > 20$
	Haematemesis	–

end of 96 h ($n = 1$). However, the majority considered it at the end of 120 h ($n = 17$). Thus, by definition secondary prophylaxis starts on day 6.

BAVENO III CRITERIA

These criteria about UGI bleeding due to portal hypertension (PHT) were defined in the Baveno II meeting [4] and validated in the Baveno III meeting [5]. They mainly described three items: (1) qualitative (active bleeding) or quantitative (clinically significant) aspects of bleeding, (2) criteria of failure to control bleeding; (3) time frames.

The criteria defining failure to control bleeding are presented in Table 4.

LIMITATIONS OF BAVENO III CRITERIA

In a previous study (1) based on data of a randomised controlled trial (RCT) [6], we reported the limitations in using Baveno III and II criteria. They are summarised as follows:

- Some of the definitions of the Baveno II criteria were either not precise enough or too impractical to be used in a clinical protocol.

• The first time point for the control of bleeding is 6 h after admission (t_{0+6} h, t_0 being the time of admission at the first medical unit). Time zero requires no change, but the starting point of time zero to assess specific therapy is impractical, for clinical trials, evaluation of specific therapy may be started after the 6 h time point.
• Specificity of tachycardia for bleeding is debatable.
• The evaluation of success or failure rates was not clearly defined. Failure rates can be calculated two ways:
– With raw data either as a yes or no within a particular time frame.
– With life table analysis described by Kaplan–Meier plots, applied to the time until therapeutic failure or death occurs.
• Evaluation of several potential end points was not defined in the Baveno II criteria:
– Survival without bleeding at 5 days. This is the main end point in several recent RCT [6,7,8]
– Transfusion rate,
– Length of hospital stay.

ADDITIONAL LIMITATIONS OF BAVENO III CRITERIA

In a recent unpublished RCT, Calès *et al.* encountered other limitations of Baveno III and II criteria:
• Tachycardia may be 'non-significant' due to delayed transfusion secondary to the unavailability or delay in blood transfusion.
• The volume in each blood unit (BU) is variable among centres and countries.
• The number of BUs is not adjusted to baseline haemoglobin (Hb) level. It would be more appropriate to consider relative variation in Hb level because this takes into account the baseline Hb of the patient, minimising 'false positive' failures based on transfusion requirements. For example, in the Baveno III criteria, pre-existing anaemia is a confounding factor, increasing the probability to declare a patient as a failure since more blood would be needed to reach the fixed Hb target.
• Another difficulty is to translate time dependent criteria of Baveno (signs not evaluated at a fixed time) in statistical language when analysing the data.
• A patient with an initial isolated failure is considered as a failure despite a final control of bleeding. This overall criterion is convenient for a trial but is debatable whether it reflects 'clinical' failure in everyday clinical practice where the main aim is to obtain final control of bleeding. Thus, the concept of failure at a single time point should be distinguished from that of final

failure, unless the initial failure criteria were to reflect a definite change in therapy in everyday clinical practice.

EXAMPLES OF DIFFICULTIES APPLYING THE PREVIOUS BAVENO CRITERIA IN ACUTE BLEEDING IN PHT

We present here simulations of different cases according to the course of variceal bleeding during the first 5 days after hospital admission (time zero).

In order to depict different clinical situations, we used a model of bleeding as a function of time, called the function of bleeding risk. These scenarios depict the different possible courses, as a function of a simulated bleeding risk. This bleeding risk is a prediction probability. So, bleeding can be defined as when the probability is ≥ 0.5. The bleeding becomes clinically significant or overt when the probability is ≥ 0.75. Thus, the severity of bleeding is proportional to that probability. In Figs. 12–16, we describe five main examples. In certain cases, especially with an early failure, the judgement as a final failure is debatable in clinical practice. These simulations argue for a late estimation of control of bleeding reflecting more the reality in day to day clinical practice. They also suggest that the failure can be defined in different ways.

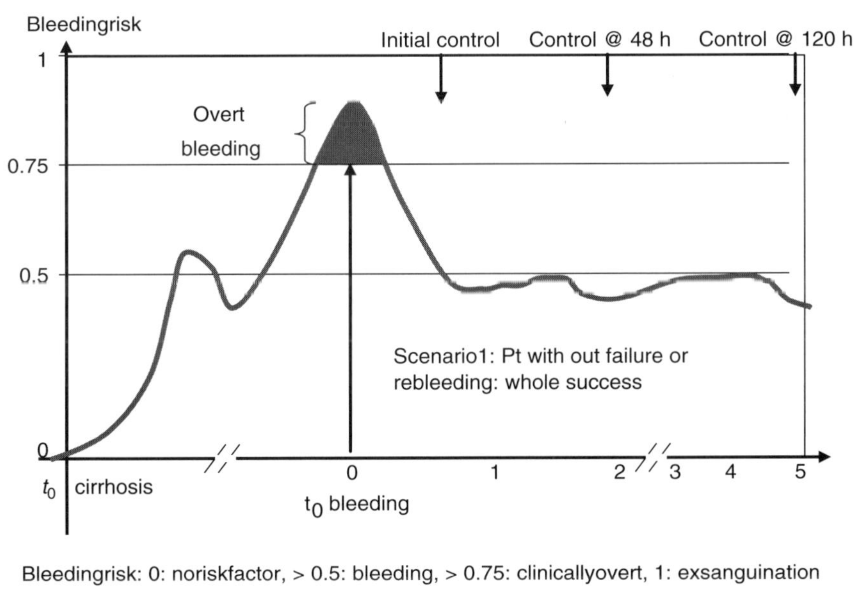

Fig. 12 Simulation of bleeding risk and definition of failure as a function of time. Scenario 1.

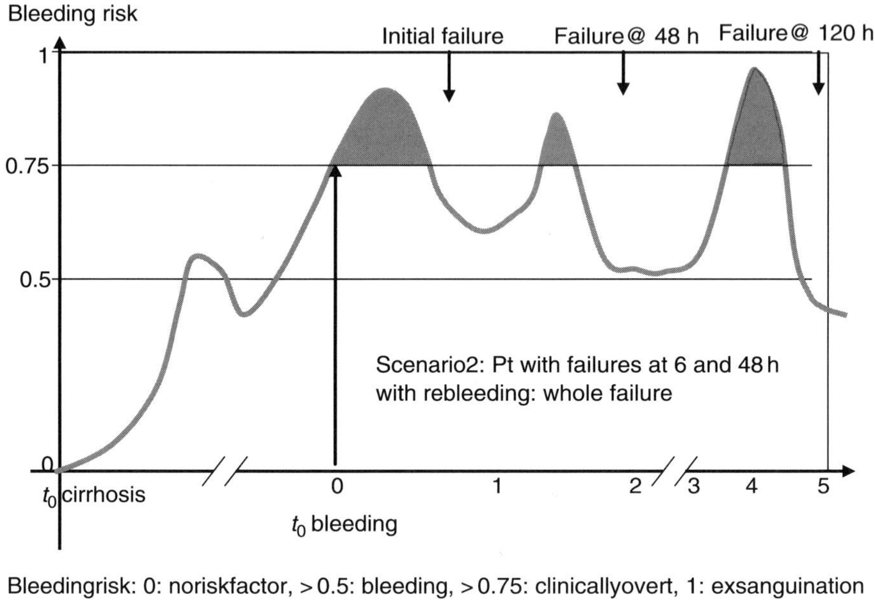

Fig. 13 Simulation of bleeding risk and definition of failure as a function of time. Scenario 2.

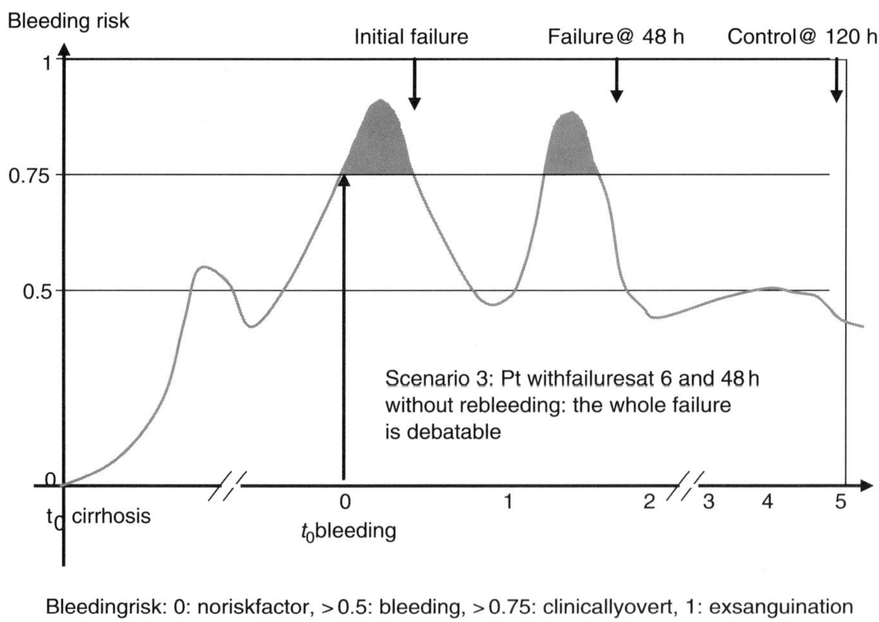

Fig. 14 Simulation of bleeding risk and definition of failure as a function of time. Scenario 3.

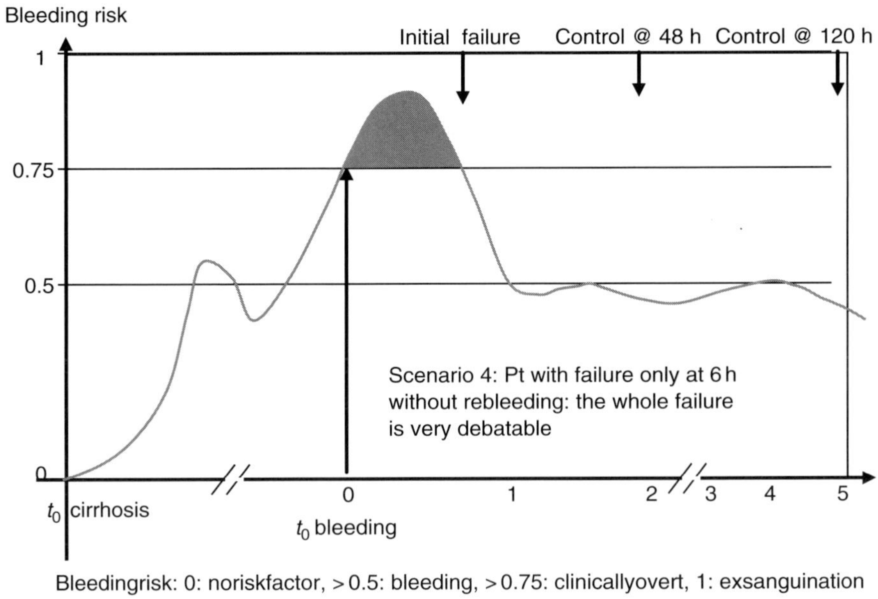

Fig. 15 Simulation of bleeding risk and definition of failure as a function of time. Scenario 4.

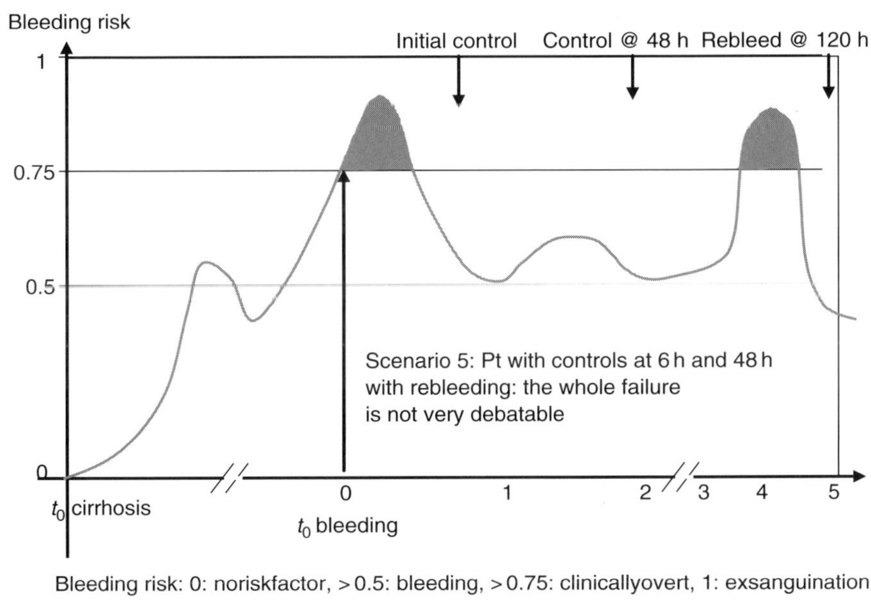

Fig. 16 Simulation of bleeding risk and definition of failure as a function of time. Scenario 5.

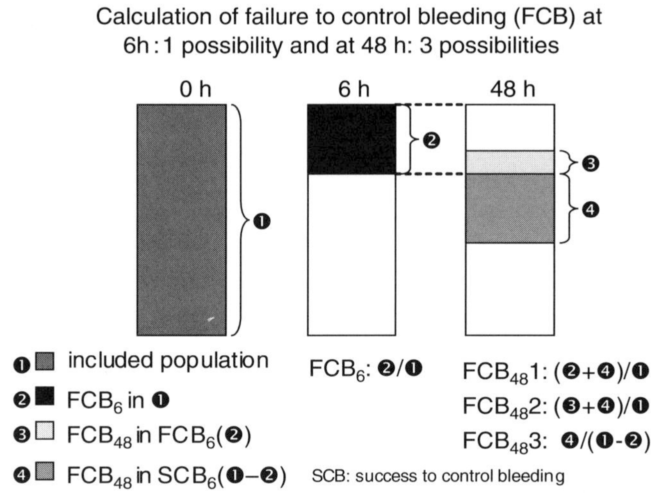

Fig. 17 Simulations of calculation of failure to control variceal bleeding as a function of cumulative judgement by clinicians and not at 6 and 48 h.

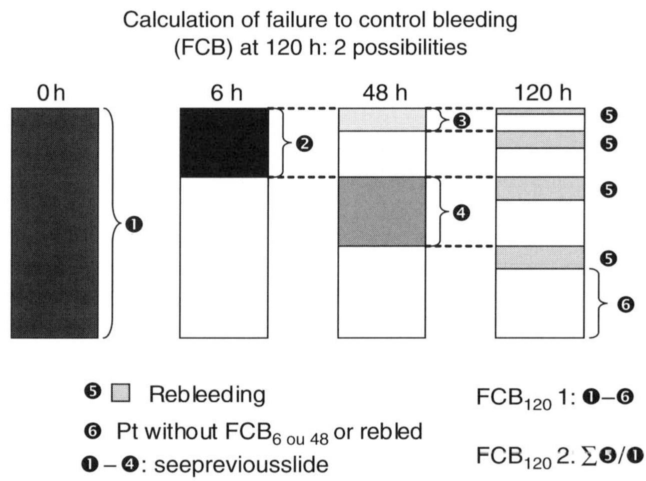

Fig. 18 Simulations of calculation of failure to control acute variceal bleeding (FCB) as a function of cumulative judgement of clinicians or not at 120 h.

Indeed, we can simulate different calculations of failure to control bleeding during the first 5 days. The calculation of failure to control bleeding shows 1 possibility at 6 h, 3 possibilities at 48 h (Fig. 17) and 2 possibilities at 120 h (Fig. 18) whether the calculation is cumulative or not.

LIMITATIONS OF BAVENO III CRITERIA: CASE-CONTROL STUDY

The previous study [1] led us to evaluate the predictors of bleeding in a case-control study (unpublished): 365 cirrhotic patients admitted in emergency for a complication of liver cirrhosis – variceal bleeding, ascites, jaundice or encephalopathy – were prospectively included into three groups:

- Controls without bleeding ($n = 163$);
- Variceal bleeding treated by endoscopic therapy only ($n = 99$);
- Early vapreotide followed by endoscopic therapy ($n = 103$).

Predictors of bleeding

We first evaluated the independent predictors of bleeding. Baseline variables were compared between the bleeding and control groups: no significant differences were observed for arterial pressure and haematocrit (Hct) between controls and bleeders treated by vapreotide.

We then evaluated the independent predictors of all bleeding episodes. Eleven variables independently predicted the bleeding group compared to controls without bleeding with a diagnostic accuracy (DA) = 92.3% and Area under the Receiver Operating Characteristic Curve (AUROC) = 0.968. No haemodynamic variable was selected, and Hb was selected at the second step (DA = 68.2%). Finally, we evaluated the independent predictors of all significant bleeding episodes defined by the transfusion of at least two BU: nine variables independently predicted significant bleeding with DA = 95.8% and AUROC = 0.982 compared to controls. No haemodynamic variable was selected, and Hb was selected at the first step with DA = 83.7% and AUROC = 0.899 compared to control group.

Evaluation of the specificity of Baveno III criteria

In a first step, the composite variables of Baveno criteria defining the control of bleeding (as defined in Table 4) were studied as crude (quantitative) variables at 6 and 48 h by comparing the three groups.

Discriminant variables (in univariate analysis) were:

- At 6 h: heart rate (HR), Hct and BU;
- At 48 h: HR, systolic arterial pressure (SAP), Hct and BU.

In a second step, the overall failure to control bleeding (according to Baveno definitions) was considered, as well as its composite variables together (quantitative variables transformed in binary variables); the significant differences between the three groups were:

- At 6 h: HR ($\geq$ 100/min) and overall failure;
- From 6 to 48 h: HR ($\geq$ 100/min), BU ($\geq$ 2) and overall failure.

Independent predictors of failure to control bleeding

We evaluated the relative role of composite variables in the definition of overall failure. In a first step, at 6 h HR $\geq$ 100/min was the only significant independent variable predictive of failure with DA = 99%. In a second step, (after exclusion of the binary composite variables of failure criteria), failure was independently predicted by HR and BU with DA = 98.7%.

Summary

At baseline, haemodynamic parameters (HR, SAP) are neither specific nor very discriminant to diagnose bleeding with current recommended treatment (early vasoactive drug followed by endoscopic treatment). On the contrary, haematological parameters (BU transfused, Hct) are very specific and discriminant. The only independent predictor of failure, as defined by Baveno criteria, at 6 and 48 h is HR > 100/min suggesting that other criteria of Baveno have no role. Since HR is not predictive of bleeding, this suggests that all the composite variables of Baveno definition of failure have little interest. The results of this study contribute to the proposal to define new criteria according to the following assumption: the predictors of failure to control bleeding should be those which are predictors of bleeding, that is Hb.

PROPOSALS

The previous results and consideration of answers to the questionnaire, as well as discussion with the panellists, have led us to propose new criteria for failure to control bleeding and to define the time frames of acute bleeding. We should keep in mind that the judgement criterion is a composite one and is a surrogate marker of success, that is prevention of death. We agree and recommend that failure criteria should reflect a change of therapy, that is the management of the patient changes, thus, making failure criteria very close if not the same as in day to day clinical practice.

Definitions of failure to control acute variceal bleeding

We propose two kinds of clinical setting for criteria for failure to control acute variceal bleeding.

1 A time dependent variable analysed by Kaplan–Meier plots: the patient is censored at time of failure. This judgement criterion is sensitive and is convenient for trials. The new end point is time to failure and is called t_f. Patient is censored at this time (t_f) when he or she meets the failure criteria. Death is a failure criterion, and removes the problem of competing end points.
2 A time fixed variable analysed by simple comparison: the patient is considered at the end of surveillance, that is at 120 h. This means failure criteria may have occurred at any time from 6 to 120 h. This judgement criterion is more convenient for clinical practice.
The sensitivity of the time dependent criterion compared to the time fixed criterion is shown by an example provided by a previous randomised trial [1,6]. Testing with comparison of proportions did not show any significant difference ($p = 0.09$) in survival without bleeding for the period from 6 to 48 h, whereas the difference was very significant ($p = 0.003$) with life table analysis between treatment groups, taking into account time to failure.

Criteria for failure to control bleeding

New composite criteria (Table 5)

We propose two kinds of criteria: non-transfusion criteria and transfusion-related criteria.

Non-transfusion criteria. These criteria are particularly applicable to around 20% of patients who do not need blood transfusion [9].

We propose the following main criteria:

- Fresh haematemesis ($\geq$ 6 h after t_0 and $\geq$ 2 h after diagnostic endoscopy, or $>$ 2 h after start of specific therapy or therapeutic endoscopy).
- 3 g drop in Hb ($\approx$ 9% Hct), if no blood transfusion is given.
- Death.

Table 5 New Baveno IV criteria defining failure to control bleeding. One criterion defines failure, which ever occurs first.

- (New) fresh haematemesis $\geq$ 2 h after start of specific drug treatment or therapeutic endoscopy.
- 3 g drop in Hb ($\approx$ 9% Hct) in those not transfused.
- Death.
- Index of blood transfusion requirement: ABRI $\geq$ 0.75.

One criterion defines failure, whichever occurs first.

Minor criteria could be the following:

- Blood aspiration could be considered equivalent to haematemesis at a certain threshold (e.g. $\geq$ 100 ml/h of fresh blood for two consecutive hours) – this should be used by groups that use nasogastric aspiration.
- Rectorragia ($\geq$ 6 h after t_0 and $\geq$ 2 h after endoscopy).
- Tachycardia $\geq$ 120 with no other plausible cause.
- SAP $\geq$ 20 mmHg decrease despite transfusion.

Two minor criteria could define failure. However, a consensus was not reached among panellists for these minor criteria. Consequently, these were not part of the final proposals.

Transfusion-related criteria. Transfusion requirement is an independent surrogate marker of mortality in variceal bleeding [10]. This criterion can be applied in patients requiring transfusion since blood requirement is a quantitative and sensitive variable.

The patients that should be transfused are defined by an initial Hct $\leq$ 22% since the target is 24% [11] and one BU usually corresponds to a 2–3% gain in Hct.

The predictive value of blood transfusion has been already emphasised. Moreover, blood transfusion reflects the severity of bleeding. However, we have observed that use of a crude rate of transfusion can be biased since a patient with an initial dramatic low level in Hb would be automatically classified as a failure according to transfusion requirement even if initial control was obtained. Finally, it has been shown that Hct levels are significant predictors of 5-day failure [10].

Thus, failure should be constituted by the number of BU transfused to achieve target Hb or Hct corrected by baseline Hb or Hct.

So, we propose an adjusted blood requirement index (ABRI):

$$\text{ABRI} = \text{BU}/[(\text{final Hct} - \text{initial Hct}) + 0.01]$$

with BU: blood units, Hct: haematocrit.

The constant is introduced to discard impossible calculations due to null denominator and is fixed at 0.01 since it is lower than the sensitivity of Hct measurement. It also allows exclusion of the influence of this constant on the result when two decimals are used (Table 6). Hct is suggested instead of Hb since this parameter may be available at bedside in ICU.

The assumptions are the following:

- 1 BU = 2% Hct.
- The target Hct is 24%.

- The usual transfusion rate is 1 BU/h in a patient with non-immediate life threatening-conditions.
- The transfusion rate should be $\leq$ 1 BU/2 h.

Issues related to ABRI. A normal ABRI is 0.5 based on the assumption that 1 BU induces an increase of 2% in Hct.

Thus over-requirement of transfusion is above 0.5.

Under-requirement is less than 0.5.

Failure is defined by ABRI $\geq$ 0.75. In calculations, the figure used should be 0.745 to account for the difference due to the constant, the corresponding figure for the 0.5 threshold should be 0.495 (see Table 6), since this means one additional BU compared to the expected requirement without ongoing bleeding. Case examples are shown in Table 6.

This index has to be validated, especially its threshold. The influence of haemodilution by plasma substitutes has to be taken into account in trials. So, this variable should be measured and comparison of ABRI should be adjusted for this variable, when validating its use.

The count of BU is cumulative from time zero (t_0).

The target Hct when transfusion is used is proposed at 24% for the following reasons. This is the choice of most panellists. This is also suggested by two RCTs. One large RCT including 418 ICU patients concluded that a restrictive strategy of red-cell transfusion (7 to 9 g/dL of Hb) is at least as effective and possibly superior to a liberal transfusion strategy in critically ill patients, with the possible exception of patients with acute myocardial infarction and unstable angina [12].

Table 6 Examples of ABRI calculation showing different transfusion requirements.

Requirement	Under	Normal	Over*	Over
Initial Hct (%)	20	20	20	20
Final Hct (%)	24	24	24	24
Blood units (n)	1	2	3	6
ABRI $\approx$†	0.25	0.5	0.75	1.5
ABRI =‡	0.244	0.489	0.732	1.463
ABRI = §	0.249	0.499	0.748	1.496

* With 1 additional BU compared to normal or expected requirement

† Or = without constant or with two decimals

‡ Constant = 0.1

§ Constant = 0.01

Table 7 Randomised study of transfusion in cirrhotic patients with severe variceal bleeding (ref 13).

	Group according to target Hct		
	1	2	p
Patients (n)	43	47	–
Target Hct (%)	25 ± 2	32 ± 2	–
Blood units (n)	2.6	4.4	0.001
Rebleeding (%)	40	48	NS
Death (%)	14	12	NS

Table 8 Comparison of haematocrit (Hct), blood units and ABRI in an RCT [6].

	Treatment		
	Placebo	Vapreotide	p
Initial Hct (%)	26.6 ± 6.3	27.9 ± 6.6	0.17
Final Hct (%)	27.9 ± 3.5	29.6 ± 4.4	0.005
Variation in Hct (%)	11 ± 30	11 ± 28	0.98
Blood units (n)	3.0 ± 3.0	1.9 ± 2.2	0.006*
ABRI score	1.13 ± 4.94	0.46 ± 3.02	0.25
ABRI ≥ 0.5 (%)	37.6	30.0	0.26
ABRI ≥ 0.75 (%)	31.2	16.0	0.02

$*p = 0.04$ by log-rank test for Kaplan–Meier estimates

One small RCT was performed in PHT including 90 cirrhotic patients with severe variceal bleeding defined by initial Hct $< 27\%$ [13]. The rebleeding rate and death rate were similar between the two Hct target groups (25% and 32%) as shown in Table 7.

Finally, a systematic review concluded that the limited published evidence supports the use of restrictive transfusion triggers in patients who are free of serious cardiac disease [11].

Application of ABRI in a trial. The specificity of ABRI index was evaluated in the previous case-control study performed in 365 cirrhotic patients. Failure defined by ABRI index ≥ 0.75 was observed in 1.9% of controls versus 22.3% of bleeders, $p < 10^{-4}$.

The sensitivity of ABRI score was evaluated in the RCT (Table 8) corresponding to the bleeding group mentioned above [6]. Failure defined by ABRI index ≥ 0.75 was observed in 31% in the placebo group versus 16% in the vapreotide group, $p = 0.02$. This RCT clearly shows that there was an imbalance for Hct between treatment groups so that crude comparison of BU is not appropriate. This RCT also shows that ABRI used as a score is not sensitive, due to negative values in patients with an under-requirement for transfusion especially with a final Hct superior to initial Hct. However, the use of ABRI as a dichotomous (binary) index is sensitive provided the threshold is fixed at 0.75.

Time frames

Time is divided in periods of 6 h for the first 48 h and 12 h from 48 to 120 h. Blood pressure, HR, Hb or Hct are recorded at the end of each period (Table 9).

The reference time (t_r) for the first period begins with the start of specific treatment provided it is begun within 4 h after admission (t_0). The reference values (Hb, Hct) have to be recorded at ± 4 hourly intervals based on t_r. These values are called 'initial'.

Clinical settings of failure

There are two ways to define the failure to control bleeding, which depend on time (see the section on time frames):

Table 9 Different times used in Baveno IV criteria.

Variable	Abbreviation	Meaning	Conditions
Time zero	t_0	Admission to the first medical unit*	Haematemesis and/or melaena within previous 24 h
Reference time	t_r	Start of specific treatment	Within 4 h after t_0
Time to failure	t_f	End point	From 6 h to 120 h after t_r
Periods	–	Measurement of Hct	Every 6 h for the first 48 h after t_r and every 12 h from 48 to 120 h after t_r
(New) fresh haematemesis	–	Criterion of failure	$\geq$ 2 h after t_r or therapeutic endoscopy

* or bleeding start when bleeding occurs in an inpatient

• a time dependent criterion defining time to failure suitable for trials or clinical practice;
• a time fixed criterion at 120 h suitable for clinical practice – when there is a yes/no evaluation for failure.

The failure criteria at 120 h are the same as the previous four major criteria (Table 5).

Summary

There are two kinds of criteria for failure of control of acute variceal bleeding, each of which is not mutually exclusive.

• Non-transfusion or clinical;
• Transfusion related.

Clinical settings of failure:

• Time dependent criterion defining time to failure suitable for trials and clinical practice;
• Time fixed criterion at 120 h suitable for clinical practice.

Each setting is not mutually exclusive, and in both the criteria for failure are the same.

Both time dependent and time fixed criteria should be reported in future studies in PHT.

Calculation of transfusion rate and length of hospitalisation

The crude comparisons of blood requirements between treatment groups are biased since these data are apt to be censored earlier in the placebo group (or group with the worst prognosis) due to a higher failure rate, unless a time factor is considered.

To compensate for this, life table analysis could be applied to the number of BU transfused as suggested in an RCT [7]. See an example in Table 8.

The same bias may exist for the length of hospital stay, so that the duration could be reported in survivors only, or the life-table analysis could be applied to the number of days in hospital.

However, experts did not reach a consensus so that this issue should be evaluated in the future.

Clinically significant bleeding (CSB)

A CSB episode is be defined by transfusion $\geq$ 2 BU as in Baveno II and III statements.

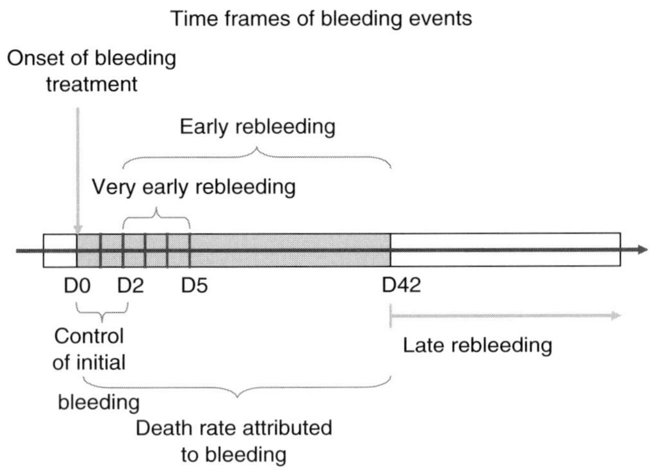

Fig. 19 Time frames for acute variceal bleeding.

Time frames of bleeding events

Rebleeding should be defined as *early* rebleeding between the 3rd day (from 48 h) and 42nd day, that is the end of the follow-up period after bleeding where the hazard of death appears to return to baseline. Late rebleeding is after 42 days.

Early rebleeding should be separated into *very early* rebleeding between 48 and 120 h when treatment, especially pharmacological, is usually the same as that for the index bleed. The period between 120 h and 6 weeks is the first period for secondary prevention (Fig. 19).

On the other hand, it would be simpler to define early rebleeding as between 3 and 5 days and late rebleeding afterwards. As long as time intervals are specified, comparison can be made between trials.

The time point of reference for the control of bleeding (t_0 in Baveno II criteria) should be fixed, not only to t_0 but also to the time when the first specific treatment is used, especially when treatment is started before admission. This time point could be called t_r. The different times used are listed in Table 9.

Applications

We propose that both time dependent and time fixed criteria should be used in parallel in trials and that time fixed criteria are sufficient in clinical practice, although some units may also wish to use time dependent criteria.

In trials there have been frequent debates on the failure criteria as applied to individual patients. We recommend failure should be classified according to the above criteria and independently by a senior clinician during a trial. In trials, the steering committee should validate all discordant cases of failure. At least two clinicians with expertise in current practice should be included in this committee.

FOR THE FUTURE

The above criteria need validation in prospective studies. They need to be compared to Baveno II/III criteria and also to any independent judgement of steering committees in randomised therapeutic trials. The latter will be allocating treatment failures in cases of dispute, and verifying whether failure criteria were met.

In addition, assessment of failures and successes independent of treatment allocation will allow an evaluation of whether failure criteria are sufficiently discriminatory to identify patients who have a poorer outcome following acute variceal bleeding.

Future studies should address the following:

1 Blood transfusion management in randomised studies.
2 The threshold for the ABRI index.
3 The ABRI index for other sources of upper gastrointestinal bleeding.

SECONDARY PROPHYLAXIS

Variceal rebleeding occurs frequently after controlling acute variceal bleeding in patients with cirrhosis and PHT [14–16]. Thus, prevention of a rebleeding episode is mandatory [17–19]. However, in clinical trials, due to the lack of a commonly used definition of failure of secondary prophylaxis, comparison between studies and/or interpretation of outcomes research is very difficult.

Time frame for start of secondary prophylaxis

In Baveno III there was no consensus regarding when the secondary prophylaxis of variceal rebleeding should be started, as well as disagreement concerning the definition of treatment failure. In an attempt to clarify these issues the first question investigated was:

Q: In your centre when do you consider secondary prophylaxis to start?

R: A total number of 38 responses were obtained, and the results can be seen in Table 10.

Again no consensus could be reached. For this reason, the results of a recent randomised, controlled clinical trial [20] comparing the efficacy of

Table 10 Criteria selected by 38 responders to define the appropriate to start secondary prophylaxis.

	Yes (%)	No (%)
At admission	16	84
End day 2 (48 h)	16	84
End day 3 (72 h)	24	76
End day 5 (120 h)	45	55

Table 11 Interval between index bleeding and randomisation in the trial.

Days after index bleeding	Drugs *n* (%)	Banding *n* (%)
6–15	28 (49)	26 (50)
16–30	14 (25)	14 (27)
> 30	15 (26)	12 (23)

pharmacological treatment against endoscopic band ligation for the prevention of variceal rebleeding were evaluated. The difference between this clinical trial and similar published trials [21–23], is that the patients included in the former trial [20] were randomised after a longer period of time from the acute variceal bleeding episode. Consequently, an analysis of the efficacy of both treatments, according to intervals to randomisation after admission for the acute variceal bleeding episode was performed.

There were a total of 109 cirrhotic patients followed for a mean of 18 months. The patients were randomised in two groups: (1) nadolol plus 5 isosorbide mononitrate (57 patients) and (2) endoscopic band ligation plus one or two sessions of sclerotherapy at the end of the banding ligation (52 patients).

One of the inclusion criteria was that the index variceal bleeding episode, demonstrated by emergency endoscopy, was within 3 months of randomisation and that there was no other evidence of bleeding within this time. No significant differences in gastrointestinal and variceal rebleeding, treatment failure, complications and survival were observed between groups. Both treatment groups were similar at the time of inclusion for all the demographic characteristics, Child–Pugh class and score, interval of follow-up and loss of follow-up. The interval to randomisation was divided into three different periods and the results were analysed between groups, as shown in Table 11.

During the three periods of time the proportion of Child A patients were similar as well as for Child B and Child C patients (Table 12).

Table 12 Distribution of patients among Child–Pugh classes in relation to the interval between index bleed and randomisation.

Days	Child A (%)	Child B (%)	Child C (%)
6–15	33.3	55.6	11.1
16–30	39.3	46.4	14.3
> 30	40.7	44.4	14.8

The evaluation of rebleeding from all sources and from varices alone did not show any significant differences between groups. In addition, the cumulative probability of being free of gastrointestinal and variceal bleeding at 2 years was also similar. When treatment failure was analysed in relation to the time of inclusion, no significant difference was observed between groups in relation to treatment failure rate and or with respect to the probability of being free of rebleeding at 2 years. Furthermore, the survival analysis performed between the three groups demonstrated no significant differences with a similar cumulative probability of survival at 2 years.

A commonly used definition for failure of secondary prophylaxis and for a minimum start date would be useful for the analysis of clinical trials, and for clinical practice. It is important that the definition should have wide applicability.

Additional issues were considered before the definition was agreed upon, as follows: (1) the time frame for acute variceal bleeding episode is 5 days (120 h); (2) the results presented above in relation to different time intervals for starting the secondary prophylaxis and; (3) the knowledge that many centres adopt a 2-week interval between therapeutic endoscopic sessions (from the one or two performed as an emergency to the next elective one), due to the problem in performing further endoscopic treatment sooner because of the presence of multiple ulcers [23]. Thus, the consensus definition on when the secondary prophylaxis should be started is as soon as possible from day 6 of the index variceal bleeding.

Criteria for failure of secondary prophylaxis

In the Consensus of Baveno III the accepted definitions were [4,24] as follows.

- Rebleeding: A new haematemesis or new melaena after a period of 24 h of stable vital signs, Hct/Hb.
- Failure of secondary prophylaxis: a single episode of clinically significant rebleeding together with a systolic blood pressure < 100 mmHg or postural change of > 20 mmHg and/or pulse rate of > 100 bpm at time zero.
- CSB: at least 2 U/blood within 24 h of time zero.

Table 13 Criteria selected by 38 responders to define failure of secondary prophylaxis.

	YES (%)	NO (%)
1 CSB	63	37
1 CSB potentially needing another therapy	76	24
2 CSB	63	37
2 bleeding only 1 CSB	55	45

However, many doubts we raised concerning these definitions. With the addition of new data the following question was posed:

Q: In your centre what do you consider to be failure of secondary prophylactic therapy?

The answers from 38 respondents can be seen in Table 13.

Again no consensus could be obtained after consulting all the experts of Baveno IV conference. As previously discussed in this chapter, the haemodynamic parameters do not necessarily define CSB in cirrhotic patients. Furthermore the units of blood (BU) transfused alone do not necessarily identify the severity of a bleeding episode [3,4,24]. For these reasons the following definition for failure of secondary prophylaxis was agreed upon: one single episode of clinically significant rebleeding from portal hypertensive sources.

Moreover, a new definition for clinically significant rebleeding was presented. In addition to the amount of blood transfused a new index was incorporated.

The new definition is as follows:

New haematemesis and/or new melaena within the previous 24 h of hospital admission that requires $\geq$ 2 U/blood plus the ABRI $\geq$ 0.5 or a decrease of 3 g/dL of Hb if no transfusion is given.

However it is important to observe that the $\geq$ 2 U/blood transfused is the main point of the definition, and the ABRI and a fall of 3 g of Hb should be further validated. For this purpose it was recommended that all the necessary data should be included in the results of clinical trials in order to be able to compare this index with the previous parameters defining CSB.

The incidence of complications observed with pharmacological and endoscopic treatments for secondary prophylaxis of variceal bleeding is variable and in general mild with both treatments. However, although the percentage of overall side effects is similar, the rate of severe complications is usually significantly lower among patients who receive medical therapy, compared to those treated with endoscopic measures. The overall incidence

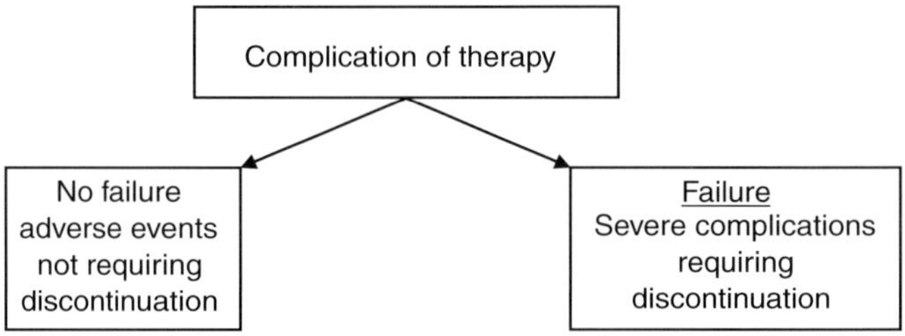

Fig. 20 Complications of therapy and treatment failure.

observed with β-blocker is between 15% and 20%, and this number slightly increases when nitrates are added. In relation to endoscopic treatment, band ligation has significantly fewer side effects than sclerotherapy [25]. The overall complication rate observed in band ligation groups is between 20% and 30%. With sclerotherapy the rate and severity of complications increases up to 40%, with 1–2% resulting in death [26]. However, the distinction between side effects and severe complications is not well defined. Furthermore, this discordance makes it difficult to compare the results of the different clinical trials in relation to treatment failure. Due to this discrepancy and in order to clarify this point the following question was posed:

Q: Are therapy complications requiring changes of treatment considered treatment failure? From only 18 answers, 61% said no and 39% said yes.

Due to the small number of answers and the lack of consensus a proposal shown in Fig. 20 was put forward.

Examples of severe complications are as follows:

- Endoscopy: perforation, severe bleeding due to treatment, stricture requiring dilation
- β-blockers: heart block, severe hypotension and syncope.

SUMMARY KEY EVENTS BAVENO IV

Acute variceal bleeding

1 The time frame for the acute variceal bleeding episode is 5 days (120 h).
2 Failure to control bleeding signifies change in therapy.
3 Failure to control bleeding is defined by the following whichever occurs first.

(a) death,
(b) fresh haematemesis 2 h or more after the start of specific drug therapy or therapeutic endoscopy,

(c) a drop of Hb from baseline of 3 g/dL (Hct of 9%) or more if no blood transfusion is given,
(d) index of blood transfusion requirement defined as ABRI > 0.75 at any time point.
The ABRI is:

$$\frac{\text{Blood units}}{(\text{final Hct} - \text{initial Hct}) + 0.01}$$

The Hct or Hb should be measured at least every 6 h during the first 48 h and 12 hourly from day 3 to day 5.

1 Transfusion target should be a Hct of 24% or Hb of 8 g/dL.

2 For analysis of therapeutic effect during acute bleeding:
(a) The time to failure is the first occurrence of any of the failure criteria (Kaplan–Meier analysis). Although death is not a competing end point with these definitions, logistic or Cox modelling should be evaluated with respect to the end point.
(b) Failure occurring at any time within 120 h is considered as either yes or no. Again regression modelling should also be evaluated.
(c) All specific therapeutic procedures should be documented with time points related to their first use.
(d) Intentions to use further specific therapy should be documented even if not used.
(e) Transfusion requirements should be recorded as a function of time for the whole interval of acute bleeding if no failure has occurred for example units transfused/120 h, or units transfused to time of failure if failure has occurred.

3 The new definitions regarding acute variceal bleeding need to be validated in appropriate studies. In particular:
(a) the criteria for failure to control variceal bleeding need to be evaluated as valid surrogate markers of outcome;
(b) the threshold of ABRI defining failure needs validation;
(c) failure and success should be evaluated independently of treatment allocation to establish that failure criteria do discriminate for those patients who have a worse outcome.

4 Current and future studies should incorporate both Baveno III and IV criteria, and evaluate end points using both sets of criteria.

Secondary prophylaxis

1 The start of secondary prophylaxis is from day 6 after day 0, or later, and the specific time point should be recorded.

2 Failure of secondary prophylaxis is defined by the occurrence of the first clinically significant rebleeding episode related to PHT.

3 Clinically significant rebleeding is defined as haematemesis or melaena with a transfusion requirement of an ABRI > 0.5 and/or decrease of 3 g/dL Hb (9% Hct) if no blood transfusion is given.

4 Complications and side effects should be documented more accurately:

(a) cumulatively per patient and not per episode of therapy;

(b) to distinguish those complications that do not result in stopping therapy versus those who do.

REFERENCES

1 Cales P, Lacave N, Silvain C *et al.* Prospective study on the application of Baveno II criteria in patients with cirrhosis and gastrointestinal bleeding. *J Hepatol* 2000;**33**: 738–741.

2 Burroughs AK, Patch D. Therapeutic benefit of vasoactive drugs for acute variceal bleeding: a real pharmacological effect or a side effect of definition in trials? *Hepatology* 1996;**222**: 737–739.

3 Burroughs AK ed. Assessment of value of consensus definitions in acute variceal bleeding. *Lancet* 2001;**357**: 1147–1148.

4 de Franchis R. Developing consensus in portal hypertension. *J Hepatol* 1996;**25**: 390–394.

5 de Franchis R. Updating consensus in portal hypertension: report of the Baveno III consensus workshop on definitions, methodology and therapeutic strategies in portal hypertension. *J Hepatol* 2000;**33**: 846–852.

6 Calès P, Masliah C, Bernard B *et al.* Early administration of vapreotide for variceal bleeding in patients with cirrhosis. *N Engl J Med* 2001;**344**: 23–28.

7 Avgerinos A, Nevens F, Raptis S, Fevery J and the ABOVE Study Group. Early administration of somatostatin and efficacy of sclerotherapy in acute esophageal variceal bleeds: the European acute bleeding esophageal variceal episodes (ABOVE) randomised trial. *Lancet* 1997;**350**: 1495–1499.

8 Bosch J, Thabut D, Bendtsen F *et al.* European Study Group on rFVIIa in UGI Haemorrhage. Recombinant factor VIIa for upper gastrointestinal bleeding in patients with cirrhosis: a randomized, double-blind trial. *Gastroenterology* 2004;**127**: 1123–1130.

9 Sorbi D, Gostout CJ, Peura D *et al.* An assessment of the management of acute bleeding varices: a multicenter prospective member-based study. *Am J Gastroenterol.* 2003;**98**: 2424–2434.

10 D'Amico G, De Franchis R, Cooperative Study Group. Upper digestive bleeding in cirrhosis. Post-therapeutic outcome and prognostic indicators. *Hepatology* 2003;**38**: 599–612.

11 Hill SR, Carless PA, Henry DA *et al.* Transfusion thresholds and other strategies for guiding allogeneic red blood cell transfusion. *Cochrane Database Syst Rev* 2002;**2**: CD002042.

12 Hebert PC, Wells G, Blajchman MA *et al.* A multicenter, randomized, controlled clinical trial of transfusion requirements in critical care. Transfusion requirements in Critical Care Investigators, Canadian Critical Care Trials Group. *N Engl J Med* 1999;**340**: 409–417.
13 Hochain P, Mele V, Tuil S *et al.* Transfusion for variceal bleeding in cirrhotic patients. *Gut* 1996;**38**: 154.
14 Graham DY, Smith JL. The course of patients after variceal hemorrhage. *Gastroenterology* 1981;**80**: 800–809.
15 Pagliaro L, D'Amico G, Pasta L *et al.* Portal hypertension in cirrhosis: natural history. In Bosch J Groszmann RJ eds. *Portal Hypertension. Pathophysiology and Treatment.* Oxford: Blackwell,1994; 72–92.
16 Lebrec D, Stiegmann G. Prevention of recurrent variceal haemorrhage (secondary prophylaxis). *Portal hypertension. Proceedings of the third baveno international consensus workshop.* Oxford, Blackwell Science, 2001.
17 D'Amico G, Pagliaro L, Bosch J. The treatment of portal hypertension: a meta-analytic review. *Hepatology* 1995;**22**: 332–354.
18 Bosch J, Abraldes JG, Groszmann R. Current management of portal hypertension. *J Hepatol* 2003;**38**: 554–558.
19 Bernard B, Lebrec D, Mathurin P, Opolon P, Poynard T. Beta-adrenergic antagonists in the prevention of gastrointestinal rebleeding in patients with cirrhosis: a meta-analysis. *Hepatology* 1997;**25**: 63–70.
20 Romero G, Kravetz D, Argonz J *et al.* Comparative study between nadolol and 5 isosorbide mononitrate vs. endoscopic band ligation plus sclerotherapy in the prevention of variceal rebleeding in cirrhotic patients. A randomized controlled trial. *Hepatology* 2004;**40** (suppl 1): 204 A.
21 Villanueva C, Minana J, Ortiz J *et al.* Endoscopic ligation compared with combined treatment with nadolol and isosorbide mononitrate to prevent recurrent variceal bleeding. *N Engl J Med* 2001;**345**: 647–655.
22 Lo G H, Chen W C, Chen M H *et al.* Banding ligation versus nadolol and isosorbide mononitrate for the prevention of esophageal variceal rebleeding. *Gastroenterology* 2002;**123**: 728–734.
23 Patch D, Sabin CA, Goulis J *et al.* A randomized, controlled trial of medical therapy versus endoscopic ligation for the prevention of variceal rebleeding in patients with cirrhosis. *Gastroenterology* 2002;**123**: 1013–1019.
24 de Franchis R, Primignani M. Endoscopic treatment for portal hypertension. *Sem Liver Dis* 1999;**19**: 439–455
25 Stiegmann GV, Goff JS, Michaletz-Onody PA *et al.* Endoscopic sclerotherapy as compared with endoscopic ligation for bleeding esophageal varices. *N Eng J Med* 1992;**326**: 1527–1532.
26 Infante-Rivard C, Esnaola S, Villeneuve JP. Role of endoscopic variceal sclerotherapy in the long-term management of variceal bleeding: a meta-analysis. *Gastroenterology* 1989;**96**: 1087–1092.

Baveno IV Consensus Statements: Definition of Key Events

Andrew K. Burroughs, Patrick S. Kamath (Chairpersons), Paul Calès, David Kravetz, Oliviero Riggio, Dominique Thabut and Henk R. van Buuren

Baveno IV definitions and criteria for failure to control bleeding

1 The time frame for the acute bleeding episode should be 120 h (5 days).

2 Failure signifies need to change therapy: one criterion defines failure, whichever occurs first:

(a) Fresh haematemesis $\geq$ 2 h after start of specific drug treatment or therapeutic endoscopy. In the minority of patients who have a nasogastric tube in place, aspiration of greater than 100 mL of fresh blood represents failure;

(b) 3 g drop in Hb ($\approx$ 9% drop in Hct) if no transfusion is administered;

(c) Death;

(d) Adjusted blood transfusion requirement index (ABRI, see Box 1) $\geq$ 0.75 at any time point. (The threshold of ABRI defining failure requires validation.)

Box 1 ADJUSTED BLOOD REQUIREMENT INDEX (ABRI)

$$\text{ABRI} = \frac{\text{Blood Units transfused}}{[(\text{final Hct} - \text{initial Hct}) + 0.01]}$$

- Hct (or Hb) is measured at least every:
- 6 h for the first 2 days
- 12 h for days 3–5
- The transfusion target should be a Hct of 21% or a Hb of 8 g/dL

Notes for the Baveno IV definitions and criteria

For the purposes of analysis the following criteria should be adopted:

- Time to failure – first occurrence of any of the above criteria for failure; (cumulative hazard plots and Cox regression analysis)
- Failure occurring at 120 h is considered as YES or NO;
- The use of both time to failure and final evaluation at 120 h is encouraged;

- All specific therapeutic procedures should be documented with time points;
- Intention to use further specific therapy should be documented even if not used;
- Transfusion requirements should be recorded as a function of time for the whole interval of acute bleeding if no failure has occurred for example units transfused/120 h or units transfused up to time of failure.

Baveno IV definitions and criteria for failure of secondary prophylaxis

Failure to prevent rebleeding is defined as a single episode of clinically significant rebleeding from portal hypertensive sources

Clinically significant rebleeding:

1. Haematemesis/melaena. In the minority of patients who have a nasogastric tube in place, aspiration of greater than 100 mL of fresh blood represents failure;

   plus

2. ABRI ≥ 0.5 (the threshold of ABRI defining failure requires validation);

   or

3. Decrease 3 g of Hb if no transfusion is given.

LECTURE

Abnormalities of Haemostasis Tests in Chronic Liver Disease: Clinically Relevant?

Pier Mannuccio Mannucci

INTRODUCTION

The main components of the haemostatic system are primary haemostasis (platelet–vessel wall interactions), blood coagulation and fibrinolysis. The majority of activators and inhibitors of the haemostatic system are proteins synthesised by the hepatocytes (with the notable exception of factor VIII, a key component of the intrinsic coagulation system, and von Willebrand factor, the main determinant of platelet adhesion to the damaged vessel wall) [1,2]. With this as background, it is not surprising that the majority of the components of the haemostatic system are abnormally reduced in plasma as soon as the synthetic capacity of the hepatocyte is impaired [1,2]. The epitome of the abnormalities of haemostasis in severe liver disease is the prolongation of the prothrombin time, which is a key component of the Child–Pugh score widely used to classify and grade the severity of liver disease. The other point of the matter is that patients with severe liver disease bleed frequently from the gastrointestinal tract, mainly but not exclusively from ruptured oesophageal varices [3]. Accordingly, it has become only too natural and consequential to link these two abnormalities and to imply that one (impaired haemostasis) is the cause of the other (abnormal variceal bleeding). The astute hepatologist is aware that the anatomic and haemodynamic consequences of portal hypertension are the main determinants of variceal bleeding in severe liver diease [3]. Yet, the impairment of haemostasis has long been considered an important cofactor, as witnessed by the abundant literature on the value of haemostasis test in the prediction of bleeding, on the clinical evaluation of haemostatic drugs as adjuvants in the prevention and control of bleeding. With this as background, I shall first review critically the past literature on the relationship between haemostasis abnormalities and the bleeding tendency in severe liver disease. Then I shall demonstrate how the recent adoption of haemostasis tests that are truly more capable than those available in the past to reflect *in vitro* what is happening *in vivo* leads to the conclusion that *in vivo* haemostasis is not truly abnormal in patients with severe liver disease. This reassessment of the problem has implications on treatment, and particularly on whether or not it is warranted to look for haemostatic drugs as adjuvants to the treatments currently used to control portal hypertension and its anatomical consequences.

THE PAST AS A PROLOGUE

In every haematology or haemostasiology textbook, liver disease is listed as an important cause of acquired bleeding. Liver disease is indeed a cause of abnormal haemostasis tests, spanning from low count and abnormal function of blood platelets (some reflected by a prolonged skin bleeding time) to low coagulation factors (reflected by such prolonged coagulation screening tests as the prothrombin time and activated partial thromboplastin time) (Table 14). There is also evidence that the fibrinolytic activity is heightened in chronic liver disease, with the implication of a contribution of this system to the derangement of haemostasis through the increased tendency of formed clots to lyse (Table 14). Yet, the evidence that the abnormalities of haemostasis tests are associated with an increased tendency to bleed is meagre. To make this point, it is appropriate to distinguish spontaneous bleeding from oesophageal varices from bleeding provoked by surgical operations or by such invasive manoeuvres as liver biopsy. Two small but innovative studies by Ewe [4] and Dillon *et al.* [5] did observe that an array of haemostasis tests performed in peripheral blood correlate poorly with the actual duration of bleeding and the amount of blood loss measured directly at laparoscopy

Table 14 Haemostasis in severe liver disease.

- Multiple coagulation factor deficiencies
- Thrombocytopenia and thrombocytopathy
- Hyperfibrinolysis (tissue plasminogen activator, thrombin activatable fibrinolysis inhibitor)

BUT

- Deficiency of naturally occurring anticoagulants (antithrombin, thrombomodulin/protein C/protein S system, tissue factor pathway inhibitor)
- Deficiency of profibrinolytic factors (plasminogen) and increase of the principal inhibitor of plasminogen activation (PAI-1)

from the biopsy puncture. In an editorial accompanying one of these articles, MacGill [6] concluded that abnormal bleeding after liver biopsy is a random event that cannot be predicted by the methods used to explore the haemostatic system. Other studies indicating little or no association between the risk of bleeding after liver biopsy and the degree of abnormal haemostasis tests are those of McVay and Toy [7] and Caturelli *et al.* [8]. The only significant exception comes from Boberg *et al.* [9], who showed that among 219 patients undergoing percutaneous liver biopsy those with a prolonged skin bleeding time carried a five-fold greater risk of significant bleeding, defined by a decrease in haemoglobin of > 2 g/dL. Moreover, in a study of patients with 'decompensated' liver disease Bok *et al.* [10] concluded that while there was an association between the abnormality of coagulation and fibrinolysis tests and the development of soft tissue haematomas, variceal bleeding was not related to the impairment of coagulation and fibrinolysis [10].

On the whole, these data indicate that haemostasis tests are not important predictors of the tendency to bleed from varices or even after surgical procedures (including biopsies) in patients with liver disease. However, the aforementioned data on the skin bleeding time make the clinician uneasy when there is a prolonged bleeding time during such a blind procedure as liver biopsy. Therefore, when a bleeding time is longer than 10 min, it is our practice to avoid biopsy or to attempt a pharmacological correction of the prolonged bleeding time with a pre-biopsy infusion of 0.3 μg/kg of desmopressin, that helps to shorten the prolonged bleeding time in approximately 40% of patients [11]. Another peculiar situation is orthotopic liver transplantation, which is known to be accompanied by substantial intraoperative bleeding and that in the past required a huge use of transfusional blood products [12]. During liver transplantation major changes in the already disturbed haemostatic system do indeed occur, but it not certain that these abnormalities play a key role in the determination of excessive bleeding, because the major improvements that took place in the last few years in surgical techniques have substantially reduced the amount of blood losses in spite of no significant change in the adoption of medical interventions and, in particular, of haemostatic drugs.

TESTING HAEMOSTASIS IN LIVER DISEASE WITH NEW HAEMOSTASIS TESTS

The time honoured paradigm that haemostasis is abnormal in liver disease has been supported by methods that explore haemostasis functions but have obvious limits of clinical significance. For instance, such coagulation tests as the prothrombin time and the activated partial thromboplastin time (and other tests specifically designed to evaluate the capacity of liver to synthesise coagulation factors, that is the Normotest, HepatoQuick and Thrombotest) suffer from the fact that they explore only the early phase of the formation of thrombin, the final and key enzyme of the coagulation system. Thrombin formation is a dynamic process in which the forming coagulation enzyme is continuously neutralised by such naturally occurring anticoagulant proteins as antithrombin, thrombomodulin, activated protein C and tissue factor pathway inhibitor (Table 14). Standard coagulation tests do not measure global thrombin as it is formed and then neutralised, but only the small amounts that are needed to form a first visible clot. In patients with severe liver disease this process is slowed by the presence of low plasma levels of coagulation factors, and hence standard coagulation tests are abnormally prolonged. In a recent study, Tripodi *et al.* [13] have shown that when thrombin formation is globally measured using a thrombin generation assay, modified by the addition of thrombomodulin and hence sensitive not only to the low plasma levels of coagulation factors but also to the reduced levels of naturally occurring inhibitors [14], patients with liver cirrhosis did form thrombin in amounts similar to those of healthy individuals taken as controls. The study of Tripodi *et al.* [13] was designed as a cross-sectional study of patients presenting with varied degrees of severity of liver cirrhosis, so that no attempt could be made to correlate their bleeding tendency to the results of the thrombin generation assay. A prospective study is warranted to establish whether or not such an association exists. It would be useful also to evaluate thrombin generation using platelet rich plasma instead of platelet poor plasma (as it was done by Tripodi *et al.* [13]), in order to establish the role of platelets in securing haemostasis in chronic liver disease [15]. On the whole, Tripodi's study [13] supports the views that the coagulopathy of liver cirrhosis is less important than it does appear from the abnormal results of the prothrombin and partial thromboplastin times, which were indeed abnormal in these patients [13]. By the same token, it would be of interest to see whether or not the use of the thrombin generation test is preferable to that of the traditional coagulation tests and of the skin bleeding time in the evaluation of the safety of percutaneous liver biopsy in patients with chronic liver disease.

Another challenge to the concept of an abnormal haemostatic system is given by the study of Lisman *et al.* [16] on the behaviour of the fibrinolytic system in patients with severe liver disease. Some of the components of the fibrinolytic system are altered in the direction of hyperfibrinolysis (high plasma levels of tissue plasminogen activator and low levels of α2-plasmin inhibitor) but others are altered in the direction of hypofibrinolysis (low plasminogen, high plasminogen activation inhibitor type 1), so that it is possible that a balance does ultimately exist also for this haemostatic system [17] (Table 14). Lisman *et al.* [16] have shown that a recently discovered inhibitor of fibrinolysis, that is the thrombin-activatable fibrinolysis inhibitor, is reduced in patients with severe liver disease to a degree proportional to the severity of the disease (mean levels were 66% in Child A, 55% in Child B, 47% in Child C cirrhosis and 26% in acute liver failure). The decrease of this principal fibrinolysis inhibitor should in principle cause an excess of fibrinolysis. However, when the fibrinolysis potential was explored with a global test sensitive to both activators and inhibitors of the system, the results obtained in cirrhotics were no different from those obtained in healthy controls [16]. Most importantly, an elegant *in vitro* experiment included in Lisman's study showed convincingly that the interplay of decreased activators and inhibitors eventually leads to normal fibrinolysis in severe liver disease [16]. By artificially reducing to half-normal the plasma levels of thrombin activatable fibrinolysis inhibitor, lysis of the clot was as expected more accelerated than in a sample containing normal plasma levels of the inhibitor. On the other hand, a sample with half-normal levels of antithrombin made the lysis time slower than normal, but plasma containing at the same time half-normal levels of fibrinolysis inhibitor and of antithrombin had a lysis time that was identical to that of normal plasma, indicating that the two decreases are balanced and eventually yield normal results [16].

THERAPEUTIC IMPLICATIONS

In the past, and even in more recent years, there have been attempts to evaluate the role of haemostatic agents in the management of the most frequent bleeding problem of patients with severe liver disease, that is bleeding from oesophageal varices. Several types of haemostatic agents have been evaluated, spanning from such antifibrinolytic amino acids as epsilon aminocaproic acid or tranexamic acid to, more recently, potent procoagulant agents such as recombinant activated factor VII [18]. The results of these trials have been in general negative or inconclusive, and there are perhaps two possible reasons for this. The first is that the weapons currently used in the prevention and treatment of variceal bleeding (β-blockers, vasoactive agents, banding and sclerotherapy) are so effective that little space is left for adjuvant haemostatic agents that obviously must be evaluated on top of these effective treatments. As a result of this situation, very large series of patients need to be included in clinical trials in the attempt to find out a modest improvement. Second, for all the reasons that were mentioned above and that cast serious doubts on the relevance of abnormal haemostasis in the causation of variceal bleeding, it is at least uncertain that the evaluation of these haemostatic drugs, some of whom are outrageously expensive, has a solid rationale.

REFERENCES

1 Rapaport SI. Coagulation problems in liver disease. *Blood Coagul Fibrinolysis* 2000;**11**(suppl)1: S69–S74

2 Lisman T, Leebeek FW, de Groot PG. Haemostatic abnormalities in patients with liver disease. *J Hepatol* 2002;**37**: 280–287.

3 Roberts LR, Kamath PS. Pathophysiology and treatment of variceal hemorrhage. *Mayo Clin Proc* 1996;**71**: 973–983.

4 Ewe K. Bleeding after liver biopsy does not correlate with indices of peripheral coagulation. *Dig Dis Sci* 1981;**26**: 388–393.

5 Dillon JF, Simpson KJ, Hayes PC. Liver biopsy bleeding time: an unpredictable event. *J Gastroenterol Hepatol* 1994;**9**: 269–271.

6 McGill DB. Predicting hemorrhage after liver biopsy. *Dig Dis Sci* 1981; **26**: 385

7 McVay PA, Toy PT. Lack of increased bleeding after liver biopsy in patients with mild haemostatic abnormalities. *Am J Clin Pathol* 1990;**94**: 747–753.

8 Caturelli E, Squillante MM, Andriulli A *et al.* Fine-needle liver biopsy in patients with severely impaired coagulation. *Liver* 1993;**13**: 270–273.

9 Boberg KM, Brosstad F, Egeland T, Egge T, Schrumpf E. Is a prolonged bleeding time associated with an increased risk of hemorrhage after liver biopsy? *Thromb Haemost* 1999;**81**: 378–381.

10 Boks AL, Brommer EJ, Schalm SW, Van Vliet HH. Haemostasis and fibrinolysis in severe liver failure and their relation to hemorrhage. *Hepatology* 1986;**6**: 79–86.

11 Mannucci PM, Vicente V, Vianello L *et al.* Controlled trial of desmopressin in liver cirrhosis and other conditions associated with a prolonged bleeding time. *Blood* 1986;**67**: 1148–1153.

12 Porte RJ, Knot EA, Bontempo FA. Haemostasis in liver transplantation. *Gastroenterology* 1989;**97**: 488–501.

13 Tripodi A, Salerno F, Chantarangkul V *et al.* Evidence of normal thrombin generation in cirrhosis despite abnormal conventional coagulation tests. *Hepatology* 2005;**41**: 553–558.

14 Hemker HC, Giesen P, Al Dieri R *et al.* Calibrated automated thrombin generation measurement in clotting plasma. *Pathophysiol Haemost Thromb* 2003;**33**: 4–15.

15 Bosch J, Reverter JC. The coagulopathy of cirrhosis: myth or reality? *Hepatology* 2005;**41**: 434–435.

16 Lisman T, Leebeek FW, Mosnier LO *et al.* Thrombin-activatable fibrinolysis inhibitor deficiency in cirrhosis is not associated with increased plasma fibrinolysis. *Gastroenterology* 2001;**121**: 131–139.

17 Leebeek FWG. Hyperfibrinolysis in liver cirrhosis. In: Greenwalt P. (ed.) *Fibrinolysis in disease*. Vol. 2, Boca Raton, FL, CRC Press, 1995; 194–201.
18 Bosch J, Thabut D, Bendtsen F *et al.* Recombinant factor VIIa for upper gastrointestinal bleeding in patients with cirrhosis: a randomized, double-blind trial. *Gastroenterology* 2004;**127**: 1123–1130.

SESSION 2

Predictive Models in Portal Hypertension

Guadalupe Garcia-Tsao, Gennaro D'Amico*, Juan G. Abraldes, Filippo Schepis, Manuela Merli, W. Ray Kim and Erik Christensen*

BACKGROUND AND DEFINITION OF DIFFERENT CIRRHOTIC STATUS

Natural history of cirrhosis

The natural history of cirrhosis is characterised by an asymptomatic phase, designated as 'compensated' cirrhosis, followed by a rapidly progressive phase marked by clinical signs of liver dysfunction designated as 'decompensated cirrhosis' (Fig. 21). In the compensated phase, portal pressure may be normal or below the threshold level identified for the development of varices or ascites ('clinically significant portal hypertension') [1], As the disease progresses, portal pressure increases and liver function decreases, resulting in the development of ascites, portal hypertensive gastrointestinal bleeding, encephalopathy and jaundice. The development of any of these complications marks the transition from a compensated to a decompensated phase. Progression may be accelerated by the development of other complications such as (re)bleeding, renal impairment (refractory ascites, hepatorenal syndrome) and sepsis (spontaneous bacterial peritonitis). The development of hepatocellular carcinoma (HCC) may accelerate the course of the disease in any stage.

Definition of compensated and decompensated cirrhosis

Ideally, a staging system should be simple and reproducible and should identify patients with a similar rate of disease progression or survival

* The first authorship of this chapter is shared by Dr Garcia-Tsao and Dr D'Amico.

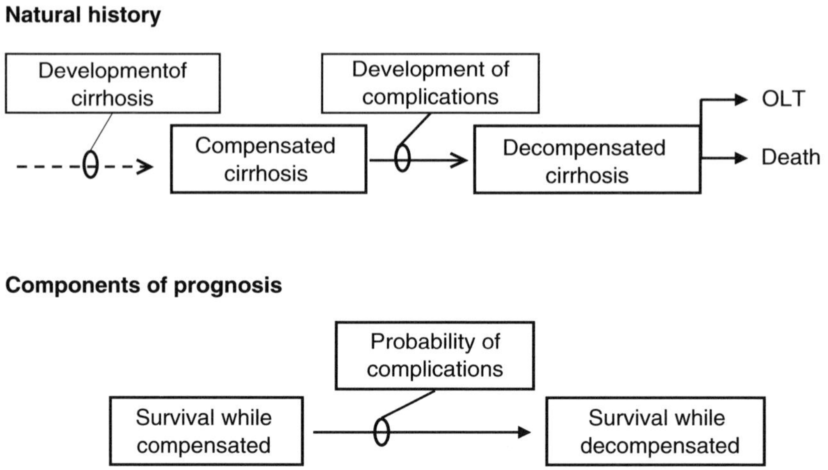

Fig. 21 The natural history of cirrhosis and components of prognosis. A simplified view.

expectancy. Classification of cirrhosis into compensated and decompensated stages satisfies this requirement. Decompensated cirrhosis is defined by the presence of ascites, bleeding, encephalopathy and/or jaundice [2,3]. Moreover, since ascites is most frequently the first of these signs to appear [4], it is usually considered a landmark sign of decompensated cirrhosis.

Survival of patients with compensated cirrhosis is significantly longer than survival of patients with decompensated cirrhosis. In a systematic review of 93 prognostic studies of cirrhosis, the median 1-year survival for compensated and decompensated cirrhosis was 98% (range 88–100%) and 71% (range 48–85%), respectively [5]. In a prospective inception cohort study of 494 patients with cirrhosis followed for 25 years, the median survival for patients with compensated and decompensated cirrhosis at diagnosis is 14 years and 20 months, respectively ($p = 0.00001$) (Fig. 22) [6]. Patients with compensated cirrhosis die mostly after transition from a compensated to a decompensated stage. The rate of transition is ~5% per year and ascites represents the most frequent decompensating event. Survival while in the compensated stage is calculated by censoring data at the first manifestation of decompensation. This approach allows for the assessment of survival probability while patients remain at a compensated stage (Fig. 22b). This probability is quite different from the probability of survival of a given clinical stage at a given point along the course of the disease, for example at diagnosis (Fig. 22a).

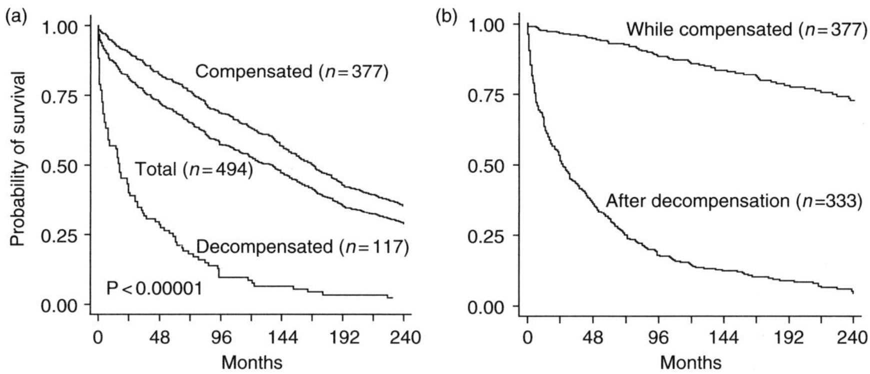

Fig. 22 Survival according to decompensation at diagnosis (a) and while remaining in the compensated or decompensated stages (b).

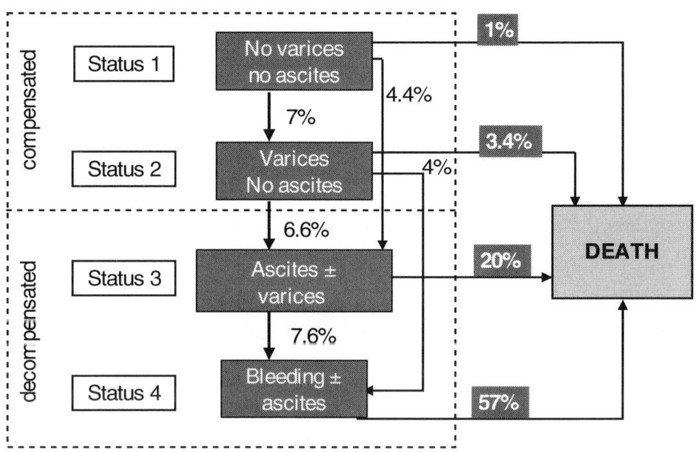

Fig. 23 Clinical course of cirrhosis: 1-year outcome probabilities according to clinical stages.

Clinical states of cirrhosis

By combining data from two large natural history studies including over 1,600 patients, D'Amico identifies four clinical states or status of cirrhosis, each with distinct clinical features and a markedly different prognosis (Fig. 23) [4,6].

Status 1 is characterised by the absence of oesophageal varices (OV) and of ascites. While patients remain in this status, the mortality rate is as low as 1% per year. Patients exit this status at a cumulative rate of 11.4% per year: 7% because of the development of varices and 4.4% because of the development of ascites (with or without varices).

Status 2 is characterised by the presence of OV without ascites and without bleeding. While patients remain in this status, the mortality rate is 3.4% per year. Patients leave this status by developing ascites (6.6% per year) or by developing bleeding before or at the time of development of ascites (rate 4% per year).

Status 3 is characterised by ascites with or without OV in a patient who has never bled. While patients remain in this status, the mortality rate is 20% per year, significantly higher than in the two former states. Patients exit this stage by bleeding (7.6% per year).

Status 4 is characterised by GI bleeding with or without ascites. In this stage the one-year mortality rate (OYM) is 57% (nearly half of these deaths occur within 6 weeks from the initial episode of bleeding).

Status 1 and 2 refer to patients with compensated cirrhosis while status 2 and 3 refer to decompensated cirrhosis. HCC develops at a fairly constant rate of 3% per year and it is associated with worse outcome in whatever status it develops.

Prognostic indicators

Many prognostic indicators and more than 20 prognostic scores have been proposed to predict mortality from cirrhosis. In a systematic review of 93 prognostic studies published between 1980 and 2003, 172 candidate prognostic variables were identified [5]. Those confirmed in at least five studies within the first five levels of statistical significance are reported in Table 15. Among the proposed prognostic scores, only the Child–Pugh [7] and the Model for End-Stage Liver Disease (MELD) scores [8] are currently used in clinical practice. The only advantage of the MELD score is the appropriate selection of liver transplant candidates [9] while the Child–Pugh score (CPS) is still more useful in clinical practice.

Since different clinical states of cirrhosis are associated with very different survival rates, it is expected that prognostic indicators will differ according to the clinical state. In fact, in a systematic review of prognostic studies [5], it was shown that prognostic indicators differ in patients with compensated and decompensated cirrhosis (Table 16).

Moreover in an ongoing study of the clinical course of cirrhosis, D'Amico has shown that while the predictive accuracy of both Child–Pugh and MELD scores is fairly satisfactory when validated in the whole population, it is much less accurate when separately assessed in compensated and decompensated patients (Fig. 24).

Table 15 Significant prognostic indicators in the first five levels of significance in at least 5 of 93 prognostic studies published between 1980 and 2003 [4].

Variable	Significant/assessed	
	n/N	%
HVPG	5/6	83
Pugh	20/29	69
Eps	19/37	51
Bilirubin	25/58	43
Albumin	24/55	43
Ascites	17/41	41
Varices	9/23	39
Bleeding	6/19	32
Creatinine	6/19	32
Age	20/55	36
Prothrombin %	13/54	24

Table 16 Prognostic indicators that have been shown to be significant in at least 5 of 93 studies.

Compensated cirrhosis	Decompensated cirrhosis
Age	Age
Bilirubin, albumin, prothrombin	Child–Pugh or components, aminopyrine breath test, pseudocholinesterase
Varices	Varices, bleeding
	BUN or creatinine

Summary

1 Compensated cirrhosis: absence of ascites, portal hypertensive gastrointestinal bleeding, encephalopathy and jaundice.
2 Decompensated cirrhosis: presence of any of ascites, bleeding, encephalopathy or jaundice.
3 Clinical stage (or status): a clinical stage of cirrhosis should be a condition defined by few, simple and reproducible criteria easy to be verified, allowing to identify patients with a very similar disease progression or survival probability.
4 Outcome of a clinical stage: the outcome for a given clinical stage is the transition to a different stage, death or liver transplant.
5 The presence or absence of varices, ascites and bleeding identify four clinical states of cirrhosis characterised by increasing severity from status 1 to status 4.

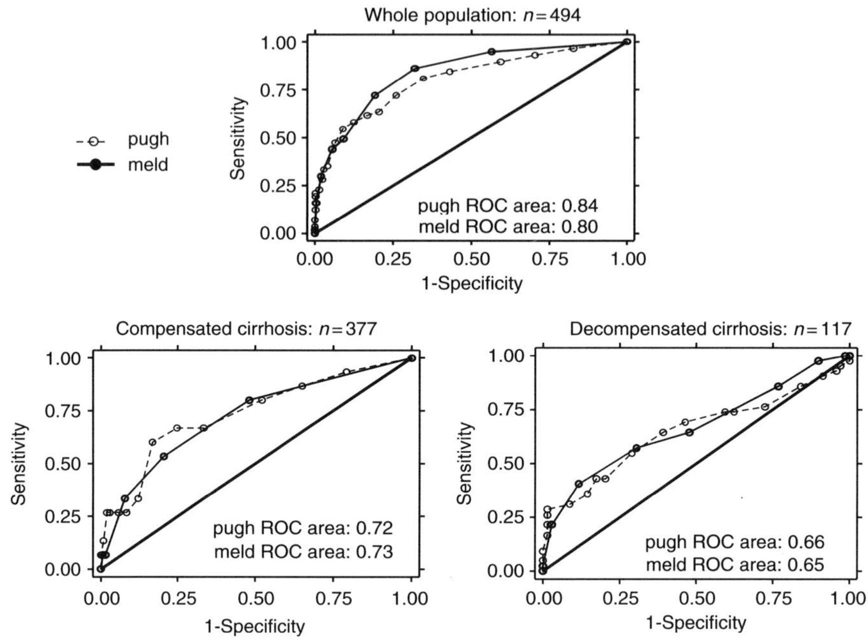

Fig. 24 Child–Pugh and MELD for 1-year mortality prediction in the whole population and respectively in compensated and decompensated patients in a prospective study of the natural history of cirrhosis.

6 Status 1 and 2 refer to compensated cirrhosis while status 3 and 4 refer to decompensated cirrhosis.
7 The development of HCC may accelerate the course of cirrhosis at any of its states.
8 Prognostic indicators of cirrhosis associate differently with the outcome depending on the clinical status of the disease, and their predictive accuracy may vary accordingly.
9 Prognostic indicators of each clinical status of cirrhosis should be assessed separately.

Conclusions

The clinical course of cirrhosis is largely dependent on the development of decompensation. Before that time, mortality is low and usually determined by causes not related to cirrhosis. For this reason, prognostic indicators assessed in the whole patients population may be unsatisfactory when applied separately in patients with compensated and decompensated cirrhosis. Therefore, predictors of the outcome according to clinical stages of the disease may allow a more accurate prognostic assessment of patients. A staging system based on varices, ascites and bleeding is proposed for future prognostic studies.

WHERE DO WE NEED PROGNOSTIC MODELS? – RESULTS OF A SURVEY

In order to get a consensus of the experts invited to participate in Baveno IV, a 'questionnaire' was sent to all participants in the form of a table. The predictors of the development of the following complications of cirrhosis were evaluated (columns): varices, variceal enlargement, variceal haemorrhage (VH), ascites, refractory ascites, spontaneous bacterial peritonitis, hepatorenal syndrome, survival in compensated cirrhosis and survival in decompensated cirrhosis. The specific parameters listed (rows) were: CPS, MELD score, North Italian Endoscopic Club (NIEC) index, alcoholic or viral aetiology, presence of varices, presence of ascites, presence of encephalopathy, variceal size, red signs on varices, albumin, International Normalised Ratio (INR), bilirubin, platelet count, ascites protein, Aspartate Aminotransferase/Alanine Aminotransferase (AST/ALT), creatinine and HVPG. The responders had the opportunity of adding other (unlisted) parameters.

Responders were asked to check those parameters that they considered as having been identified as predictive of each of the above-mentioned complications of cirrhosis. At the end of the questionnaire, participants were asked whether further work was necessary in improving current predictive models, whether new predictive models were needed, whether they were satisfied with current models or whether models were not really needed for that specific complication of cirrhosis.

Of the 67 questionnaires that were sent out, 40 responses (60%) were received. The predictors most frequently identified (i.e. identified by > 50% of the respondents) are shown in Table 17. As can be seen, almost total consensus (> 90% of respondents agreed) was achieved on HVPG being a predictor of the development of varices, on variceal size being a predictor of VH and on CPS being a predictor of death in decompensated cirrhosis. HVPG and size of varices were recognised as isolated parameters. Regarding predictive *models*, the only one recognised by > 90% of respondents was the CPS (for survival in decompensated cirrhosis), although both the NIEC score and the MELD score were recognised by > 75% as being predictive of variceal bleeding and survival, respectively.

To the provided list of predictors, there were several others that were added: bacterial infections and variceal pressure (for VH), blood pressure (for ascites, refractory ascites and survival in decompensated cirrhosis),

Table 17 Most frequently recognised predictors of the different complications of cirrhosis by Baveno IV participants.

	Predictors of each complication classified by reported frequency		
	> 90%	75–90%	50–75%
Varices	HVPG	Platelet count	
Variceal enlargement			HVPG Child–Pugh score
Variceal haemorrhage	Variceal size	Red signs HVPG NIEC	
Ascites			
Refractory ascites			Child–Pugh score
SBP			
HRS			Ascites
Survival (compensated)			Child–Pugh score HVPG MELD score
Survival (decompensated)	Child–Pugh score	MELD score	HVPG

HVPG, hepatic venous pressure gradient; NIEC, North Italian Endoscopic Club score; MELD, Model for End-Stage Liver Disease; SBP, Spontaneous bacterial peritonitis; HRS, Hepatorenal syndrome.

plasma renin activity (for refractory ascites and hepatorenal syndrome) and serum sodium (for refractory ascites, hepatorenal syndrome and survival in decompensated cirrhosis).

Responses to the questions regarding satisfaction (or not) or need for models are summarised in Table 18. Although the highest number of respondents who were satisfied with current models were in the area of VH and survival in decompensated cirrhosis, practically all respondents thought that models for all parameters were needed, particularly in the areas of development of varices and variceal enlargement (i.e. in compensated cirrhosis).

Summary

1 HVPG and variceal size were isolated parameters recognised by the majority of respondents as being predictive of the development of varices and VH, respectively.

Table 18 Satisfaction with currently available predictive models in cirrhosis (number of respondents).

	Satisfied	Require further study	Models not needed
Varices	5	**29**	3
Variceal enlargement	2	**32**	1
Variceal haemorrhage	**8**	20	3
Ascites	2	25	4
Refractory ascites	2	25	4
SBP	3	27	2
HRS	3	27	2
Survival (compensated)	7	27	2
Survival (decompensated)	**9**	27	2

2 Of predictive models, only the CPS was identified by the majority as being predictive of survival in decompensated cirrhosis.
3 Practically everybody identified the need to develop further predictive models in cirrhosis.

HVPG AS A PREDICTOR OF OUTCOME

Hepatic venous pressure gradient (HVPG) accurately reflects portal pressure gradient in the most common causes of cirrhosis and portal hypertension (i.e. alcoholic and hepatitis C virus (HCV) related cirrhosis) [10,11]. Technical requirements for reliable measurements have been recently reviewed [12]. Since most complications of cirrhosis are related to portal hypertension it would be expected that portal pressure measurements would be of prognostic value. Indeed, cross-sectional studies show that portal pressure (estimated by the HVPG) must reach a certain threshold of 10–12 mmHg for the development of complications of portal hypertension, specifically ascites [13], varices [14] and variceal bleeding [14,15]. However, there are difficulties in interpreting studies evaluating its predictive value. First, since HVPG correlates with the severity of liver disease [16–19], its independent prognostic value should be assessed in the context of multivariable analyses. Second, HVPG can decrease spontaneously with improvements in liver function [20] or it can decrease with pharmacological therapy independent of changes in liver function [21], which questions the prognostic value of a single HVPG measurement and hinders the comparison of studies including patients subjected to different therapies. Third, the relation between HVPG and prognosis might not be linear, for example a 1 mmHg-difference may not have the same prognostic significance in the range of HVPG values. This leads to the question of how this variable should be used in prognostic models. In many studies it has been analysed as a continuous variable, without taking into account the linear gradient assumption. Dichotomisation by the estimated 'best' cut-off or by the median value probably reduces the predictive potential of HVPG. Further, the use of different cut-offs impairs the comparability of different studies, and it is possible that different cut-offs might apply for patients at different stages of the disease, and for the prediction of different outcomes.

Prognostic value of HVPG in patients with compensated cirrhosis without varices

Only one study evaluated the prognostic value of HVPG in patients without varices (Table 19) [22]. In this large randomised controlled trial (RCT) evaluating the efficacy of β-adrenergic blockers in preventing the development of varices (status 1 patients), HVPG was measured at baseline and yearly. A baseline HVPG > 10 mmHg (clinically significant portal hypertension) is independently associated with an increased risk of developing varices, and with an increased risk of developing a composite end point (varices, VH, ascites, encephalopathy, transplant or death). Further analyses including information on the individual events of the composite and on the value of sequential HVPG measurements are expected.

Prognostic value of HVPG in patients with varices without previous variceal bleeding

Six studies selectively include patients with varices without previous bleeding (Table 20) [20,21,23–26]. Additional information is drawn from studies that include patients with and without previous variceal bleeding in which previous bleeding is analysed as a covariate (Table 21) [17,18,27–34].

Risk of bleeding. A single HVPG measurement has been associated with risk of variceal bleeding in some studies [17,18,27,28], but others show no association. In these, a substantial number of patients received pharmacological therapy to reduce portal pressure [21,23–25], an intervention to promote alcohol abstinence [20] or treatment was not reported [34]. In four of these studies HVPG was repeated after pharmacological treatment [21,23,25] or after alcohol abstinence [20]. HVPG reduction (either absolute or relative) is invariably associated with the risk of bleeding. A decrease in HVPG to less than 12 mmHg is associated with a negligible risk of first variceal bleeding. Further, a 15–20% decrease in HVPG from baseline values markedly

Table 19 Studies in patients with cirrhosis without varices.

Study	Type of study	Patients	Follow-up	Outcome (number of events)	HVPG measurement	Analysis	Treatment of the patients	Results
Groszmann 2003	Prospective cohort study embedded in a multicentre RCT	213 pt. 100% HVPG > 5 mmHg. 24% alcoholics. Child A/B/C (%): 89/11/0. 63% HVPG ≥ 10 mmHg	54.9 months (0–99.4)	1 Development of varices or variceal bleeding (84) 2 Development of varices or variceal bleeding or ascites or encephalopathy or liver transplantation or death (128)	At entry into the study, and every year	HVPG ≥ 10 mmHg. Cox model	Timolol versus placebo (no differences in the outcome) No patient received antiviral treatment	HVPG ≥ 10 mmHg independent predictor of end point 1 (Covariate: AST) and end point 2. No quantitative information

Table 20 Studies in patients with varices without previous variceal bleeding.

Study	Type of study	Patients	Follow-up	Outcome (number of events)	HVPG measurement	Analysis	Treatment of the patients	Results
Groszmann 1990	Prospective cohort study embedded in a multi centre RCT	84 pt. 100% HVPG > 12 mmHg. 76% alcoholics. Child A/B/C (%): 60/34/8. 52% ascites	16 ± 12 months	**1** First variceal bleeding (13) **2** Death (12)	HVPG measured at baseline, and at 3, 12 and 24 months after randomisation	HVPG ≤ 12 mmHg in the follow-up. Univariate survival analysis	Propranolol versus placebo	HVPG ≤ 12 mmHg in the follow-up was associated with decreased risk of variceal bleeding (0/21 versus 13/63) and death (1/21 versus 11/63). No adjusted values
Moller 1994	Prospective cohort study embedded in an RCT	55 pt. 83% alcoholics. Child A/B/C (%): 56/29/15. 54% ascites	15 months (0–40)	Composite end point: bleeding or death (19)	HVPG measured at baseline	HVPG (continuous variable). Cox model	RCT: no treatment versus propranolol, versus sclerosis versus propranolol+ sclerosis	HVPG predictor at univariate, but not an independent predictor. Independent predictors: nutritional status, alb, bil, coagulation, central circulatory time

Vorobioff 1996	Prospective cohort study	30 pt. 100% HVPG $\geq$ 12 mmHg. 100% alcoholics. Child A/B/C (%): 60/34/8. 60% ascites	39 months (11–120)	**1** First portal-hypertension related bleeding (8 variceal bleeding, 2 portal-hypertensive gastropathy) **2** Death (17)	HVPG measured at baseline, and at 1, 2, 3 and 4 years	HVPG at baseline and at 1 year. Cox model. HVPG decrease of > 15% from baseline. Univariate survival analysis	No vasoactive drugs. Interven tions to promote alcohol absti-nence	HVPG at 1 year independent predictor of bleeding (+age and abstinence) and death (+variceal size). No adjusted HR provided HVPG decrease of > 15% from baseline: predictor of bleeding and death at univariate analysis
Zimmerer 1996	Retrospective cohort study	190 pt. 100% alcoholics. Mean Child 6.19. *(40% of patients with HVPG < 8 mmHg had varices)*	47 months	Death (64)	HVPG measured at baseline	HVPG as a continuous variable. Cox model	Unknown	HVPG associated with the risk of death in univariate, but not an independent predictor of death (independent were cholinesterase, variceal size, albumin)

Table 20 (Continued).

Study	Type of study	Patients	Follow-up	Outcome (number of events)	HVPG measurement	Analysis	Treatment of the patients	Results
Merkel 2000	Prospective cohort study	49 pt. 37% alcoholics. 45% ascites. Child A/B/C (%): 43/49/8	Up to 5 years. Median follow-up not reported	1 Variceal bleeding (9) 2 Death (11)	HVPG measured at baseline and 1–3 months after drug therapy	Baseline HVPG. Good haemodynamic response (HVPG decrease of > 20% or to < 12 mmHg). Cox model. HVPG ≥ 16 mmHg univariate survival analysis	59% nadolol 41% nadolol + IMN	Baseline HVPG not predictive of bleeding. Good haemodynamic response independent predictor of bleeding. Adj HR: 6.8 (covariates: red weal marks) Baseline HVPG independent predictor of death. Adj HR: 1.17 (covariate: Child)
Turnes 2005	Retrospective cohort study	71 pt. 26% alcoholics. Child A/B/C (%): 80/20/0. 35% ascites	68 months (8–96)	1 Variceal bleeding (16) 2 Death (24) 3 Ascites (26) 4 SBP or bacteraemia (14) 5 Encephalopathy (25)	HVPG measured at baseline and 4 months (2–6) after drug therapy	Baseline HVPG. Good haemodynamic response (HVPG decrease of > 20% from baseline or to < 12 mmHg). % Change in HVPG. Cox model	70% propranolol. 30% propranolol+ IMN	Good haemodynamic response independent predictor of bleeding. HR: 10.3 (covariates: platelets). % change in HVPG independent predictor of SBP or bacteraemia. HR: 1.07 (covariates: GGT and Na). Not an independent predictor of death

Table 21 Studies that included patients with and without previous variceal bleeding.

Study	Type of study	Patients	Follow-up	Cutcome	HVPG measurement	Analysis	Treatment of the patients	Results
Lebrec 1980	Cross-sectional+ prospective cohort study	100 pt. 47% ascites and/or jaundice. 53% previous gastrointestinal bleeding (only half of them variceal bleeding)	Up to 1 year	GI Bleeding (source not specified) (17)	HVPG measured within 2 weeks from admission from decompensation	HVPG was handled as continuous variable. Baseline HVPG in patients that bled in the follow-up was compared with baseline HVPG in those that did not (*t*-test)	Unknown	Baseline HVPG was not different between patients that bled in the 1 year follow-up and patients that did not
Tage-Jensen 1988	Retrospective cohort study	81 pt. 94% alcoholics. Child A/B/C (%): 13/36/71. 73% ascites. 30% previous bleeding (not 'recent')	38 months (1–97)	Death (47)	In patients with previous bleeding, HVPG was measured 'well after' the bleeding episode	HVPG categorised in three levels: ≤ 12 mmHg versus 12–20 mmHg versus > 20 mmHg. Cox model	32% of patients included in an RCT comparing testosterone versus placebo. 30% included in an RCT comparing peritoneovenous shunting versus diuretics	HVPG independent predictor of death. Adjusted HR: 1.15 (covariates: plasma noradrenaline, bil, ascites, cardiovascular disease)

Table 21 (Continued).

Study	Type of study	Patients	Follow-up	Outcome	HVPG measurement	Analysis	Treatment of the patients	Results
Gluud 1988	Prospective cohort study embed-ded in an RCT	58 pt. 100% alcoholics. 45% varices (only 53% had initial endoscopy). 16% previous bleeding. Child A/B/C (%): 26/38/36	31 months (2–51)	1 Variceal bleeding (12) 2 Death (17)	At least 1 month after a variceal bleeding episode	HVPG (continuous variable). Various cut-offs. Cox model	RCT: Testos-terone/placebo	HVPG independent predictor of bleeding. Adjusted HR: 1.22 (covariates age, Child, incapaci-tation index, testosterone treatment). HVPG independent predictor of death. Adjusted HR: 1.13 (covariates: age, Child, incapaci–tation index, testosterone treatment)
Merkel 1992	Prospective cohort study	129 pt. 71% alcoholics. Median Child–Pugh: 7. 100% varices. 45% previous variceal bleeding. 56% ascites	45 months (2–60)	1 GI bleeding (44) 2 Death due to liver disease (47)	In previous bleeders HVPG was measured > 14 days after the bleeding episode	HVPG (continuous variable). Cox model. HVPG $\geq$ 16 mmHg. Univariate survival analysis	11% β-blockers	HVPG independent predictor of GI bleeding. Adjusted HR: 1.11 (covariates: previous bleeding, Child, size of varices). HVPG independent predictor of death. Adjusted HR: 1.11 (covariates Child, ICG clearance, previous bleeding)

Urbain 1993	Prospective cohort study	99 pt. 100% alcoholics. Child A/B/C (%): 31/43/22. Unknown number of patients with varices, previous bleeding or ascites	Up to 48 months	1 Variceal bleeding (31) 2 Death due to liver disease (41)	Measured at entry	HVPG dichotomised by 8, 12, 15, 20, 25, 30 mmHg. Log-rank test. Multivariate analysis not performed.	Apparently, no patient received vasoactive medication of prophylaxis for variceal bleeding	HVPG > 12 mmHg predictive of bleeding. Not quantitative information. HVPG not predictive of death
Stanley 1998	Retrospective cohort study	96 pt. 25% previous bleeding. 100% alcoholics. Child A/B/C (%): 16/37/47	19 ± 2 months	1 Variceal bleeding (16) 2 Death (38)	At least more than 10 days after the bleeding episode	HVPG > 12 mmHg for bleeding analysis, HVPG > 16 mmHg for bleeding and survival analysis. Cox model	28% banding ligation	HVPG > 12 mmHg or HVPG > 16 mmHg were the only independent predictors of bleeding. HVPG > 16 mmHg independent predictor of death (covariates: Child–Pugh). Quantitative estimates not provided
Escorsell 2000	Prospective cohort study	47 pt. 36% alcoholics. Child A/B/C (%): 60/38/2. 44% previous variceal bleeding. 27% ascites	28 months (4–36)	1 Variceal bleeding (16) 2 Death (10)	HVPG measured at baseline and 4 months after propranolol treatment	Good haemodynamic response (HVPG decrease of > 20% from baseline or to < 12 mmHg). Logistic regression	100% propranolol. 2% propranolol + IMN	Good haemodynamic response independent predictor of variceal bleeding. Adjusted OR: 10.6 (covariates: fall in variceal pressure > 20%). Good haemodynamic response not predictive of death
Deltenre 2002	Retrospective cohort study	89 pt. 100% alcoholics. Child A-B/C (%): 60/40. 93% ascites. 77% varices. 18% previous variceal haemorrhage	35 months (1–76)	Death (56)	HVPG measured at the time patients were submitted for liver biopsy	HVPG ≥ 12 mmHg. HVPG ≥ 16 mmHg. Cox model	Unknown	HVPG not predictive of death

Table 21 (Continued).

Study	Type of study	Patients	Follow-up	Outcome	HVPG measurement	Analysis	Treatment of the patients	Results
Bureau 2002	Prospective cohort study	34 pt. 76% alcoholics. Mean Child 8.1.38% ascites. 41% previous variceal bleeding	24 months (1–96)	Variceal bleeding (11)	HVPG measured at baseline, 4 days (1–60) after propranolol, and 16 days (3–47) after IMN in initial non-responders	Good haemo-dynamic response (HVPG decrease of > 20% from baseline or to < 12 mmHg). Logistic regression	100% propranolol. IMN was added in non-responders (/). Previous bleeders non-responding to propranolol + IMN were shifted to banding ligation (8)	Good haemodynamic response was the only independent predictor of variceal bleeding. OR: 6.4
Dittrich 2003	Prospective cohort study	83 pt. 61% alcoholics. 98% varices. 69% previous variceal bleeding. No data on liver function	17 ± 16 months	1 Bleeding (?) 2 Death (27) 3 Death or liver transplantation or bleeding or need for porto-caval shunt (54)	HVPG measured at baseline	HVPG > 12 mmHg. Chi-square. HVPG > 16 mmHg. Chi-square. HVPG means in patients with/without outcomes (*t*-test)	Unknown	HVPG > 12 mmHg predictive of bleeding (unadjusted RR 1.52). HVPG > 16 mmHg not predictive of any event. HVPG mean was higher in patients with any event than in patients with no events

reduces the risk of bleeding [20,23,25]. In patients treated with β-adrenergic blockers ± nitrates, the 3-year incidence of first variceal bleeding is less than 10% in patients in whom HVPG decreases by more than 20% from baseline or to less than 12 mmHg (good responders), and between 20% and 40% in non-responders.

Risk of death. Baseline HVPG has been consistently associated with the risk of death [17,18,23,27,29]. Most importantly, at multivariable analysis the influence of HVPG on survival is independent of baseline liver function, indicating that HVPG can potentially classify patients at increased risk within each Child–Pugh class. There are a number of conflicting studies, mainly in series including only alcoholic patients without information on abstinence [26,28,32], reporting unreliable HVPG measurements [26] or with insufficient information on the baseline characteristics of patients [26,28]. In alcoholic patients who become abstinent, HVPG is predictive of survival only if it is measured after alcohol abstinence [20]. In patients on drug therapy, an HVPG reduction to < 12 mmHg seems to be associated with an improved survival [21]. However, a good haemodynamic response was not found to predict survival [25,35].

In most studies HVPG is analysed as a continuous variable, both in the assessment of the risk of bleeding and the risk of death, but some authors propose 16 mmHg as the best cut-off to predict survival. This value, originally derived in a cohort that included both patients with and without previous bleeding [27], was subsequently validated in a cohort of patients without variceal bleeding [23], and in a series with a small number of previous bleeders [18]. However, the use of a single cut-off value probably decreases the potential predictive value of HVPG.

Prognostic value of HVPG in patients with acute variceal bleeding (Table 22)

An initial study, measuring portal pressure gradient instead of HVPG, suggested that the degree of portal hypertension could influence the short-term outcome of acute variceal bleeding [36]. Subsequent studies showed that HVPG measurement within 48 h from admission can predict the short-term prognosis of these patients [37–40]. Moitinho *et al.* found that HVPG (best cut-off of 20 mmHg) is the only independent predictor of 5-day failure (rebleeding or death) [38]. The 20 mmHg cut-off was validated in two subsequent studies [39,40], but the initial 80% sensitivity to predict 5-day failure was reduced to 62%, with a specificity of 75–80% [40]. In this latter study CPS was also an independent predictor of failure, indicating that the

Table 22 Studies that included only patients with previous variceal bleeding: short-term prognosis.

Study	Type of study	Patients	Follow-up	Outcome	HVPG measurement	Analysis	Treatment of the patients	Results
Ready 1991	Prospective cohort study	22 pt. 100% alcoholics. Child A/B/C (%): 32/50/18	4 days	Failure in the initial control of bleeding + rebleeding in the first 4 days (9).	From admission for variceal bleeding, every 2 h for 72 h	HVPG > 16 mmHg at day 1. Chi-square	No active treatment	9/17 of patients with HVPG ≥ 16 continued bleeding or rebled versus 0/5 of patients with HVPG < 16
Moitinho 1999	Prospective cohort study	65 pt. 45% alcoholics. Child A/B/C (%): 26/54/20. 50% ascites	Up to 1 year	**1** 5-day failure (23) **2** 1 year mortality (27)	Within 48 h of admission. Without vasoactive drugs	HVPG as continuous variable: logistic regression. HVPG > 20 mmHg: Chi-square	Initial treatment: 66% sclerotherapy. 44% somatostatin	HVPG (continuous) was the only independent predictor of 5-day failure. OR 1.28. HVPG independent predictors of 1-year mortality. Adjusted OR: 1.16 (covariate: Child–Pugh)
Villanueva 2001	Prospective cohort study embedded in an interventional experimental study	40 pt. 73% alcoholics. 70% ascites. Child A/B/C (%): 17/58/25.	5 days	5-day failure (10)	Within 24 h from admission, before drug therapy, atleast 6 h after sclerotherapy. Repeated six times in the first 24 h	Baseline HVPG ≥ 20 mmHg. HVPG decrease ≤ 10%. Logistic regression	All patients received injection sclerotherapy from admission. Patients were randomised to receive somatostatin or placebo (2:1)	HVPG > 20 (OR: 4.5) and decrease in HVPG ≤ 10% (OR: 14) independent predictors of 5-day failure

Monescillo 2004	Prospective cohort study embedded in a multicentre RCT	90 pt. 67% alcoholics. 53% ascites. Child A/B/C (%): 19/44/35	Up to 1 year	1 5-day failure (21) 2 6-week mortality (13) 3 1-year mortality (?)	Within 24 h from admission. Without vasoactive treatment	HVPG as continuous variable. Logistic regression for 5-day failure. Cox model for 6-week and 1-year mortality HVPG ≥ 20 mmHg: univariate survival analysis	All patients received injection sclerotherapy	HVPG (continuous variable) independent predictor of – 5-day failure: adjusted OR: 1.27 (covariate: Child) – 6-week mortality: adjusted HR: 1.36 (covariates: active bleeding, Child) – 1-year mortality: adjusted HR: 1.36 (covariates: Child, creatinine, infection or encephalopathy in the first week)
Avgerinos 2004	Prospective cohort study embedded in an interventional experimental study	50 pt. 64% alcoholics. 74% ascites. Child A/B/C (%): 26/28/46	Up to 42 days	1 Rebleeding in the 42-day period (13) 2 6-week mortality (12) 3 Rebleeding or death (19)	Within 24 h of admission. Repeated every day up to 5 days	Baseline HVPG > 16 mmHg. Changes not analysed. Cox regression	Randomised to receive banding or injection sclerotherapy	HVPG > 16 predictive of death and of rebleeding or death. Not an independent predictor at multivariate analysis (no adjusted HR provided)

predictive value of HVPG can be improved if included in a model together with liver function. An HVPG decrease of < 10% on somatostatin has also been reported as a predictor of poor outcome, and the combination of this criterion with the 20 mmHg cut-off achieved a 90% sensitivity to predict 5-day failure [39]. HVPG is also an independent predictor of 6-week (38% versus 5% in patients with HVPG < 20 mmHg) [40] and 1-year mortality (65% versus 20%) [38,40]. An HVPG > 20 mmHg was used in a single RCT to select high-risk patients who were subsequently randomised to receive conventional therapy or aggressive therapy (transjugular intrahepatic portosystemic shunts, TIPS) [40], showing for the first time that tailoring therapy according to HVPG values can decrease overall mortality of acute variceal bleeding.

Prognostic value of HVPG in patients who have recovered from an episode of acute variceal bleeding (Table 23)

Risk of bleeding. It is controversial whether a single HVPG measurement predicts rebleeding in patients surviving an episode of variceal bleeding. Merkel *et al.* reported that an HVPG ≥ 16 mmHg was an independent predictor of bleeding both in patients with and without previous bleeding [27]. In contrast, in the study by Patch *et al.* (all previous bleeders) a single HVPG measurement was not predictive of rebleeding [41]. In this study 63% of the patients received β-adrenergic blockers, as compared with 11% in the study by Merkel. This could account for the lack of predictive value since a reduction in HVPG [42–46] has been shown to be a robust predictor of the risk of rebleeding. Four studies from two different groups have shown that a good HVPG response (defined as a decrease of > 20% from baseline values or to < 12 mmHg) is an independent predictor of rebleeding [43–46]. Two additional studies including patients with and without previous bleeding validate these haemodynamic targets [30,31]. Two studies from the same group failed to find a significant association between good haemodynamic response and the risk of rebleeding [47;48]. An unpublished meta-analysis by D'Amico shows that a good haemodynamic response markedly decreases the risk of bleeding in the follow-up [OR: 0.17 (0.05–0.32)]. Significant heterogeneity was found, but was attributable to a single trial [48]. Meta-regression showed that the time between measurements was the only factor associated with the reported odds ratios. The longer the time between measurements, the lower the proportion of poor responders experiencing rebleeding. The only clear outlier [48] had the longest time between measurements.

Risk of death. HVPG measured within two weeks after variceal bleeding is controlled has independent prognostic value for survival [41]. Patients

Table 23 Studies that included only patients with previous variceal bleeding: long term prognosis.

Study	Type of study	Patients	Follow-up	Outcome	HVPG measurement	Analysis	Treatment of the patients	Results
Feu 1995	Prospective cohort study	69 pt. 59% alcoholics. Child A/B/C (%): 54/40/6. 38% ascites	28 months (1–69)	1 Rebleeding (25) 2 Death (9)	HVPG measured within the first week after bleeding, and at 3 months	Good haemodynamic response (HVPG decrease of > 20% from baseline). Cox model	100% propranolol	Good haemodynamic response independent predictor of rebleeding. Adjusted HR: 11.1 (covariates: decrease in cardiac output, active alcoholism). Good haemodynamic response not predictive of death
Villanueva 1996	Prospective cohort study embedded in an RCT	62 pt. 57% alcoholics. Child A/B/C (%): 22/58/20. 45% ascites	18 months (1–36)	1 Rebleeding (34) 2 Death (13)	HVPG measured within the first week after bleeding, before randomisation, and at 3 months	HVPG as continuous variable, at baseline and at 3 months. Cox model. Good haemodynamic response (HVPG decrease of > 20% from baseline or to < 12 mmHg). Univariate survival analysis	Randomised to receive injection sclerotherapy or nadolol+ IMN	HVPG at 3 months independent predictor of rebleeding (covariate: treatment group) and death (covariates: Child at 3 months, rebleeding). No quantitative estimates. Good haemodynamic response predictive of rebleeding at univariate analysis

Table 23 (Continued).

Study	Type of study	Patients	Follow-up	Outcome	HVPG measurement	Analysis	Treatment of the patients	Results
Mc Cormick 1998	Prospective cohort study	44 pt. 70% Alco-holics. Child A/B/C (%): 54/36/9	24 months (0.1–60)	1 Rebleeding (16)	HVPG measured at least 5 days after control of the bleeding episode. Repeated at 5.3 ± 0.9 months	Good haemo-dynamic response (HVPG decrease of > 20% from baseline or to < 12 mmHg). Univariate survival analysis	100% propra-nolol + IMN	Good haemodynamic response not predictive of rebleeding. The frequency of rebleeding was higher in responders
Patch 1999	Retrospective cohort study	105 pt. 100% previous portal hypertensive bleeding (94% varices) 65% alcoholics. Child A/B/C (%): 27/39/34. 41% ascites	18.7 months (0–84.5)	1 Rebleeding (54) 2 Death (33)	0–372 days after the bleeding episode (median 11). 67% within first 2 weeks.	HVPG as continuous variable: Cox model. HVPG > 16 mmHg. Univariate survival analysis	63% β-blockers 37% sclerotherapy	HVPG independent predictor of death. Adjusted HR: 1.11 (covariates: PT, Bil, ascites, previous long-term endoscopic treatment). HVPG as a continuous variable or HVPG > 16 mmHg not predictive of rebleeding

Villanueva 2001	Prospective cohort study embedded in an RCT	95 pt. 44% alcoholics. Child A/B/C (%): 21/57/22. 67% ascites	21 months (1–68)	1 Rebleeding (59) 2 Death (62)	HVPG measured within the first week after bleeding, before randomisation, and at 1–3 months	Good haemodynamic response (HVPG decrease of > 20% from baseline or to < 12 mmHg). Cox model	Randomised to banding ligation or nadolol+ IMN	Good haemodynamic response independent predictor of rebleeding (covariates: treatment group, Child at 3 months). Good haemodynamic response predictor of survival at univariate. Not an independent predictor
Patch 2002	Prospective cohort study embedded in an RCT	102 pt. 67% alcoholics. Child A/B/C (%): 13/36/51	11 months (0–46)	1 Rebleeding (46) 2 Death (34)	HVPG measured 5 days after bleeding, before randomisation. Follow-up HVPG repeated in 26 pt. at 2–3 months in the drugs arm. Repeated at 1 year in 31 pt.	HVPG as continuous variable: Cox model	Randomised to 'A la carte' drug therapy (propranolol, to which IMN was added in non-responders) versus banding ligation	Baseline HVPG was the only independent predictor of rebleeding. HR: 1.08. Baseline HVPG. Not an independent predictor of survival. Longitudinal HVPG values not predictive of events

Table 23 (Continued).

Study	Type of study	Patients	Follow-up	Outcome	HVPG measurement	Analysis	Treatment of the patients	Results
Abraldes 2003	Retrospective cohort study with patients from 3 RCTs	73 pt. 52% alcoholics. A/B/C (%): 45/48/7. 32% ascites	70 months (1–96)	1 Rebleeding (26) 2 Death (15) 3 Ascites (22) 4 SBP (9) 5 Encephalopathy (15)	Baseline HVPG: 5–14 days after index bleeding. Follow-up HVPG: 111 days (34–164) after	Good haemodynamic response (HVPG decrease of > 20% from baseline or to < 12 mmHg). Cox model	39% propranolol. 61% propranolol + IMN	Good haemodynamic response independent predictor of 1 Rebleeding. Adj HR: 2.8 (covariates: albumin) 2 Survival. Adj HR: 12.3 (covariates: age, albumin) 3 Ascites. Adj HR: 3.5 (covariates: platelets) 4 SBP. HR: 8.6 (covariates: prothrombin rate). Not predictive of encephalopathy
Villanueva 2004	Retrospective cohort study	132 pt. (41 previously included in Villanueva 2001). 46% alcoholics. Child A/B/C (%): 23/56/21	16 months (1–48)	1 Rebleeding (37) 2 Death (33) 3 Ascites (55) 4 Encephalopathy (28)	Baseline HPVG: within 5 days of control of variceal bleeding. Follow-up HVPG: 58 days (26–123) after	Good haemodynamic response (HVPG decrease of > 20% from baseline or to < 12 mmHg). Univariable analysis for bleeding, ascites and encephalopathy. Cox model. For survival	100% nadolol+ IMN	Good haemodynamic response independent predictor of survival. Adj HR: 1.5 (covariates: Child, rebleeding, encephalopathy, hepatocarcinoma in the follow-up). Good haemodynamic response predictor of bleeding, ascites and encephalopathy at univariate analysis

with HVPG $\leq$ 16 mmHg have a 35% 2-year survival versus 15% in those with HVPG $>$ 16 mmHg. In patients receiving vasoactive medication, absolute HVPG values after drug therapy [42] or a good HVPG response (>20% decrease from baseline or to less than 12 mmHg) are independent predictors of survival [45,46], while baseline HVPG is not. Further, a good haemodynamic response predicts survival after adjusting for liver function [45,46], and this survival benefit cannot be attributed to an improvement in liver function [49]. Additionally, a good haemodynamic response is independently associated with a decreased risk of ascites and spontaneous bacterial peritonitis during follow-up [45,46], indicating that overall prognosis in patients with cirrhosis surviving a variceal bleeding episode can be improved by decreasing portal pressure.

Prognosis in patients undergoing liver surgery for HCC (Table 24)

In a series of compensated cirrhotic patients (Child A) undergoing liver surgery for a single HCC, HVPG was the only variable independently associated with decompensation at 3 months [50]. No patient with an HVPG $<$ 10 mmHg had liver decompensation. The same group analysed the long-term outcome of 43 patients with Child A cirrhosis and resectable HCC. An HVPG $\geq$ 10 was the only independent predictor of survival [51].

Summary

1 HVPG must increase over 10 mmHg for the development of varices, and above 12 mmHg for the development of variceal bleeding.
2 HVPG is a prognostic indicator of bleeding in patients with compensated cirrhosis (status 1), in patients with varices without bleeding (status 2) and in patients after a variceal bleeding (status 4). In status 3 and 4 patients, HVPG is a prognostic indicator of death. The predictive value of HVPG is independent of liver function.
3 In patients receiving drug therapy to reduce portal pressure or in alcoholics who become abstinent, HVPG must be repeated to maintain its prognostic value. A decrease in portal pressure of 20% or to $<$ 12 mmHg achieves effective protection from variceal bleeding, and in stage 4 patients it leads to a better overall prognosis.

Recommendations

1 Models combining Child–Pugh or MELD with HVPG should be elaborated for the use in centres in which HVPG measurement is available.

Table 24 HVPG as a prognostic indicator in patients undergoing liver resection for hepatocellular carcinoma (HCC).

Study	Type of study	Patients	Follow-up	Outcome (number of events)	HVPG measurement	Analysis	Treatment of the patients	Results
Bruix 1996	Prospective cohort study	29 pt. 100% Child A. Single HCC < 5 cm	Up to 3 months	Unresolved liver decompensation (jaundice, ascites, ecephalopathy) or death at 3 months (11)	Within 10 days before surgery	HVPG (continuous variable). Logistic regression	Surgical resection of HCC	HVPG was the only independent predictor of decompensation. OR: 1.90. No patient with HVPG < 10 mmHg had liver decompensation
Llovet 1999	Retrospective cohort study	43 pt. (presumably 29 belonged to Bruix 1996 study). 96% Child A. 75% single HCC < 5 cm	32 months	Death (49% of the series)	Before surgery	HVPG ≥ 10 mmHg. Cox regression	Surgical resection of HCC	HVPG ≥ 10 mmHg was the only preoperatory independent predictor of survival

2 Further studies are required to model the relationship between HVPG and different outcomes within each stage of cirrhosis. HVPG should not be dichotomised unless clearly justified by the analysis of large samples with a sufficient number of strata or by clinical usefulness.

NON-INVASIVE INDICATORS OF OESOPHAGEAL VARICES

The Baveno III consensus conference recommended universal endoscopic screening for oesophagus varices (OV) in patients with newly diagnosed cirrhosis [52]. Furthermore, in patients without varices, it was recommended that endoscopy be repeated at 2–3 years intervals to evaluate the development of OV, and in patients with small varices, yearly endoscopies were recommended [52]. However, these recommendations imply a considerable burden of endoscopies and related costs. In particular, they require that patients undergo repeat unpleasant procedures, even though up to 50% of them might be free of OV 10 years from diagnosis [53].

A recent analysis of cost-effectiveness [54] suggests that universal treatment of cirrhotics with β-blockers, avoiding any screening procedure (i.e. both universal endoscopic screening and endoscopy reserved to patients with the highest likelihood of OV presence), represents the most advantageous strategy in terms of bleeding prevention. However, these conclusions seem to be merely speculative since the available evidence on the efficacy of β-blockers in pre-primary prophylaxis does not support yet their use in patients without varices, even in those with a demonstrated increase of portal pressure [22,55]. In addition, data on the efficacy of β-blockers in delaying variceal enlargement are still conflicting [55,56]. Therefore, since both β-blockers [57] and endoscopic prophylaxis [58] can be considered effective in preventing bleeding only in patients with high-risk varices (i.e. patients with large OV), it would be ideal to confine endoscopic screening programs to those patients with the highest likelihood of having OV.

Several studies evaluated different clinical, radiological and laboratory parameters as predictors of the presence of OV (Table 25) and/or large OV (LOV) (Table 26) in viral or alcoholic cirrhosis [59–69]. However, only two of them [63,66] attempted to identify indicators of OV in compensated cirrhotics, which represent the target population of the guidelines and that would benefit most from a 'non-invasive' follow-up. Moreover, two studies [70,71] assessing non-invasive indicators of OV in patients with primary sclerosing cholangitis (PSC) and primary biliary cirrhosis (PBC) were recently published (Tables 25 and 26). Interestingly, the study by Zein *et al.* [70], besides providing information on the prevalence of OV in patients with PSC (Tables 25 and 26), also shows that only 53% of patients with OV had

Table 25 Studies assessing non-invasive indicators of oesophageal varices (OV).

Author	Year	No. Pts	EtOH (%)	Child A/B/C (%)	No. with OV (%)	Predictors	LR + (−)	Post test P + (−) %
Fook-Hong *et al.**	1999	92	30	41/47/12	53 (58)	PLT < 150.000 and/or ascites (or Bil > 40 mmol/L)	1.9 (0.4)	71 (33)
Pilette *et al.*	1999	116	57	50/24/26	83 (72)	PLT < 160.000 (and/or PT)	NA	NA
Schepis *et al.*	2001	143	15	59/41/0	63 (44)	PLT < 100.000 and PT < 70% and PV > 13 mm	13.9 (0.6) [7.3]†	94 (45) [86]†
Schepis *et al.* (compensated)	2001	112	15	73/27/0	53 (47)	PLT < 100.000 and PT < 70% and PV > 13 mm	NA	NA
Schepis *et al.* (validation cohort)	2001	105	0	68/32/0	45 (43)	PLT < 100.000 and PT < 70% and PV > 13 mm	NA	NA
Giannini *et al.* (1st)‡	2003	145	17	37/36/27	89 (61)	PLT/Splenic LD > 909	18.6 (0)	96 (0)
Giannini *et al.* (2nd)	2003	121	24	41/42/17	59 (71)	PLT/Splenic LD > 909	1.7 (0)	68 (0)
Giannini *et al.* (compensated)	2003	145	Nr	69/31/0	53 (37)	PLT/Splenic LD > 909	3.4 (0)	81 (0)
Thomopoulos *et al.*§	2003	184	43	65/27/8	92 (50)	PLT < 118.000 and Splenic LD > 135 mm and ascites on US¶	5 (0.9) [6.8]†	86 (51) [85]†

Zein *et al.* (PSC)	2004	183	–	Nr	47 (26)	PLT < 150.000 (or Alb < 3.3 g/dL or stage 3–4)	5.9 (0.4)	73 (16)
Zein *et al.* (valid.) (PSC)	2004	72	–	Nr	27 (37)	PLT < 150.000 (or histologic stage 3–4)	3.8 (0.4)	63 (18)
Bressler *et al.* (PBC/PSC)	2005	87	–	Nr	26 (30)	PLT < 200.000 and/or Alb < 40 g/L and/or Bil > 20 mm/L	NA	NA
Bressler *et al.* (viral cirr.)	2005	104	0	Nr	38 (37)	PLT < 110.000	NA	NA
Bressler *et al.* (other cirr.)	2005	45	0	Nr	21 (47)	PLT < 105.000	NA	NA
Dragoni *et al.* (HCV cirr. in Haemoph. HIV+)	2005	40	Nr	Nr	13 (32)	PV and splenic LD	3.8 (0.2)	65 (9)

LR + (−), Likelihood ratio for the presence (absence) of OV; Post test P + (−), probability of correctly (erroneously) diagnosing OV presence. The pre-test probability is the OV prevalence (55%) reported by D'Amico *et al.*; PLT, platelet count; Bil, bilirubin; PT, prothrombin index (%); PV, portal vein diameter; Splenic LD, Splenic longitudinal diameter; US: ultrasound; Alb, albumin; Nr, not reported; NA, not applicable

* Included patients with different aetiologies between the two groups and those that had been treated with diuretics

† In square brackets are reported the LR+ and the post-test probability for absence of OV when all the indicators are absent

‡ Albumin missing at univariate analysis

§ 7 years to collect the patients (26/year); This study groups patients without OV and those with small OV

¶ Univariate/multivariate comparison on no + small varices versus large varices —» conclusion on varices overall (83.3% of patients with PLT < 118.000 and Spleen > 135 mm and ascites had OV; 12.8% of patients with PLT ≥ 118.000 and spleen ≤ 135 mm and no ascites had small sized OV

Table 26 Studies assessing non-invasive indicators of *large* oesophageal varices (LOV).

Author	Year	No. Pts	EtOH (%)	Child A/B/C (%)	No. with LOV (%)	Predictors	LR + (−)	Post test P + (−) %
Cottone *et al.*	1986	213	23	Nr	43 (20)	PV > 13 mm and no respiratory variations in SV and MV	2 (0.2)	31 (5)
Chalasani *et al.*	1999	346	22	22/48/30	20 (6)	PLT < 88.000 and splenomegaly*	2 (0.6)	31 (12)
Pilette *et al.*	1999	116	57	50/24/26	51 (44)	PLT < 160.000 (and/or PT and/or spider naevi)	1.9 (0.3)	30 (7)
Zaman *et al.*	1999	98†	13	34/51/15	20 (20)	PLT < 88.000	1.8 (0.6)	29 (11)
Fook-Hong *et al.*	1999	92	30	41/47/12	19 (20)	PLT < 150.000 and ascites	2 (0)	31 (0)
Madhotra *et al.*	2002	184	18	43/34/23	24 (13)	PLT < 68.000 and splenomegaly‡	3.4 (0.5)	43 (10)
Thomopoulos *et al.*§	2003	184	43	64/28/8	33 (18)	PLT < 118.000 or splenic LD > 135 mm or ascites on US¶	1.7 (0.9) [nc]**	28 (17) [nc]**
Zein *et al.*‖	2004	183	–	Nr	20 (11)	PLT < 150.000 (or Alb < 3.3 g/dL)	4.1 (0.3)	33 (4)
Zein *et al.* (valid.)	2004	72	–	Nr	9 (12)	PLT < 150.000 (or histologic stage 3–4)	3.1 (0.3)	27 (4)
Vanbiervliet G#	2005	146	100	Nr	23 (16)	PT ≤ 60% and hyaluronate > 100 g/L and Alk Ph > 110 IU/L	8.4 (0.5)	65 (11)

LR + (−), Likelihood ratio for the presence (absence) of OV; Post test P + (−), probability of correctly (erroneously) diagnosing OV presence. The pre-test probability is the mean LOV prevalence (18%) reported in the listed studies; PV, portal vein diameter; SV, splenic vein diameter; MV, mesenteric vein diameter; PLT, platelet count; PT, prothrombin index (%); Splenic LD, Splenic longitudinal diameter; US: ultrasound; Alb, albumin; Alk Ph, alkaline phosphatase; nc, not calculable; Nr, not reported

* Splenomegaly was diagnosed by physical examination or CT scan: no definition of the parameters used was provided

† Pretransplant patients

‡ Splenomegaly was diagnosed by US or CT scan: no definition of the parameters used was provided

§ 7 years to collect the patients (25/year)

¶ Univariate/multivariate comparison on no + small varices versus large varices —» conclusion on varices overall (83.3% of patients with PLT < 118.000 and spleen > 135 mm and ascites had OV; 12.8% of patients with PLT ≥ 118.000 and spleen ≤ 135 mm and no ascites had small sized OV). No clear final conclusion on the positive predictive value of the rule on LOV)

‖ Only three patients with large OV (8 moderate)

** In square brackets are reported the LR+ and the post-test probability for absence of OV when all the indicators are absent

Only 40.4% of patients had severe fibrosis at liver biopsy

cirrhosis on liver biopsy. This finding, whatever the cause (i.e. sampling error or pre-sinusoidal portal hypertension), underscores the need of non-invasive indicators of OV in patients with cholestatic liver disease.

Overall, these studies have identified variables related to liver function (i.e. prothrombin time or PT, albumin, bilirubin, Child–Pugh class), liver fibrosis (i.e. PT, hyaluronate), clinical stage (i.e. ascites, Child–Pugh class, cirrhosis on liver biopsy), portal hypertension (i.e. portal vein diameter, spleen size) and hypersplenism (i.e. low platelet count, platelet count/spleen diameter ratio) that significantly correlate with the presence or size of OV. However, a broad range of predictive values of the OV indicators has been reported (Tables 25 and 26) together with different cut-off values for discriminating low platelet count, which represents the finding most commonly associated with OV presence in the published studies (Tables 25 and 26) [72].

Quality assessment of these studies (Tables 27 and 28 and Figs 25 and 26) shows that the majority of them present many sources of bias, which contribute to invalidate the 'diagnostic' efficacy of their results. Only one study [63] presents with a prospective design (i.e. predefined criteria with consecutive enrolment of newly diagnosed patients), blinding of disease stage and results of diagnostic tests to clinicians managing the patients, adequate reference standard (i.e. use of a definite classification system of OV; recorded endoscopy performed and revised by the same team), and, finally, an attempt of external validation of results. Selection bias arises in retrospective studies [61,64–66,68] and in those with very specific referral pattern (i.e. liver transplant units) [61,64,68]. Another bias, likely explaining the different cut-off levels of platelets reported in the published studies, is the spectrum bias, which may occur when the study population has a different clinical spectrum than the population in whom the test will be applied [59,61,64–66]. Selection and spectrum bias are likely acting together in the analysed studies. High interobserver and intraobserver variability in diagnosing the presence and size of OV or in reporting radiological (i.e. portal vein diameter, spleen longitudinal axis and Doppler parameters) measurements together with observer bias (i.e. prior knowledge of the patients clinical status) are likely to be very common in all the studies without *a priori* planning design and without adequate blindness of all the diagnostic procedures [60–62,64–69,71]. Therefore, no study has reached a high enough level of evidence to warrant the widespread use of non-invasive markers of OV (Fig. 27).

An additional issue that further explains the inefficiency of the proposed markers is the inclusion of cirrhotic patients at different stages. There are at least three different populations of cirrhotic patients with a different prevalence of OV that have been included in an overlapping fashion in these studies. The first is a population of asymptomatic patients with

Table 27 Quality analysis of the studies assessing non-invasive indicators of oesophageal varices (OV).

Author	Year	Study design	Patients	Pre-defined pro forma	Validation	Reference standard	Level of evidence
Fook-Hong *et al.*	1999	Cross-sectional	Consecutive	Yes*	No	Good†	2b
Pilette *et al.*	1999	Cross-sectional	Consecutive	Yes*	No	Good†	2b
Schepis *et al.*	2001	Cross-sectional	Consecutive (incident)	Yes	Internal/External	Good	2b
Schepis *et al.* (compensated)	2001	Cross-sectional	Consecutive (incident)	Yes	–	Good	
Schepis *et al.* (validation cohort)	2001	Cross-sectional	Consecutive	–	–	Good	
Giannini *et al.* (1st)	2003	Retrospective	Nr	–	External†	Poor	3b
Giannini *et al.* (2nd) (validation cohort)	2003	Cross-sectional	Consecutive*	Nr	–	Poor	
Giannini *et al.* (compensated)	2003	Mixed	–	–	–	Poor	
Thomopoulos *et al.*	2003	Cross-sectional	Consecutive (incident*)	Yes*	No	Good†	2b
Zein *et al.* (PSC)	2004	Cross-sectional	Consecutive* (first visit)	Yes*,‡	External	Good†	2b
Zein *et al.* (validation cohort) (PSC)	2004	Retrospective	First visit§	–	–	Poor	
Bressler *et al.* (**PBC**/PSC)	2005	Retrospective	Consecutive*	–	No	Poor	3b
Bressler *et al.* (viral cirrhosis)	2005	Retrospective	Consecutive*	–	No	Poor	
Bressler *et al.* (other cirrhosis)	2005	Retrospective	Consecutive*	–	No	Poor	
Dragoni *et al.* (HCV cirrhosis in haemophilic HIV+)	2005	Cross-sectional	Consecutive	Nr	No	Good†	3b

PSC, primary sclerosing cholangitis; PBC, primary biliary cirrhosis
* Not clearly stated
† Uncertainty about blindness and reliability of endoscopic classification of OV
‡ 80 patients collected between 1995 and 1998 compared with 203 collected between 1991 and 1994
§ Data were probably collected with a pre-defined pro forma, but for another study

Table 28 Quality analysis of the studies assessing non-invasive indicators of large oesophageal varices (LOV).

Author	Year	Study design	Patients	Pre-defined pro forma	Validation	Reference standard	Level of evidence
Cottone *et al.*	1986	Cross-sectional	Consecutive	Yes†	No	Good*	2b
Chalasani *et al.*	1999	Retrospective	No	–	Internal	Poor	3b
Pilette *et al.*	1999	Cross-sectional	Consecutive	Yes†	No	Good*	2b
Zaman *et al.*	1999	Retrospective	No	–	No	Poor	3b
Fook-Hong *et al.*	1999	Cross-sectional	Consecutive	Yes†	No	Good*	2b
Madhotra *et al.*	2002	Retrospective	Consecutive†	–	No	Poor	3b
Thomopoulos *et al.*	2003	Cross-sectional	Consecutive (incident†)	Yes†	No	Good*	2b
Zein *et al.* (PSC)	2004	Cross-sectional	Consecutive† (first visit)	Yes†, §	External	Good*	2b
Zein *et al.* (validation cohort) (PSC)	2004	Retrospective	First visit‡	–	–	Poor	3b
Vanbiervliet G (alcoholics)	2005	Cross-sectional	Consecutive	Nr	No	Good*	3b

PSC, primary sclerosing cholangitis; PBC, primary biliary cirrhosis

* Uncertainty about blindness and reliability of endoscopic classification of OV.

† Not clearly stated

‡ 80 patients collected between 1995 and 1998 compared with 203 collected between 1991 and 1994

§ Data were probably collected with a pre-defined pro forma, but for another study

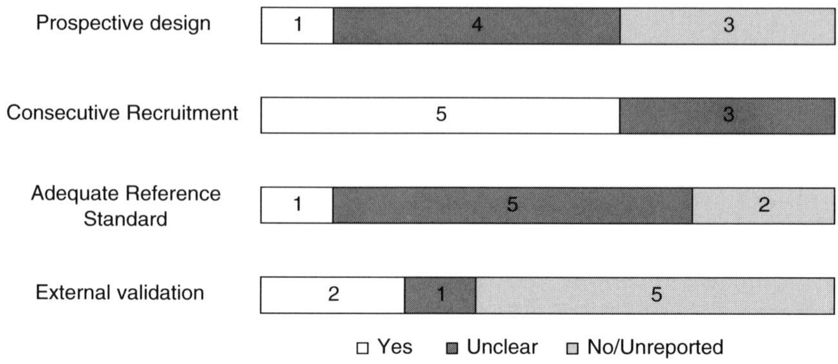

Fig. 25 Summary description of quality analysis of studies on non-invasive indicators of oesophageal varices (OV) ($n = 8$).

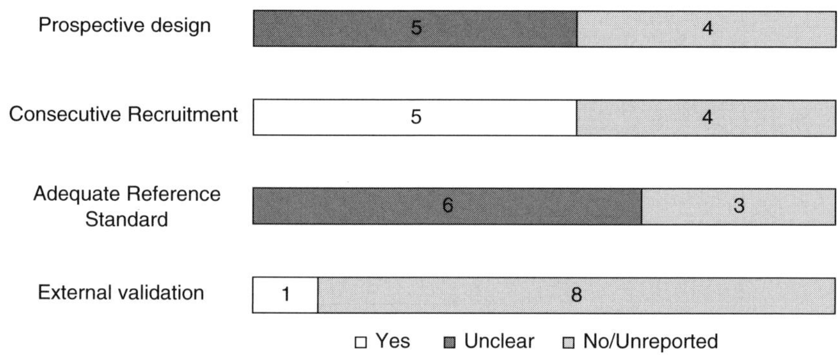

Fig. 26 Summary description of quality analysis of studies on non-invasive indicators of large oesophageal varices (LOV) ($n = 9$).

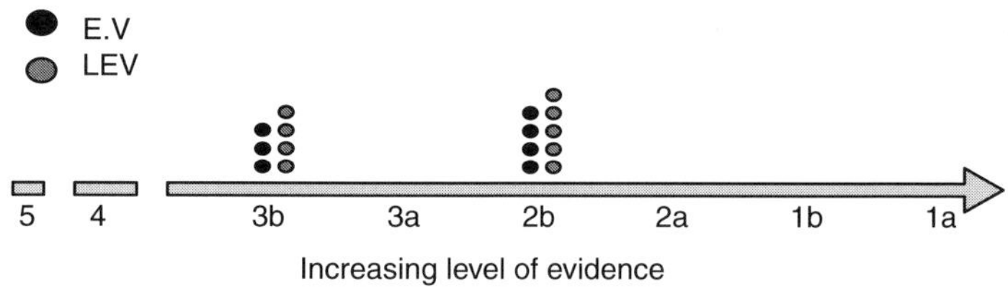

Fig. 27 Summary description of the levels of evidence reached by the studies on non-invasive indicators of oesophageal varices (OV; $n = 8$) and large oesophageal varices (LOV; $n = 9$).

biopsy-proven cirrhosis (i.e. mostly, cohorts of HCV positive patients or with a history of alcohol abuse) [60,62,67,70,73]. The second population is that of patients with or without biopsy-proven cirrhosis who have clinical features diagnostic of cirrhosis (low platelet count, low albumin, prolonged

PT and/or compatible radiological features) but who do not have ascites or encephalopathy [60,63,68,70]. These two different populations are usually joined in a group of Child class A cirrhotics under the statement 'diagnosis of cirrhosis was based on liver biopsy or history, physical examination, biochemical and radiological parameters'. The third population is that of patients with decompensated cirrhosis. These patients are usually classified as belonging to Child–Pugh class B or C depending on liver function tests [59,61,64–67]. Furthermore, the existence of a pre-cirrhotic target population of patients at risk of OV could also be postulated (the fourth population?). This population, which includes both asymptomatic and symptomatic patients, presents with different degrees and location of fibrosis [62,70,71,73–75] likely depending on the aetiology and pathogenesis of the disease (e.g. PSC/PBC versus alcoholic versus cryptogenic versus viral) and on the biopsy false negative rate.

Conclusion

There are no satisfactory non-endoscopic indicators of the presence of varices. While further studies are awaited, endoscopic screening is still the best practice to detect the presence and size of varices. The design of future studies assessing non-invasive indicators of OV should:

1 include compensated patients and should be designed as prospective with blinding of the diagnostic procedures and adequate reference standard – patients with cholestatic liver disease may require a separate evaluation;

2 be large enough to identify specific indicators or cut-off levels of the same indicator in different subgroups of patients;

3 evaluate indicators that have already been identified and include others that take into account the multifactorial origin of OV;

4 include HVPG measurements in order to identify indicators that best relate to portal pressure levels and OV presence in various subgroups of patients;

5 be presented in a way that allows calculation of the probability of having OV for each level or combination of the indicators included in the analysis;

6 be externally validated.

PREDICTORS OF VARICEAL DEVELOPMENT, ENLARGEMENT AND BLEEDING

Oesophageal varices develop in cirrhotic patients when the HVPG threshold of 10–12 mmHg is reached [14]. Varices increase in size progressively and large varices are related with an increased bleeding risk. Since prophylactic therapy is effective in reducing the risk of VH, particularly in those with large varices, patients with cirrhosis undergo periodic endoscopic examination to determine the presence and size of varices [1].

Prospective studies have shown that patients without varices develop new varices at a rate of 5–10% per year [1,76]. These percentages differ depending on the severity of liver disease. While the incidence of OV may be as low as 4% per year in patients with compensated cirrhosis [53], it is significantly higher in patients with severe PBC [77] (12% per year), in those with cirrhosis of alcoholic origin [55] (44% in 16 months) and in patients with decompensated cirrhosis [53] (25% per year).

A low platelet count [78], a prolonged PT [78], worsening liver function during follow-up [55] or continued alcohol abuse have been shown to be predictive of the development of new varices. A decreased platelet count is a good indicator of portal hypertension, while worsening liver function and alcohol abuse may parallel increases in HVPG in patients with alcoholic cirrhosis [20].

In the only prospective study of consecutive cirrhotic patients without varices and portal hypertension (HVPG > 5 mmHg), the majority of patients had hepatitis C (68%) and were Child–Pugh A (88%) with a mean score of 5.4. The primary end point was the development of varices or VH. Median follow-up was 4.6 years. Patients developed a primary end point at a rate of approximately 8% per year. On multivariable analysis (that included treatment group, that is, β-blocker or placebo), the only parameters predictive of development of a primary end point were AST ($p = 0.007$) and a baseline HVPG > 10 mmHg ($p = 0.005$) [22].

Regarding enlargement of varices, prospective studies have shown a rate of progression from small to medium or large varices ranging from 5% to 20% per year [1,56,76,79]. Factors influencing the enlargement of OV are similar to those causing their development. Alcoholic aetiology [76], severity of liver disease at the time of initial observation [55,76] or a worsening liver function during follow-up [79] are associated with a more rapid variceal progression rate. Endoscopic parameters such as the presence of small OV and red weal marks at initial endoscopy have also been reported as predictive of variceal enlargement [55,76].

It has been suggested that changes in HVPG may induce variations in the size of OV [20]; however extensive data on this topic are lacking. In alcoholic cirrhotic patients who abstain from alcohol, OV may even disappear (associated to a reduction in HVPG), however patients achieving a significant HVPG reduction with pharmacological treatment with β-blockers may or, more frequently, may not reduce their variceal size [56]. Other factors such as variceal wall tension or formation of other portosystemic collaterals may play a role in determining variceal size progression.

The probability of bleeding from OV is variable and depends on cirrhosis status. In patients with no varices at endoscopy, the risk of bleeding is as low as 3% in 4.6 years [22] or 2–4% at 2 years [76], while patients with small varices have a 2 years risk of 12% (CI: 5–19%) [76]. Several predictors have been proposed to identify patients at higher risk of bleeding. Variceal size, red weal marks and Child–Pugh class have been combined to obtain a valid risk score after one screening endoscopy [35,80]. Other authors have suggested identifying patients at high risk of bleeding by using only endoscopic criteria [81]. Whatever the prediction system adopted, it should be noted that only a relatively small proportion of the patients presenting with VH have risk factors predictive of bleeding [80]. The continuous changes in the predictive parameters that cannot be submitted to real time monitoring may be one of the causes for this low accuracy. To improve prediction of bleeding it is necessary to add other parameters or information derived from a dynamic evaluation. In a recent multicentre study including patients with large oesophageal varices (LOV), the risk of first bleeding was higher when PT was prolonged and when the percentage of patients receiving β-blockers was lower, while in a Cox model the presence of tense ascites (RR: 3.4, CI: 2.5–5.9) and prior history of haemorrhage (RR: 4.4, CI: 2.6–7.5) were independent predictors of variceal bleeding [82]. Variceal pressure measured at endoscopy has also been proposed to be an independent predictor of variceal bleeding at 1 year [83].

As mentioned in the section on 'HVPG as a Predictor of Outcome', therapeutic trials have shown that the bleeding risk is abolished when HVPG is decreased below 12 mmHg by pharmacological treatment or is significantly reduced when HVPG decreases > 20% from pretreatment values.

Summary

1 HVPG is presently the most reliable predictor of variceal development.
2 Liver dysfunction or a worsening liver function are the most commonly described predictors of variceal growth.
3 The NIEC score is presently the most reliable predictor of variceal rupture; the contribution of HVPG and other predictors should be investigated.

Recommendations

1 Endoscopic surveillance of cirrhotic patients to ascertain the presence of varices and their size can be considered the first line screening for the risk of bleeding.

2 Follow-up endoscopies should be performed every 1–2 years in compensated cirrhosis patients with small varices and at 2–3 year intervals in those without varices [1]. Severity of liver disease is a predictor of variceal enlargement and therefore endoscopy should be repeated more frequently in patients who develop decompensation.

PROGNOSTIC MODELS FOR SURVIVAL IN PATIENTS WITHOUT ASCITES OR BLEEDING

The course of disease of cirrhosis is usually one of progression with minor fluctuations unless the underlying factor(s) such as alcoholism or viral replication can be successfully controlled. Even though the process of progression is continuous, various stages have been defined. Thus it is common to classify patients as being in compensated or decompensated, decompensation being defined by the presence of ascites, jaundice, variceal bleeding or encephalopathy. Prognostic models particularly useful for decompensated cirrhosis patients such as the Child–Pugh and MELD scores have been recently reviewed [84]. However, since patients in the decompensated stage already have advanced disease with a poor prognosis, it is of major interest to assess the course and outcome or the prognosis prior to this stage, that is in the compensated stage.

In patients who have no ascites and no varices (status 1), mortality is low and in a large multicentre study that included 212 patients, death occurred in 25 patients in a mean follow-up period of 45 months [22]. Of the 25 patients who died, 64% had developed ascites and/or encephalopathy. Of the 9 patients who did not have ascites or encephalopathy at time of death, the cause of death was bacterial infection in 4 (44%), 4 had a non-hepatic malignancy and 1 had a cardiac-related death. The probability of survival in patients who did not develop varices (censored) or who did not develop decompensation during follow-up was 100% at 1 year and 97% at 3 years. Therefore, in patients without varices or ascites, predicting survival is not an issue as survival is directly related to the development of decompensation. As mentioned previously, in this patient population an HVPG > 10 mmHg was the most important predictor of the development of a composite end point (varices, VH, ascites and encephalopathy, transplant or death) [22].

Over the years a number of important prognostic models have been developed in various groups of patients with compensated cirrhosis (that encompass status 1 an 2). In a large study including 435 patients with compensated cirrhosis of various aetiologies D'Amico *et al.* identified male gender, HBsAg-positivity, old age, prolonged PT and the presence of OV as significant predictors of reduced survival [4].

Ginés studied the prognosis of 293 patients with compensated cirrhosis of whom 42% were alcoholics and 9% were HBsAg positive [3]. They found high bilirubin, high gamma globulin, presence of hepatic stigmata, long PT, male gender, old age and elevated alkaline phosphatase to be significantly associated with a reduced survival.

In a group of 100 patients with compensated cirrhosis of mixed aetiology (44% alcoholic, 29% HBsAg positive), Zoli *et al.* found low albumin, high bilirubin, low cholesterol and low liver volume to be independent predictors of reduced survival [85]. In a subsequent study performed in 50 patients with compensated cirrhosis the prognostic influence of portal haemodynamics measured by pulsed echo-Doppler was also investigated [86]. CPS and reduced portal blood velocity were found to be independent predictors of reduced survival.

In a large European study including 366 patients with compensated cirrhosis due to hepatitis B followed for up to 17 years, old age, low albumin, low platelets, splenomegaly, high bilirubin and presence of HBeAg had significant, independent association with a reduced survival [87]. In the subgroup of 200 patients who had information on delta virus infection, old age, low albumin and high gamma globulins had independent significant association with a reduced survival but the delta status had no significant influence [88].

In another large European study including 384 patients with compensated cirrhosis due to hepatitis C followed for up to 13 years, high bilirubin, the presence of hepatic stigmata, old age and low platelets had independent significant association with a reduced survival [89]. In a subgroup of 297 patients with compensated cirrhosis fulfilling stricter inclusion criteria, the influence of hepatitis B and C virus infections on the natural history was studied [90]. Age, male gender, low platelets and low albumin were significantly associated with a reduced survival. After adjusting for these variables, hepatitis B infection tended to be associated with poorer survival than hepatitis C infection ($p = 0.17$).

Conclusion

In various prognostic studies of survival in compensated cirrhosis there is some overlap in identified prognostic variables with relatively little influence of the aetiology. From the performed studies it can be concluded that a reduced survival depends on a combination of *host factors* (old age, male gender), *viral activity* (HBeAg positivity, HBsAg positivity), the *degree of reduced liver function* (high bilirubin, low albumin, prolonged PT, high alkaline phosphatase, low cholesterol, reduced liver volume), the *presence of hepatic stigmata*, the *degree of portal hypertension* (OV, low portal blood velocity, splenomegaly, low platelets) and its *effect on the immune system* (high gamma globulins). Another factor, which influences survival significantly, is the current alcohol consumption, see the time-dependent Cox model for both compensated and decompensated cirrhosis referred to in Reference [84].

There is a need for a common prognostic model for survival, which can obtain general acceptance as the model of reference. Such a model could be obtained by an analysis based on a combined database comprising all the data from the various larger studies performed. Importantly, in compensated patients the development of ascites and portal hypertensive bleeding are the most relevant outcomes.

PROGNOSTIC MODEL FOR PATIENTS WITH UPPER GASTROINTESTINAL HAEMORRHAGE

Upper gastrointestinal haemorrhage (UGIH) is an important complication of cirrhosis. The most common cause of UGIH in this setting is rupture of oesophageal or gastric varices, directly related to portal hypertension. As mentioned above, the risk of bleeding correlates with the severity of portal hypertension assessed by the HVPG [37–40].

The prognosis in patients presenting with UGIH is determined by factors, namely the severity of liver disease and the magnitude of bleeding. The severity of liver disease determines long-term prognosis in patients with cirrhosis. In addition, it affects the integrity of the patient's overall physiology and thus the ability to withstand the haemodynamic insults brought on by the acute haemorrhage. Massive UGIH not only puts the patient at risk of exsanguinations but also causes hypoxic damage to the liver, further compromising the hepatic functional reserve and, by compromising renal perfusion, may cause renal dysfunction [91].

Prognostic factors that represent severity of liver disease

It is interesting to remember that both of the well-known disease severity scales in patients with end-stage liver disease, namely the Child–Turcotte and the MELD scores were derived from patients who had experienced UGIH.

The purpose of the original Child–Turcotte score was to assess the operative risk in patients undergoing surgical portosystemic shunt [92]. It was based on five variables, including ascites, encephalopathy, nutritional status, and serum bilirubin and albumin. In 1973, Pugh and colleagues used a modified version of the Child–Turcotte classification in describing the outcome

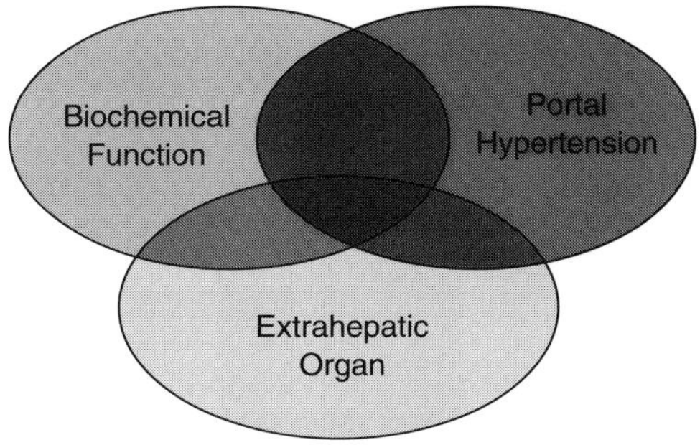

Fig. 28 Three conceptual components that determine survival in patients with end-stage liver disease.

of patients undergoing surgical ligation of OV [7]. Nutritional status in the Child–Turcotte classification was replaced with PT, this constitutes the CPS or the Child–Turcotte–Pugh (CTP) score. MELD was originally developed as a tool to assess the short-term prognosis of patients with liver cirrhosis undergoing the TIPS procedure [93]. The model incorporated serum creatinine, total serum bilirubin, INR for PT and aetiology of cirrhosis.

In examining the variables used in the CTP and MELD systems, one realises that they may be grouped into three overlapping categories (Fig. 28). First, a number of biochemical parameters measure the physiologic functional reserve of the liver. These include serum concentrations of albumin and bilirubin and PT. Second, the severity of portal hypertension that may not necessarily be measured by these biochemical parameters is likely to be of importance in determining the prognosis of patients with end stage liver disease. The direct measurement, HVPG, may be the most accurate means to assess this, but may be impractical for repeated measurements. Other indirect measures may include platelet count and grades of hepatic encephalopathy and ascites, although the latter variables also reflect the severity of liver dysfunction. Third variable is the integrity of extrahepatic organ systems, namely the renal function in MELD and nutritional status in the original Child score.

Prognostic factors that represent severity of haemorrhage

The magnitude of bleeding in patients with UGIH obviously has a significant impact on survival. This may be measured in a variety of ways such as vital signs (blood pressure and pulse rate) or haemoglobin concentrations at presentation and transfusion requirement. In addition, if there is sufficient haemodynamic derangement, the liver may sustain a degree of ischaemic damage, which may be measured by biochemical parameters such as AST

Table 29 Post-therapeutic predictors of 5-day failure and 6-week mortality in cirrhotic patients with upper GI haemorrhage (D'Amico and de Franchis).

5-day failure			6-week mortality		
Variable	OR	95% CI	Variable	OR	95% CI
CTP class	2.27	1.22–4.22	Albumin (per 1 g decrease)	2.33	1.32–4.00
PV thrombosis	2.75	1.25–6.04	Encephalopathy	2.30	1.39–3.70
AST (per 10 U increase)	1.03	1.01–1.06	Bilirubin (per 1 mg increase)	1.23	1.10–1.37
Transfusion in 24 h (units)	1.35	1.13–1.61	Transfusion total (units)	1.40	1.19–1.66
			Hepatocellular carcinoma	3.44	1.64–7.24

immediately, followed in more severe cases by worsening of biochemical functional parameters such as bilirubin.

A recent study by D'Amico and de Franchis [94] demonstrates the relative role of these prognostic parameters. In this multicentre, Italian study, a total of 465 patients with cirrhosis and UGIH were recruited. Prognostic variables for 5-day failure (uncontrolled bleeding, rebleeding or death) and 6-week mortality were sought. The 5-day failure rate was 13%, whereas by 6 weeks after presentation, rebleeding occurred in 17% and death in 20%.

Table 29 summarises the models to predict 5-day failure and 6-week mortality. There are three types of variables: (1) severity of underlying liver disease (CTP and its components); (2) severity of bleeding (AST, transfusion requirement) and (3) specific features of liver disease (portal vein thrombosis, HCC).

The last point of discussion is whether there are interactions between these prognostic factors, for example is the effect of two unit bleeding the same for patients with CTP of 6 as for those with CTP of 13?

Prognostic model for patients with ascites

Pathophysiologically, factors that determine the prognosis in patients with ascites are likely covered by the three components described for VH, namely biochemical synthetic function (albumin), degree of portal hypertension, and extra hepatic (renal) function (Fig. 28). Thus, in patients with ascites, the question is whether there are other variables that may better represent these three components. Recently, it has been suggested that serum sodium may provide prognostic information in addition to MELD [95,96]. Hyponatraemia has been described in associations with hepatorenal syndrome, ascites and liver related mortality. In 1956, Sheila Sherlock wrote, 'In patients with liver diseases serum-sodium levels below 130 meq/L must be regarded as serious and, if below 125 meq/L, ominous'. Like the components of the MELD score, sodium is a readily available, reproducible and objective laboratory test that predicts liver related mortality and is therefore a reasonable candidate for inclusion in a liver allocation model.

In a recent study that included 806 liver transplant candidates at six US centres, the role of sodium in addition to MELD was evaluated. The mean MELD score was 11.9 and the mean sodium 136.6 meq/L at the time of enrolment. The prevalence of ascites was 62% and 12% required therapeutic paracentesis. Of those who had hyponatraemia (< 130), 90% had ascites, although only 11% of those with ascites had hyponatraemia. There was a linear relationship between sodium level and the risk of death, after adjusting for MELD and centre. Between sodium levels of 120 and 135, each unit decrease in sodium was associated with 17% increase in 6-month mortality.

Summary

In patients who have experienced hepatic decompensation (UGIH or ascites), the severity of underlying liver disease as determined by the CTP or MELD score plays an important part in determining their overall outcome. In patients with UGIH, the magnitude of bleeding has a profound impact on the short- and longer-term outcome. Recent data show that the serum sodium level is an important additional prognostic variable in patients with hyponatraemia, most of whom have ascites. The additional role of HVPG and other potential predictors should be assessed.

WHAT ELSE DO WE NEED? PROPOSED CONSENSUS FOR TODAY'S CLINICAL PRACTICE AND FUTURE RESEARCH

Prognostic models for similar end points include somewhat different predictive variables. The causes for this include: differences between patient groups, differences in variables recorded, various sample sizes, random factors, statistical factors. Despite all these differences there tends to be a common pattern or a core of important variables, which is to some extent independent of the particular end point being studied. These common core variables may best reflect progression of the disease. The same underlying process of progression seems to be operative throughout the course of the disease.

Correlations among prognostic variables and their consequence on prognostic modelling

Frequently many variables from many of the components mentioned above will be associated with a given end point on univariate analysis. However in the normally applied multivariate regression models (including the Cox regression model) variables with *in*significant independent association with the end point will normally not be included. This is a consequence of a strong intercorrelation among predictive variables, that is they hold *partly* the same prognostic information. Only those variables with independent strong association with the end point will be included according to the statistical inclusion rules. This can imply a considerable type 2 error risk for not including potentially important predictors. To avoid this potential loss in prognostic information the choice of a variable for inclusion in a model should rely less on statistical significance and more on its *biological relevance*.

Challenges in describing the course of disease and in prognostic modelling

Patients are highly different at the time of diagnosis

Because of the insidious onset, the *starting point* of cirrhosis *is not well defined* and patients may be diagnosed at various stages along the course of disease. The time of diagnosis will depend on characteristics of the disease, non-disease-specific patient factors (when does he/she feel the necessity to go to a doctor), factors in the health service (accessibility, experience of the doctor, time of referral to a hepatologist, etc.). This means that *at the time of diagnosis the patients will be highly different* in regard to stage of disease progression, symptoms, signs and liver functionality (e.g. some patients may even present with variceal bleeding).

The courses of disease may be more homogeneous if considered according to status

For decompensated patients, Child–Pugh and MELD scores may be useful in assessing the risk of mortality. However, it is more important to assess prognosis in earlier compensated stages, so that therapy can be aimed at preventing complications and subsequent liver related death.

Based on a large cohort study of patients with cirrhosis by D'Amico *et al.*, four status of cirrhosis progression are proposed (Fig. 23): status 1: no varices and no ascites (OYM 1%); status 2: varices and no ascites (OYM 3.4%); status 3: ascites with or without varices (OYM 20%) and status 4: bleeding with or without ascites (OYM 57%). This staging is clearly an advance, because it defines much earlier stages of disease progression upon which relevant therapeutic action can be taken. Death is not a useful end point in the early stages of cirrhosis. For compensated patients time-fixed prognostic models for survival are not well-suited prognostic tools. Although they include variables statistically associated with survival, they provide very inaccurate prognostic estimates, because the status of the patient may change markedly for better or worse, making the prognosis very different. The outcome of a clinical status is transition to another status, death or OLT and prognostic models specific to each clinical status should be developed.

Utilisation of follow-up data in prognostic modelling

Although the assessment of patients at a similar stage of cirrhosis leads to a larger homogeneity and thereby improved prognostication of relevant end points, there may still be a considerable variability between individual courses of disease. *Patients in the same stage may not necessarily progress further with the same speed or show the same sequence of manifestations along the course.* This is due to considerable biological differences (genetic, environmental) among patients. The inclusion of consecutive patients is also no guarantee of homogeneity. Even with improved staging we have to accept considerable heterogeneity in a large number of dimensions as a fundamental feature of the data available to us. The task is to utilise those data in the best possible way to extract all the available prognostic information. Ideally, from the current status of the patient we need to be able to predict the occurrence of complications or death within the next few months, so that we can adjust the therapeutic strategy to prevent such events whenever possible.

Therefore, rather than models that have a long-term predictive value, models should be designed to predict a limited time-span (e.g. 1, 3, 6, 12 months) with increased accuracy. Because the status of the patient may rapidly change for better or worse, prognosis needs to be updated with each change. Time-dependent prognostic models utilising follow-up data are particularly well-suited prognostic tools in the clinical management of patients. Such models can be used repetitively during the course of the disease to update prognosis whenever changes occur in the clinical status of the patient and will therefore provide more accurate prognostic estimates.

Conclusions

Prognostic modelling is important to better understand the determinants of the course and outcome of cirrhosis. Over the years a large number of prognostic models have been developed. However, even the best prognostic models have a quite limited predictive ability. They are not sufficiently precise to be really useful for individual prognostication. The information provided by prognostic models should only be used as a supplement to any other relevant clinical information in the decision-making for the patient. To obtain better prognostic models in the future we need to identify more informative prognostic variables (molecular biology, genetics) being central to the disease process, to utilise follow-up information to a greater extent, to combine databases and models from different centres and countries and to directly involve highly qualified statisticians in the modelling process to ensure maximum validity of analyses and results.

REFERENCES

1 D'Amico G, Garcia-Tsao G, Cales P *et al.* Diagnosis of portal hypertension: how and when. In: de Franchis R (ed). *Portal hypertension III. Proceedings of the third Baveno international consensus workshop on definitions, methodology and therapeutic strategies in portal hypertension.* Blackwell Science, Oxford, 2001; 36–64.

2 Saunders JB, Walters JRF, Davies P, Paton A. A 20-year prospective study of cirrhosis. *Brit Med J* 1981;**282**: 263–266.

3 Gines P, Quintero E, Arroyo V. Compensated cirrhosis: natural history and prognosis. *Hepatology* 1987;7: 122–128.

4 D'Amico G, Morabito A, Pagliaro L, Marubini E. Survival and prognostic indicators in compensated and decompensated cirrhosis. *Dig Dis Sci* 1986; **31**: 468–475.

5 D'Amico G, Licata A, Pasta L, Rizzuto G, D'Amico M, Mocciaro F. Prognostic indicators in cirrhosis: the role of Child classification. Overview of 93 published studies and validation in a prospective cohort of patients. *Dig Liver Dis* 2005;**37**: S(29).

6 D'Amico G, Pasta L, Madonia S *et al.* The incidence of esophageal varices in cirrhosis. *Gastroenterology* 2001;**120**: A2.

7 Pugh RN, Murray-Lyon IM, Dawson JL, Pietrini MC, Williams R. Transection of the esophagus for bleeding oesophageal varices. *Br J Surg* 1973;**60**: 646–649.

8 Kamath PS, Wiesner RH, Malinchoc M *et al.* A model to predict survival in patients with end-stage liver disease. *Hepatology* 2001;**33**: 464–470.

9 Durand F, Valla D. Assessment of the prognosis of cirrhosis: Child–Pugh versus MELD. *J Hepatol* 2005;**42**(suppl.): S100–S107.

10 Boyer TD, Triger DR, Horisawa M, Redeker AG, Reynolds TB. Direct transhepatic measurement of portal vein pressure using a thin needle. Comparison with wedged hepatic vein pressure. *Gastroenterology* 1977;**72**: 584–589.

11 Perello A, Escorsell A, Bru C *et al.* Wedged hepatic venous pressure adequately reflects portal pressure in hepatitis C virus-related cirrhosis. *Hepatology* 1999;**30**: 1393–1397.

12 Groszmann RJ, Wongcharatrawee S. The hepatic venous pressure gradient: anything worth doing should be done right. *Hepatology* 2004;**39**: 280–283.

13 Morali GA, Sniderman KW, Deitel KM *et al.* Is sinusoidal portal hypertension a necessary factor for the development of hepatic ascites? *J Hepatol* 1992;**16**: 249–250.
14 Garcia-Tsao G, Groszmann RJ, Fisher RL, Conn HO, Atterbury CE, Glickman M. Portal pressure, presence of gastroesophageal varices and variceal bleeding. *Hepatology* 1985;**5**: 419–424.
15 Viallet A, Marleau D, Huet M *et al.* Hemodynamic evaluation of patients with intrahepatic portal hypertension. Relationship between bleeding varices and the portohepatic gradient. *Gastroenterology* 1975;**69**: 1297–1300.
16 Braillon A, Cales P, Valla D, Gaudy D, Geoffroy P, Lebrec D. Influence of the degree of liver failure on systemic and splanchnic haemodynamics and on response to propranolol in patients with cirrhosis. *Gut* 1986;**27**: 1204–1209.
17 Gluud C, Henriksen JH, Nielsen G and the Copenhagen Study Group for Liver Disease. Prognostic indicators in alcoholic cirrhotic men. *Hepatology* 1988;**8**: 222–227.
18 Stanley AJ, Robinson I, Forrest EH, Jones AL, Hayes PC. Haemodynamic parameters predicting variceal haemorrhage and survival in alcoholic cirrhosis. *QJM* 1998;**91**: 19–25.
19 Le Moine O, Hadengue A, Moreau R *et al.* Relationship between portal pressure, esophageal varices, and variceal bleeding on the basis of the stage and cause of cirrhosis. *Scand J Gastroenterol* 1997;**32**: 731–735.
20 Vorobioff J, Groszmann RJ, Picabea E *et al.* Prognostic value of hepatic venous pressure gradient measurements in alcoholic cirrhosis: a 10-year prospective study. *Gastroenterology* 1996;**111**: 701–709.
21 Groszmann RJ, Bosch J, Grace N *et al.* Hemodynamic events in a prospective randomized trial of propranolol vs placebo in the prevention of the first variceal hemorrhage. *Gastroenterology* 1990;**99**(5): 1401–1407.
22 Groszmann RJ, Garcia-Tsao G, Makuch RW *et al.* Multicenter randomized placebo-controlled trial of non-selective beta-blockers in the prevention of the complications of portal hypertension: final results and identification of a predictive factors. *Hepatology* 2003;**38**(suppl. 1): 206A (abstract).
23 Merkel C, Bolognesi M, Sacerdoti D *et al.* The hemodynamic response to medical treatment of portal hypertension as a predictor of clinical effectiveness in the primary prophylaxis of variceal bleeding in cirrhosis. *Hepatology* 2000;**32**: 930–934.
24 Moller S, Bendtsen F, Christensen E, Henriksen JH. Prognostic variables in patients with cirrhosis and oesophageal varices without prior bleeding. *J Hepatol* 1994;**21**: 940–946.
25 Turnes J, Garcia-Pagan JC, Abraldes JG *et al.* Pharmacological reduction of portal pressure and long term risk of first variceal bleeding in patients with cirrhosis. *Hepatology* 2003;**38**: 62A.
26 Zimmerer J, Haubitz I, Mainos D, Hadass H, Tittor W. Survival in alcoholic liver cirrhosis: prognostic value of portal pressure, size of esophageal varices and biochemical data. Comparison with Child classification. *Z Gastroenterol* 1996;**34**: 421–427.
27 Merkel C, Bolognesi M, Bellon S *et al.* Prognostic usefulness of hepatic vein catheterization in patients with cirrhosis and esophageal varices. *Gastroenterology* 1992;**102**: 973–979.

28 Urbain D, Muls V, Makhoul E, Jeghers O, Thys O, Ham HR. Prognostic significance of hepatic venous pressure gradient in medically treated alcoholic cirrhosis: comparison to aminopyrine breath test. *Am J Gastroenterol* 1993;**88**: 856–859.
29 Tage-Jensen U, Henriksen JH, Christensen E, Widding A, Ring-Larsen H, Christensen NJ. Plasma catecholamine level and portal venous pressure as guides to prognosis in patients with cirrhosis. *J Hepatol* 1988;**6**(3): 350–358.
30 Escorsell A, Bordas JM, Castaneda B *et al.* Predictive value of the variceal pressure response to continued pharmacological therapy in patients with cirrhosis and portal hypertension. *Hepatology* 2000;**31**: 1061–1067.
31 Bureau C, Peron JM, Alric L *et al.* 'A La Carte' treatment of portal hypertension: adapting medical therapy to hemodynamic response for the prevention of bleeding. *Hepatology* 2002;**36**: 1361–1366.
32 Deltenre P, Rufat P, Hillaire S *et al.* Lack of prognostic usefulness of hepatic venous pressures and hemodynamic values in a select group of patients with severe alcoholic cirrhosis. *Am J Gastroenterol* 2002;**97**: 1187–1190.
33 Dittrich S, de Mattos AA, Becker M, Goncaves DM, Cheinquer H. Role of hepatic hemodynamic study in the evaluation of patients with cirrhosis. *Hepatogastroenterology* 2003;**50**: 2052–2056.
34 Lebrec D, De Fleury P, Rueff B, Nahum H, Benhamou JP. Portal hypertension, size of esophageal varices, and risk of gastrointestinal bleeding in alcoholic cirrhosis. *Gastroenterology* 1980;**79**: 1139–1144.
35 Merkel C, Zoli M, Siringo S *et al.* Prognostic indicators of risk for first variceal bleeding in cirrhosis: a multicenter study in 711 patients to validate and improve the North Italian Endoscopic Club (NIEC) Index. *Am J Gastroenterol* 2000;**95**: 2915–2920.
36 Vinel JP, Cassigneul J, Levade M, Voigt JJ, Pascal JP. Assessment of short-term prognosis after variceal bleeding in patients with alcoholic cirrhosis by early measurement of portohepatic gradient. *Hepatology* 1986;**6**: 116–117.
37 Ready JB, Robertson AD, Goff JS, Rector WG Jr. Assessment of the risk of bleeding from esophageal varices by continuous monitoring of portal pressure. *Gastroenterology* 1991;**100**: 1403–1410.
38 Moitinho E, Escorsell A, Bandi JC *et al.* Prognostic value of early measurements of portal pressure in acute variceal bleeding. *Gastroenterology* 1999;**117**: 626–631.
39 Villanueva C, Ortiz J, Minana J *et al.* Somatostatin treatment and risk stratification by continuous portal pressure monitoring during active variceal bleeding. *Gastroenterology* 2001;**121**: 110–117
40 Monescillo A, Martinez-Lagares F, Ruiz-del-Arbol L *et al.* Influence of portal hypertension and its early decompression by TIPS placement on the outcome of variceal bleeding. *Hepatology* 2004;**40**: 793–801.
41 Patch D, Armonis A, Sabin C *et al.* Single portal pressure measurement predicts survival in cirrhotic patients with recent bleeding. *Gut* 1999;**44**: 264–269.
42 Villanueva C, Balanzo J, Novella MT *et al.* Nadolol plus isosorbide mononitrate compared with sclerotherapy for the prevention of variceal rebleeding. *N Engl J Med* 1996;**334**: 1624–1629.
43 Feu F, Garcia-Pagan JC, Bosch J *et al.* Relation between portal pressure response to pharmacotherapy and risk of recurrent variceal haemorrhage in patients with cirrhosis. *Lancet* 1995;**346**: 1056–1059.

44 Villanueva C, Minana J, Ortiz J *et al.* Endoscopic ligation compared with combined treatment with nadolol and isosorbide mononitrate to prevent recurrent variceal bleeding. *N Engl J Med* 2001;**345**: 647–655.
45 Abraldes JG, Tarantino I, Turnes J, Garcia-Pagan JC, Rodes J, Bosch J. Hemodynamic response to pharmacological treatment of portal hypertension and long-term prognosis of cirrhosis. *Hepatology* 2003;**37**: 902–908.
46 Villanueva C, Lopez-Balaguer JM, Aracil C *et al.* Maintenance of hemodynamic response to treatment for portal hypertension and influence on complications of cirrhosis. *J Hepatol* 2004;**40**: 757–765.
47 Patch D, Goulis J, Gerunda G, Greenslade L, Merkel C, Burroughs AK. A randomized controlled trial of medical therapy versus endoscopic ligation for the prevention of variceal rebleeding in patients with cirrhosis. *Gastroenterology* 2002;**123**: 1013–1019.
48 McCormick PA, Patch D, Greenslade L, Chin J, McIntyre N, Burroughs AK. Clinical vs hemodynamic response to drugs in portal hypertension. *J Hepatol* 1998;**28**: 1015–1019.
49 Villanueva C, Lopez-Balaguer JM, Aracil C, Balanzo J. Reply to letter to the editor. *J Hepatol* 2005;**42**: 147–148.
50 Bruix J, Castells A, Bosch J *et al.* Surgical resection of hepatocellular carcinoma in cirrhotic patients. Prognostic value of preoperative portal pressure. *Gastroenterology* 1996;**111**: 1018–1022.
51 Llovet JM, Fuster J, Bruix J. Intention-to-treat analysis of surgical treatment for early hepatocellular carcinoma: resection versus transplantation. *Hepatology* 1999;**30**: 1434–1440.
52 DeFranchis R. Updating consensus in portal hypertension: report of the Baveno III consensus workshop on definitions, methodology and therapeutic strategies in portal hypertension. *J Hepatol* 2000;**33**: 846–852.
53 D'Amico G. Esophageal varices: from appearance to rupture: natural history and prognostic indicators. In: Grossmann R, Bosch J (eds). Portal hypertension in 21st century, Dordrecht, The Netherlands, Kluwer Academic Publishers, 2004; 147–154.
54 Spiegel BM, Targownik L, Dulai GS, Karsan HA, Gralnek IM. Endoscopic screening for esophageal varices in cirrhosis: is it ever cost effective? *Hepatology* 2003;**37**: 366–377.
55 Cales P, Desmorat H, Vinel JP *et al.* Incidence of large oesophageal varices in patients with cirrhosis: application to prophylaxis of first bleeding. *Gut* 1990;**31**: 1298–1302.
56 Merkel C, Marin R, Angeli P *et al.* A placebo-controlled clinical trial of nadolol in the prophylaxis of growth of small esophageal varices in cirrhosis. *Gastroenterology* 2004;**127**: 476–484.
57 D'Amico G, Pagliaro L, Bosch J. Pharmacological treatment of portal hypertension: an evidence-based approach. *Sem Liv Dis* 1999;**19**: 475–505.
58 Imperiale TF, Chalasani N. A meta-analysis of endoscopic variceal ligation for primary prophylaxis of esophageal variceal bleeding. *Hepatology* 2001;**33**: 802–807.
59 Ng FH, Wong SY, Loo CK, Lam KM, Lai CW, Cheng CS. Prediction of oesophagogastric varices in patients with liver cirrhosis. *J Gastroenterol Hepatol* 1999;**14**: 785–790.

60 Cottone M, D'Amico G, Maringhini A *et al.* Predictive value of ultrasonography in the screening of non-ascitic cirrhotic patients with large varices. *J Ultrasound Med* 1986;**5**: 189–192.
61 Chalasani N, Imperiale TF, Ismail A *et al.* Predictors of large esophageal varices in patients with cirrhosis. *Am J Gastroenterol* 1999;**94**: 3285–3291.
62 Pilette C, Oberti F, Aube C *et al.* Non-invasive diagnosis of esophageal varices in chronic liver disease. *J Hepatol* 1999;**31**: 867–873.
63 Schepis F, Camma C, Niceforo D *et al.* Which patients with cirrhosis should undergo endoscopic screening for esophageal varices detection? *Hepatology* 2001;**33**: 333–338.
64 Zaman A, Becker T, Lapidus J, Benner K. Risk factors for the presence of varices in cirrhotic patients without a history of variceal hemorrhage. *Arch Intern Med* 2001;**161**: 2564–2570.
65 Madhotra R, Mulcahy HE, Willner I, Reuben A. Prediction of esophageal varices in patients with cirrhosis. *J Clin Gastroenterol* 2002;**34**: 81–85.
66 Giannini E, Botta F, Borro P *et al.* Platelet count/spleen diameter ratio: proposal and validation of a non-invasive parameter to predict the presence of oesophageal varices in patients with liver cirrhosis. *Gut* 2003;**52**: 1200–1205.
67 Thomopoulos KC, Labropoulou-Karatza C, Mimidis KP, Katsakoulis EC, Iconomou G, Nikolopoulou VN. Non-invasive predictors of the presence of large oesophageal varices in patients with cirrhosis. *Dig Liver Dis* 2003;**35**: 473–478.
68 Dragoni F, Gentile G, Cartoni C *et al.* The role of real-time ultrasonography in predicting esophageal varices in hemophiliacs co-infected with hepatitis C and human immunodeficiency virus. *Haematologica* 2005;**90**: 207–213.
69 Vanbiervliet G, Barjoan-Marine E, Anty R *et al.* Serum fibrosis markers can detect large oesophageal varices with a high accuracy. *Eur J Gastroenterol Hepatol* 2005;**17**: 333–338.
70 Zein CO, Lindor KD, Angulo P. Prevalence and predictors of esophageal varices in patients with primary sclerosing cholangitis. *Hepatology* 2004;**39**: 204–210.
71 Bressler B, Pinto R, El Ashry D, Heathcote EJ. Which patients with primary biliary cirrhosis or primary sclerosing cholangitis should undergo endoscopic screening for oesophageal varices detection? *Gut* 2005;**54**: 407–410.
72 D'Amico G, Morabito A. Noninvasive markers of esophageal varices: another round, not the last. *Hepatology* 2004;**39**: 30–34.
73 Vanbiervliet G, Rakotoarisoa C, Filippi J *et al.* Diagnostic accuracy of a rapid urine-screening test (Multistix8SG) in cirrhotic patients with spontaneous bacterial peritonitis. *Eur J Gastroenterol Hepatol* 2002;**14**: 1257–1260.
74 Burroughs AK, Groszmann RJ, Bosch J *et al.* Assessment of therapeutic benefit of antiviral therapy in chronic hepatitis C. Is hepatic venous pressure gradient (HVPG) a better endpoint? *Gut* 2002;**50**: 425–427.
75 Sanjal AJ, Fontana R, Everhart J, Di Bisceglie A, Wtight E. The presence and spectrum of varices in the absence of cirrhosis in patients with chronic hepatitis C. *Hepatology* 2003;**38**: 218A.
76 Merli M, Nicolini G, Angeloni S *et al.* Incidence and natural history of small esophageal varices in cirrhotic patients. *J Hepatol* 2003;**38**: 266–272.
77 Gores GJ, Wiesner RH, Dickson ER, Zinsmeister AR, Jorgensen RA, Langworthy A. Prospective evaluation of esophageal varices in primary

biliary cirrhosis: development, natural history, and influence on survival. *Gastroenterology* 1989;**96**: 1552–1559.

78 Gentilini P, Laffi G, La Villa G *et al.* Long course and prognostic factors of virus-induced cirrhosis of the liver. *Am J Gastroenterol* 1997;**92**: 66–72.

79 Zoli M, Merkel C, Magalotti D *et al.* Natural history of cirrhotic patients with small esophageal varices: a prospective study. *Am J Gastroenterol* 2000;**95**: 503–508.

80 North Italian Endoscopic Club for the Study and Treatment of Esophageal Varices. Prediction of the first variceal hemorrhage in patients with cirrhosis of the liver and esophageal varices. A prospective multicenter study. *N Engl J Med* 1988;**319**: 983–989.

81 Sarin SK, Lamba G, Kumar M, Misra A, Murthy NS. Comparison of endoscopic ligation and propranolol for the primary prevention of variceal bleeding. *New Eng J Med* 1999;**340**: 988–993.

82 Nidegger D, Ragot S, Berthelemy P *et al.* Cirrhosis and bleeding: the need for very early management. *J Hepatol* 2003;**39**: 509–514.

83 El Atti EA, Nevens F, Bogaerts K, Verbeke G, Fevery J. Variceal pressure is a strong predictor of variceal haemorrhage in patients with cirrhosis as well as in patients with non-cirrhotic portal hypertension. *Gut* 1999;**45**: 618–621.

84 Christensen E. Prognostic models including the Child–Pugh, MELD and Mayo risk scores – where are we and where should we go? *J Hepatol* 2004;**41**: 344–350.

85 Zoli M, Cordiani MR, Marchesini G *et al.* Prognostic indicators in compensated cirrhosis. *Am J Gastroenterol* 1991;**86**: 1508–1513.

86 Zoli M, Iervese T, Merkel C *et al.* Prognostic significance of portal hemodynamics in patients with compensated cirrhosis. *J Hepatol* 1993;**17**: 56–61.

87 Realdi G, Fattovich G, Hadziyannis S *et al.* Survival and prognostic factors in 366 patients with compensated cirrhosis type B: a multicenter study. The investigators of the European Concerted Action on Viral Hepatitis (EUROHEP). *J Hepatol* 1994;**21**: 656–666.

88 Fattovich G, Giustina G, Christensen E *et al.* Influence of hepatitis delta virus infection on morbidity and mortality in compensated cirrhosis type B. The European Concerted Action on Viral Hepatitis (EUROHEP). *Gut* 2000;**46**: 420–426.

89 Fattovich G, Giustina G, Degos F *et al.* Morbidity and mortality in compensated cirrhosis type C: a retrospective follow-up study of 384 patients. *Gastroenterology* 1997;**112**: 463–472.

90 Fattovich G, Pantalena M, Zagni I, Realdi G, Schalm SW, Christensen E. Effect of hepatitis B and C virus infections on the natural history of compensated cirrhosis: a cohort study of 297 patients. *Am J Gastroenterol* 2002;**97**: 2886–2895.

91 Cardenas A, Gines P, Uriz J *et al.* Renal failure after upper gastrointestinal bleeding in cirrhosis: incidence, clinical course, predictive factors, and short-term prognosis. *Hepatology* 2001;**34**: 671–676.

92 Child CG, Turcotte JG. Surgery and portal hypertension. *Major Probl Clin Surg* 1964;**1**: 1–85.

93 Malinchoc M, Kamath PS, Gordon FD, Peine CJ, Rank J, TerBorg PCJ. A model to predict poor survival in patients undergoing transjugular intrahepatic portosystemic shunts. *Hepatology* 2000;**31**: 864–871.

94 D'Amico G, de Franchis R. Upper digestive bleeding in cirrhosis. Post-therapeutic outcome and prognostic indicators. *Hepatology* 2003;**38**: 599–612.

95 Heuman DM, Abou-Assi SG, Habib A *et al.* Persistent ascites and low serum sodium identify patients with cirrhosis and low MELD scores who are at high risk for early death. *Hepatology* 2004;**40**: 802–810.

96 Ruf AE, Kremers WK, Chavez LL, Descalzi VI, Podesta LG, Villamil FG. Addition of serum sodium into the MELD score predicts waiting list mortality better than MELD alone. *Liver Transpl* 2005;**11**: 336–343.

Baveno IV Consensus Statements: Predictive Models in Portal Hypertension

Gennaro D'Amico, Guadalupe Garcia-Tsao (Chairpersons), Juan G. Abraldes, Erik Christensen, Pere Ginés, W. Ray Kim, Manuela Merli and Filippo Schepis

Status classification of cirrhosis

• Varices, ascites and bleeding in patients with cirrhosis identify four clinical status of increasing severity: status 1: no varices, no ascites; status 2: varices, no ascites; status 3: ascites ± varices; status 4: bleeding ± ascites.
• The outcome of a clinical status is transition to another status, death or Orthotopic Liver Transplant (OLT). Prognostic models specific to each clinical status should be developed.

Indicators of varices and predictors of their development

• There are no satisfactory non-endoscopic indicators of the presence of varices.
• While further studies are awaited, endoscopic screening is still the best practice to detect varices.
• The hepatic vein pressure gradient (HVPG) is presently the most reliable predictor of variceal development.

Outcome prediction in compensated patients

• In patients with compensated cirrhosis, the development of ascites and portal hypertensive bleeding are the most relevant outcomes.
• HVPG is the only known predictor of the development of ascites; other potential predictors should be investigated.
• The North Italian Endoscopic Club (NIEC) score is presently the most reliable predictor of variceal rupture; the contribution of HVPG and other predictors should be investigated.

Outcome prediction in decompensated patients

- Child-Pugh and Model for End-stage Liver Disease (MELD) predict overall mortality.
- The additional role of HVPG and other potential predictors (sodium, spontaneous bacterial peritonitis, hepatorenal syndrome and others) should be assessed.

SESSION 3

Prevention of the Formation of Varices (Pre-Primary Prophylaxis)

Roberto J. Groszmann, Carlo Merkel*, Yasuko Iwakiri, Vijay Shah, Benjamin L. Shneider, Marco Zoli, Annalisa Berzigotti, Julio Vorobioff and Alberto Morabito*

INTRODUCTION

In order to develop the field of pre-primary prophylaxis of gastroesophageal varices, we believe that a clear understanding of the factors leading to the development of this complication of portal hypertension is needed. Therefore, we have organised this chapter in a series of mini-chapters that hopefully will lead to the definition and present understanding of this important area.

* The first-authorship of this chapter is shared by Dr Groszmann and Dr Merkel.

Molecular markers in portal hypertension

Yasuko Iwakiri

Portal pressure plays a key role in development and progression of portal-systemic collaterals and varices, and is considered a main target for the prevention and treatment of variceal bleeding [1]. In this regard, factors that increase portal pressure (portal hypertension) may influence the development of collaterals and severity of variceal haemorrhage. Increased *vasodilation* in the arterial splanchnic circulation is one of the important factors that increases portal pressure [2] (Fig. 29). Nitric oxide (NO) is a key molecular marker that is involved in vasodilation [3–5] and the formation of collateral vessels [6,7]. Another important molecular marker is vascular endothelial growth factor (VEGF), which promotes NO production and portal-collateral vessel formation in portal hypertension [8]. This subchapter focuses on two important issues: (1) effects of portal pressure on vasodilation and collateral vessel formation; and (2) the role of NO in vasodilation and collateral vessel formation.

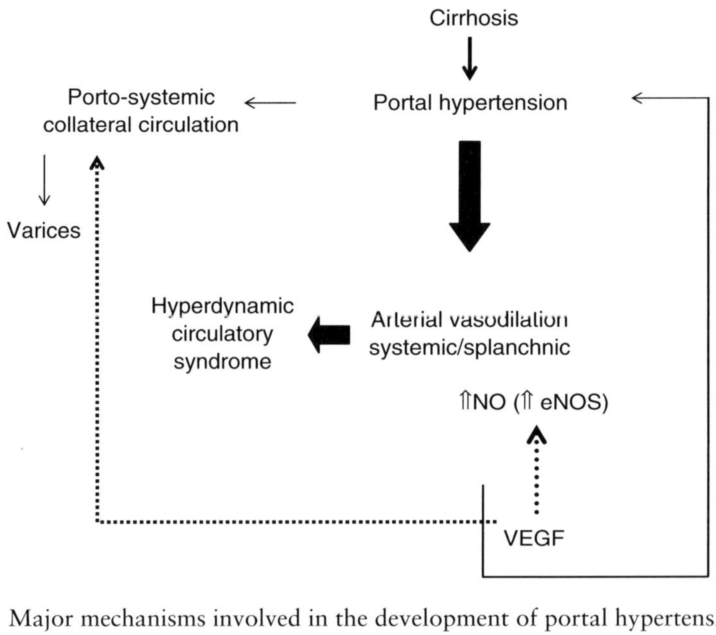

Fig. 29 Major mechanisms involved in the development of portal hypertension.

Effect of portal pressure on vasodilation

Vasodilation in arterial splanchnic circulation is the characteristic feature observed in portal hypertension (i.e. increased portal pressure). Chronic vasodilation in arterial splanchnic circulation increases blood flow to the portal venous circulation and enhances the formation of portal-systemic collateral circulation and varices [2]. NO is the most important vasodilator molecule in portal hypertension [9–11]. It has been demonstrated by us and other investigators that endothelial NO synthase (eNOS) is up-regulated in superior mesenteric arterial beds (arterial splanchnic circulation) and produces excessive NO, leading to vasodilation [12,13]. How does portal pressure induce signals that up-regulate eNOS in the splanchnic circulation?

An acute increase in portal pressure results in sudden myogenic reflex vasoconstriction in larger vessels of superior mesenteric arterial beds (artery of splanchnic circulation), which initiates eNOS activation and NO production [14]. This eNOS activation is achieved by the activation of Akt/protein kinase B, which phosphorylates and directly activates eNOS enzyme to produce NO [15]. This is an early event observed in the early stage of acute portal hypertension.

A mild portal pressure increase, on the other hand, does not cause myogenic reflex vasoconstriction in larger vessels of superior mesenteric arteries, but still ends up with the development of the portal-systemic collaterals and the hyperdynamic circulatory syndrome. Interestingly, this mild increase in portal pressure, which is similar to portal hypertension in cirrhosis, induces VEGF production at the jejunal microcirculation. This is the early signal that induces eNOS up-regulation in mild portal hypertension. This was confirmed by the finding that an inhibitor of VEGF receptor activation normalises eNOS expression to similar level as the control group, suggesting that the mild increase in portal pressure is first sensed at the intestinal microcirculation, which increases local VEGF production with a subsequent increase in eNOS (unpublished data).

Collectively, changes in portal pressure are sensed by different parts of mesenteric arterial beds and trigger different signals that induce eNOS up-regulation and NO production in the splanchnic microcirculation. In mild increase in portal pressure, similar to what happens in cirrhosis, eNOS expression is up-regulated through an increase in local VEGF production. VEGF-dependent formation of collateral vessels has also been observed in the splanchnic circulation in portal hypertensive animals [8].

Effect of portal pressure on collateral formation

Increased portal pressure is the most important risk factor for the development of portal-systemic collateral circulation and varices. In patients, varices do not develop below the threshold hepatic venous pressure gradient (a surrogate of sinusoidal portal hypertension; HVPG) value of 10–12 mmHg [16]. Furthermore, a reduction of the risk of first bleeding in patients is achieved by a reduction of HVPG, suggesting that portal pressure can be the most effective therapeutic target to reduce the development of varices [17]. Our very recent finding in an experimental model of portal hypertension clearly indicates that the formation of portal-systemic collaterals is proportional to portal pressure. We also found that the development of the hyperdynamic circulatory syndrome is associated with an increase in portal pressure (unpublished data). It is thought that *vasodilation* in arteries of systemic and particularly splanchnic circulation contributes to the development of the hyperdynamic circulatory syndrome (Fig. 29) [2,13].

The hyperdynamic circulatory syndrome, a hallmark of portal hypertension, is associated with the development of varices [2]. This syndrome consists of three main types of haemodynamic abnormalities: (1) decreased mean arterial pressure, (2) decreased systemic vascular resistance and (3) increased cardiac output [18]. Our data clearly indicate that all these features are exacerbated as portal pressure increases. NO plays a key role in vasodilation and subsequent development of the hyperdynamic circulatory syndrome that exacerbates portal hypertension [13].

The formation of portal-systemic collateral circulation is achieved by *the opening of pre-existing vessels* [19] and *angiogenesis* [8,20]. A mechanical force by the increased portal pressure and the dilation of pre-existing vessels results in the opening of pre-existing vessels. Thus, therapeutic strategies have been aimed at decreasing portal pressure [21]. In recent years, it has been demonstrated that angiogenesis is another important mechanism that is involved in the formation of the portal-systemic collateral vessels [8,20]. A study by Fernandez *et al.* [8] clearly demonstrated the occurrence of VEGF-mediated angiogenesis in the formation of portal-systemic collateral vessels in portal hypertensive animals. The administrations of a monoclonal antibody against VEGF receptor-2 and an inhibitor of VEGF receptor-2 activation both result in a marked decrease in the formation of portal-systemic collateral vessels.

The role of NO in collateral vessels formation

NO plays a key role in the formation of collateral vessels. NO was originally discovered as an endothelium-derived relaxing factor and is known to be a potent vasodilator [3–5]. In models of tumour angiogenesis, NO dilates vessels, causing sprout formation, and maintains blood flow in angiogenic vessels [6,7]. NO in the connecting vessel regulates the vessels diameter and thus, is also important for angiogenesis and haemodynamics in angiogenic vessels. Haemodynamics in angiogenic vessels is regulated by both existing vessels and angiogenic vessels themselves. Increased flow in VEGF-induced angiogenic vessels is mediated by NO-induced vasodilation [22]. NO plays a critical role in VEGF-induced angiogenesis and vascular permeability (a factor that enhances angiogenic activity). Inhibition of NO production results in reduced angiogenesis and vascular permeability induced by VEGF [23,24]. VEGF promotes NO production and also induces eNOS expression in vascular endothelial cells [25–27]. Interestingly, eNOS is the isoform among the three NO producing enzymes that plays a predominant role in VEGF-induced angiogenesis and vascular permeability [28]. Thus, besides VEGF, selective modulation of eNOS activity may be a promising strategy for preventing the development of varices.

Complete deletion of eNOS, however, induces other vasodilator molecules in portal hypertensive animals and results in the development of the hyperdynamic circulatory syndrome similar to the control animals [29]. Thus, selective and partial inhibition of eNOS may be a therapeutic strategy for the treatment of portal hypertension and the prevention of formation of varices.

Summary

The formation of portal-systemic collaterals and the severity of the hyperdynamic circulatory syndrome are proportional to portal pressure. Furthermore, different levels of portal pressure (acute versus mild) trigger eNOS up-regulation at different locations in the splanchnic circulation with different mechanisms. eNOS-derived NO plays an important role in the formation of portal-systemic collateral vessels. Increased VEGF production mediates angiogenic collateral vessel formation in the splanchnic microcirculation in portal hypertensive animals. eNOS plays an important role in VEGF-induced angiogenesis. *eNOS* and *VEGF* may be potential therapeutic targets for the treatment of varices.

Collateral formation: arterial versus venous

Vijay Shah

Collateral formation: relative role of vasodilation, angiogenesis and vascular remodelling

A major cause of complications of portal hypertension is the development of portal–systemic collateral vessels between the portal hypertensive vasculature and the lower pressure systemic venous system [30,31]. This collateral circulatory bed develops through a dynamic interplay of distinct physiological processes which include vasodilation, vascular remodelling and angiogenesis.

Vasodilation of pre-existing collateral vessels results in increased collateral blood flow and volume. This mechanism of collateral vessel regulation has probably received the greatest amount of experimental attention [19,32]. An increase in flow and pressure through pre-existing collateral vessels has also been demonstrated, and this physiological process has developed into a direction for therapy of collaterals [19]. For example, non-selective β-blockers not only reduce portal pressure but also constrict the collateral circulation. This reduction in collateral flow likely contributes to the protective effects of β-blockers from variceal haemorrhage [33].

Vascular remodelling is an adaptive response of the vessel wall that occurs in response to chronic changes in blood flow. For example, chronic increases in flow with dilation of the vascular channel result in endothelial-based signals that mediate restructuring of the vessel, thereby allowing for chronic increases in vessel diameter and capacity for high volume flow. This paradigm has been demonstrated in peripheral vessels and notably also in models of experimental portal hypertension [33–35].

Angiogenesis is the development of new blood vessels. This occurs through the traditional paradigm of angiogenesis which is mediated by proliferation of *in situ* endothelial and smooth muscle cells, as well as through a process termed vasculogenesis [36]. Vasculogenesis is mediated through the recruitment of vascular wall precursor cells from the blood [37]. This includes endothelial progenitor cells and smooth muscle progenitor cells [38]. Experimental evidence for the role of angiogenesis in collateral development is supported by a study documenting and quantifying an increase in vascular sprouts in the mesentery of portal hypertensive rats [39]. More recent studies have documented the importance of VEGF in portosystemic collaterals as well [8].

Role of nitric oxide (NO) in collateral vessel formation

Nitric oxide (NO) plays an important role in numerous vascular functions so it is not surprising that NO is important in the process of collateral vessel formation [40]. In fact, NO is implicated in each of the steps of collateral vessel formation outlined in the previous section (vasodilation, vascular remodelling and angiogenesis). Certainly the role of NO in vasodilation is well established. NO is also important in vascular remodelling as evidenced by lack of appropriate vascular remodelling in absence of NO [35]. NO is important to angiogenesis in several ways. First, NO is an important signal that mediates the endothelial effects of the growth factor, VEGF, to facilitate endothelial cell proliferation and migration. Interestingly, the effect of NO on non-endothelial, vascular type cells is quite different from that of endothelial cells, with NO inhibiting migration and proliferation of hepatic stellate cells [41,42]. Additionally, NO also stimulates the release of endothelial progenitor cells from the bone marrow, thereby contributing to vasculogenesis [43]. Thus, experimental inhibition of NO formation appears to antagonise the angiogenic response, reduce flow and shunting through existing portal–systemic collateral vessels and also inhibit the process of vascular remodelling [19,32,39,44]. Mechanical forces, most notably shear stress, stimulate NO generation and are important in collateral vessel formation. Therefore, it is likely that NO is an important signal that mediates collateral vessel development that occurs in response to changes in mechanical forces in the vasculature. These NO-dependent processes highlight the role of NO not only as a vasodilatory molecule, but also as a mediator of growth factor-induced angiogenesis, remodelling and collateralisation [34,45].

Collateral vessel formation: arteriogenesis versus 'venogenesis'

Physiological and therapeutic collateralisation is most well studied and understood for arterial vascular beds as opposed to venous systems. This includes the arterial collateralisation process that occurs in the coronary circulation and peripheral arterial circulation in response to vascular obstruction. These collateralisation processes can be termed arteriogenesis. However, within the realm of liver disease and the portal circulation, collateralisation within the venous circulation is of great relevance including the development of portosystemic collaterals and ensuing oesophageal varices as well as the cavernous transformation that occurs in response to chronic portal venous thrombosis. This process can be termed 'venogenesis'.

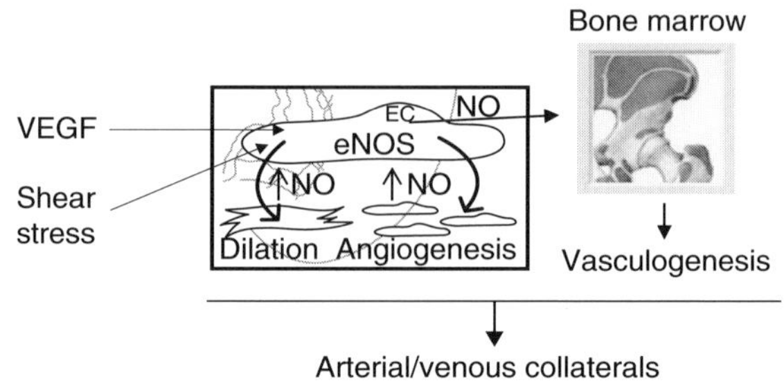

Fig. 30 Main mechanisms involved in the formation of collateral circulation.

Based on the concept of arterial and venous endothelial cell heterogeneity, an emerging concept in the field of collateralisation relates to the signals which specify arterial endothelial cell angiogenesis as opposed to venous endothelial cell angiogenesis [46,47]. This concept has received the greatest attention in the stages of vascular development; however, the concepts are also likely to be relevant for post-natal angiogenesis/vasculogenesis that occurs in response to vascular occlusion and elevated pressure.

Current concepts suggest that both arterial and venous endothelial cells probably arise from the same progenitor cell. However, there are key signals which determine whether a progenitor cell will target and develop towards an arterial or venous fate. One signalling pathway important in this process is the Notch-Jagged ligand-receptor pathway, which appears to promote arterial differentiation by repressing venous differentiation [47]. Other relevant signals include Sonic Hedgehog, VEGF, and angiopoetin, and Gridlock [47]. One major physiological process that is likely to regulate endothelial cell fate through these signals is mechanical forces, such as shear stress, flow and intraluminal pressure.

Summary (Fig. 30)

Mechanical forces such as shear stress as well as growth factors such as VEGF are critical in the steps of venous and arterial collateral vessel formation by mediating vasodilation, vascular remodelling and angiogenesis/post-natal vasculogenesis. The signalling molecules mediating these pathways are an area of active investigation.

Different experimental models have been used over the years to study the pathogenesis of portal hypertension and its complications. The bile duct ligated rat is a model of secondary cirrhosis that develops acute abnormalities very rapidly. The first day after bile duct ligation the rat already develops mild portal hypertension (Roberto Groszmann, unpublished observation). Interestingly the human counterpart is the child with biliary atresia. Probably, abnormalities that had been characterised in the rat model could well apply to biliary atresia that is the rapid development of portal hypertension and the collateralisation of the portal system.

Biliary atresia: a model of paediatric portal hypertension – opportunities for investigation and intervention

Benjamin L. Shneider

Portal hypertension and its related complications are major clinical issues in paediatric hepatology. As with adults, children develop problems as the sequelae of progressive portal hypertension. Ascites, with or without spontaneous bacterial peritonitis, and variceal haemorrhage are two of the more common and significant issues that arise in children with chronic liver disease. Failure to thrive, hepatopulmonary syndrome and neurocognitive deficits related to portal hypertension and portosystemic shunting may be relatively more important in paediatric populations where growth and development issues are so critical. In comparison to adults, there is a remarkable lack of evidence-based approaches to the management of portal hypertension in children. There have been no randomised trials of any medical therapies for portal hypertension in paediatrics and only one randomised trial of endoscopic therapy [48].

The reasons for this dearth of information are multifactorial. First and foremost is a prevailing reluctance to perform randomised blinded studies in children. This reluctance exists at the level of the patient's parents, human investigation committees, clinical investigators and the pharmaceutical industry. The second most important reason for the lack of information is related to limited numbers of patients and the wide range of disorders that lead to chronic liver disease in children. Overall, children make up less than 15% of the total number of individuals who undergo liver transplantation. Thus there are immediate problems with powering any type of clinical investigation. The spectrum of diseases that lead to chronic liver disease is broader in children than adults and the distribution amongst these disorders is more heterogeneous. Of adult liver transplants 44% are performed for either alcohol or hepatitis C related problems, while 40% of paediatric transplants are performed for biliary atresia (based on UNOS data derived from http://www.unos.org). Thus identification of relatively homogeneous and large groups of children for study is difficult. Haemodynamic physiology changes during normal development. One important change is the age dependency of basal heart rate. Normal heart rate in an infant can range between 110 and 185 beats per min, while the basal rates for an 8–12-year old range between 60 and 130 beats per min [49]. Thus the investigation of portal hypertension in children may require stratification by age. Finally, size

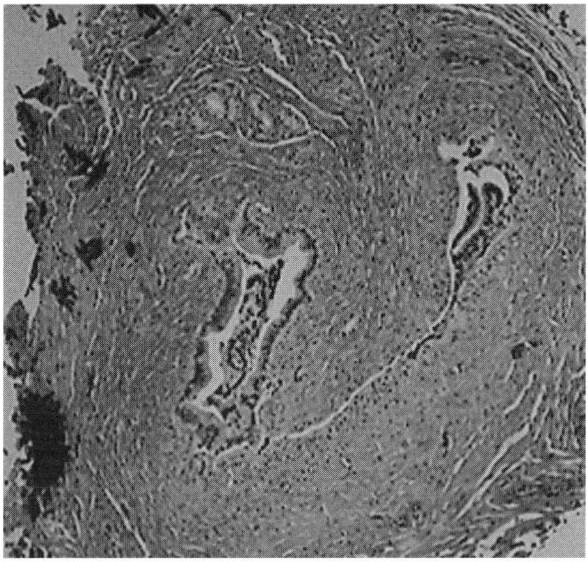

Fig. 31 Histology of the extrahepatic bile duct of a child with biliary atresia. Fibro-obliteration of the bile duct is observed in this bile duct.

and developmental issues impact on feasibility of certain types of investigations. Diagnostic and/or investigative procedures in children are associated with a relatively higher risk and often require significant sedation or anaesthesia for execution. Thus the effects of anaesthesia upon the measurement and the relative risk–benefit ratio of the activity must be taken into consideration. With the exception of studies performed during transjugular intrahepatic portosystemic shunting there are no reports of hepatic venous wedge pressure gradients in children. Thus it is not surprising that there has been little progress in developing an evidence-based literature that is applicable to children with portal hypertension.

In spite of these limitations, there is a desperate need to make progress in understanding paediatric portal hypertension. Perhaps the best opportunity in paediatrics rests with the analysis of biliary atresia, since it is the leading cause of significant liver disease in children. At the Mount Sinai Medical Center, 38% of 176 liver transplants performed in a recent 80-month period were for biliary atresia. Similar findings have been described for both US and European registries. Thus biliary atresia represents the largest single category of disease that leads to chronic liver problems in children, and as such is the best subject for clinical investigation in paediatric hepatology. The cause of biliary atresia remains enigmatic; the disease is the result of complete obliteration of the extrahepatic biliary system (Fig. 31). Thus biliary atresia in many ways may be akin to bile duct ligation models of portal hypertension [50]. Children with biliary atresia typically undergo a hepatoportoenterostomy (Kasai) procedure as treatment of their disease. In this procedure a loop of intestine is used as a replacement for the extra-hepatic biliary system. Prominent portal hypertension is often present at the time of corrective hepatoportoenterostomy and it progresses over relatively short periods of time [51]. The rate of progression of the portal hypertension is related to outcome after hepatoportoenterostomy, with more accelerated progression in children with failed procedures or with recurrent cholangitis [52]. Response to the procedure falls into three general categories. In approximately 30% to 50% of children bile flow is restored, as manifested by bilirubin levels returning to near normal. Even with this 'good' outcome, significant portal hypertension related to the development of biliary cirrhosis ensues within the first two decades of life. In approximately 35% of children there is no evidence of bile flow after the procedure and portal hypertension and its attendant complications develop over a very short time period. Variceal haemorrhage has been observed in children as young as 1 or 2 years of age. In the remaining 15% to 35% of children there is some evidence of bile drainage as bilirubin levels decrease but do not normalise. In these children severe liver injury and associated portal hypertension is often observed during school age.

The biliary injury in this disorder is associated with prominent portal hypertension at disease stages in which synthetic liver function is typically intact. Thus the relative contribution of complications of portal hypertension to morbidity and mortality in liver disease is greater in children than in adults and it occurs at an earlier stage of their liver disease. The rate of progression of the portal hypertension is fairly remarkable with complications often developing in less than 3 years. The rapid progression of disease makes biliary atresia attractive as a subject for clinical investigation, since clinical end points can be met in a relatively short period of time.

Complications that are a direct result of this portal hypertension are common in biliary atresia. Variceal haemorrhage occurs in a large percentage of children, often within the first 5 years of life [52–57]. In one cohort of 134 children with biliary atresia, variceal haemorrhage was observed in 40% of patients within 5 years of hepatoportoenterostomy [56]. In another cohort of 61 children, who did not require early liver transplantation, varices developed in 67% at a mean age of 6 years and variceal haemorrhage requiring a blood transfusion was noted in 28% of the children at a mean age of 3 years [55]. Ascites is a frequent problem in children with biliary atresia and was observed in 25% of children in the first 2 years of life in a multicentre retrospective analysis of biliary atresia in the United States [58].

Hepatopulmonary syndrome, rectal varices/colopathy, stomal haemorrhage and pulmonary hypertension have also been described in children with biliary atresia [59–64]. Bile duct ligation models have been useful as an animal model of hepatopulmonary syndrome, and intrapulmonic shunting has been prospectively demonstrated in 64% of transplant candidates with biliary atresia who underwent screening by contrast echocardiography [60,65].

Evidence-based approaches to the management of portal hypertension in children do not exist [66]. This is in stark contrast to the extensive array of randomised trials and meta-analyses that have been performed in adults [67,68]. The lack of controlled studies in paediatrics is unfortunate, but also presents ample opportunity for academic advances. The design of clinical studies in paediatrics will require creative design with somewhat modified end points due to the nature of investigation in children. It is not clear if clinicians, parents or institutional review boards will permit investigative hepatic wedge pressure measurements or surveillance endoscopy in children. β-blocker therapy is one of the current standards of care for adults with portal hypertension, yet there is clearly no similar consensus for the use of these agents in children [69]. The efficacy of β-blocker therapy in adults is typically seen only if one escalates dosing until one demonstrates adequate reduction in resting heart rate and/or a significant reduction in hepatic vein wedge pressure gradients measurements. In those patients where there is a significant drop in portal pressure, β-blocker therapy is highly efficacious in preventing recurrent or initial variceal haemorrhage [70]. β-blocker therapy has been used in children and described in 113 children in four separate anecdotal reports [71–74]. These reports provide preliminary information that this approach is safe and may be efficacious. Major adverse events were not recorded, although it is not clear that there was comprehensive screening for potential problems. Variceal bleeding episodes while on propranolol were reported to be tolerated. Typically, attempts were made to reduce heart rate in children by 25% with the requirement of variable dosing of propranolol between 1.0 and 8.0 mg/kg/day. Furthermore, high-dose β-blocker therapy has been safely utilised in children with hypertrophic cardiomyopathy. The goals of therapy in this disease are to completely eliminate variability in heart rate and very large doses of β-blockers have been well tolerated by children [75]. Doses of between 5 and 23 mg/kg with associated serum levels of 200 to 900 μg/L were utilised without significant problems.

Unfortunately, there have been no randomised trials of β-blocker therapy for either primary or secondary prophylaxis of variceal haemorrhage in children. Pivotal trials and empiric therapy are dependent upon understanding the appropriate dosing of β-blockers in children. Resting heart rate

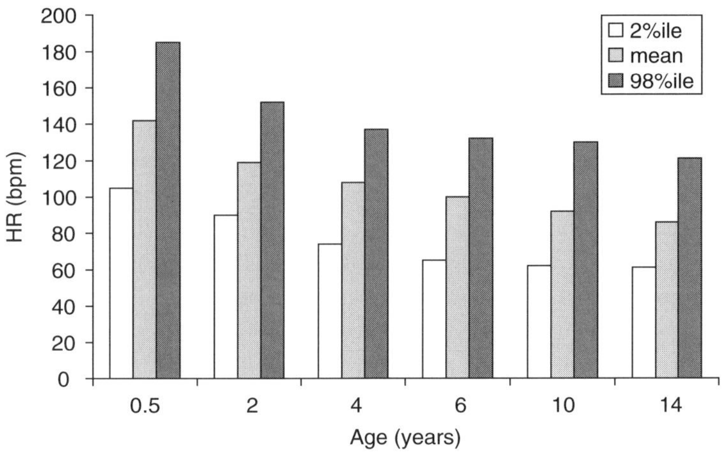

Fig. 32 Basal heart rates in children. Range of normal heart rates for different aged children are shown. Significant normal variability is observed for each age and there is a pronounced trend of reduction in basal rates as children age (adapted from Davignon *et al.* [49]).

can be very difficult to accurately assess in routine clinical practice in children. An anxious child will have a significantly elevated resting heart rate. It is unclear in children if one should seek to assess resting, active, average or exertional heart rate. In addition, as noted previously, heart rate varies significantly with age (Fig. 32). The effects of portal hypertension and its associated hyperdynamic circulation on haemodynamics in children are not known. Therefore, it is critical that these issues be prospectively addressed in a cohort of children with portal hypertension. Basic and comprehensive description of the hyperdynamic circulation in children with biliary atresia will be a significant first step.

Summary

Portal hypertension is frequently seen in children with biliary atresia. The nature of this disorder is such that the complications of portal hypertension often manifest prior to other sequelae of end-stage liver disease. Children with biliary atresia make up the largest single population of children with severe liver disease. Their disease is relatively homogeneous and is not typically impacted by other problems such as alcohol intake, steatosis and/or haemochromatosis that can complicate the analyses of adults. The relatively homogeneous nature of biliary atresia, its rapid progression and the lack of scientific information about portal hypertension in children makes this an ideal area for clinical investigation. The newly formed NIH-funded infrastructure of the Biliary Atresia Research Consortium could be an ideal mechanism for conducting an initial prospective analysis of β-blocker therapy [76]. The results of this study will have important implications not only for biliary atresia, but also for all children with chronic liver disease.

Natural history of formation and growth of oesophageal varices

Marco Zoli and Annalisa Berzigotti

Prevalence of oesophageal varices

Variceal formation is extremely frequent in cirrhosis. In the studies published in the last 20 years the prevalence of varices at diagnosis ranges from 0–10% of patients with compensated disease, to 70–80% of patients with decompensated cirrhosis; the mean figure is 40–55% of patients at diagnosis [77,78]. The analysis of the data pooled from 22 prognostic studies failed to demonstrate a significant relationship between the presence of varices and that of decompensated disease, but it indicated a statistical trend towards significance [78]. This suggests that liver failure may not influence collateral formation directly, but, since portal hypertension progresses in parallel to parenchymal liver disease, it is likely to be more severe in decompensated patients, and varices may appear more often in this group.

Since varices are not found in all patients at diagnosis, some authors [79–83] performed studies to investigate reliable non-invasive predictors of the presence of varices. The most frequently identified predictors are the Child's class, presence of spider naevi, low platelet count (< 100,000/mm^3), reduced prothrombin time (< 70%), splenomegaly and increased portal vein diameter (> 13 mm) by ultrasound; anyway the prognostic models including these variables were not reproducible in independent patients' series, and cannot be considered accurate enough [84]. As a consequence, all patients at the moment of the diagnosis of cirrhosis should undergo an upper digestive tract endoscopy for the screening of oesophageal varices.

Recently, Giannini *et al.* [85] proposed a new model based on the ratio between platelet count and spleen diameter; they found that a ratio below a cut-off value of 909 had a 100% negative predictive value for the presence of oesophageal varices. This non-invasive parameter looks promising, since it showed good results when it was applied in an independent sample of another centre [86].

Formation of oesophageal varices

Whenever portal pressure rises above normal values, collateral circulation begins to develop in an attempt to decompress the portal system;

two mechanisms have been demonstrated in the development of portal–systemic collateral circulation, namely the dilatation of pre-existent embryonic channels communicating the portal and the systemic circulation and neo-angiogenesis [87,88], which recently raised increasing interest [8]. In man, different anastomotic venous systems between portal and systemic circulation have been described [87]. Varices are a part of cephalad collaterals, formed through the dilatation of the left gastric (coronary) vein and the short gastric veins.

From a haemodynamic point of view, varices develop when the HVPG, which is equivalent to the portocaval gradient in liver cirrhosis, increases over a threshold value of 10 mmHg [16]. Above this value the median time observed to the formation of varices, or to the development of other complications of portal hypertension, is 4 years [89].

From a clinical and endoscopic point of view, most recent studies about the development of oesophageal varices agree that *de novo* formation takes place in 4–6% of patients per year [90–92]. A greater incidence has to be expected in patients with active alcoholic intake, and in patients with worsening of liver function. Accepting a risk of bleeding of 10%, patients without varices can be followed-up at 2–3 years intervals.

Growth of oesophageal varices

Once varices form, they increase in size from small to large, and they may bleed. Prospective studies showed that the progression rate is 5–12% per year [90,93,94], this variability probably depending on different criteria of patients' selection. Several factors may contribute to the dilation of varices; among them, the chronic increase in portal pressure and portal-collateral blood flow [95], and the pulses in portal pressure and blood flow associated with meals [96], ethanol consumption [97] and circadian rhythms [98] are thought to be central. The risk of bleeding depends on variceal wall tension, which increases with the increase of variceal radius and variceal transmural pressure according to Frank's modification of the Laplace's law. This explains why large varices (diameter more than 5 mm) carry a higher haemorrhagic risk than small varices (in mean 30% versus 10% at 2 years) [99,100]. The prevalence of large varices in unselected compensated cirrhotics is approximately 35% [101]. Some non-invasive predictors of the presence of large varices have been suggested [102,103]; anyway, as the detection of large varices indicates the need of a treatment aimed to reduce the haemorrhagic risk by the reduction of portal pressure, the experts' consensus is to follow-up the patient by endoscopy at 1–2 years intervals to recognise the enlargement of varices.

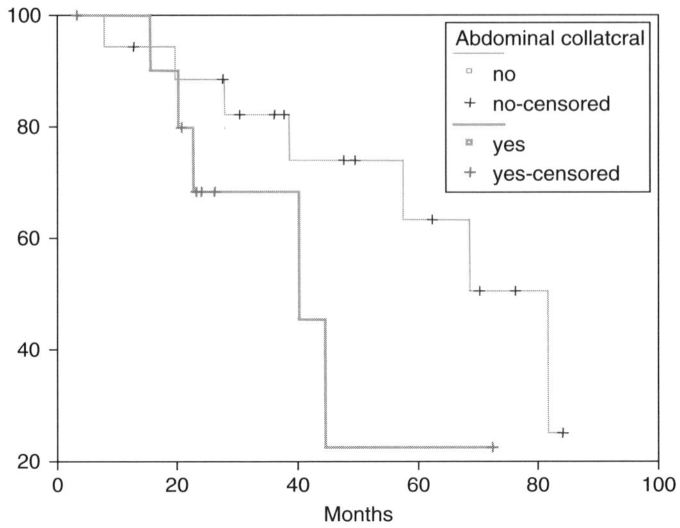

Fig. 33 Formation of oesophageal varices in patients with and without abdominal collaterals at ultrasound examination.

The role of non-variceal portal-collateral shunts, such as a patent paraumbilical vein (PUV) at ultrasound examination, on the natural history of oesophageal varices is still debated. Some authors [104–106] suggested that they may play a protective role but the data are not conclusive. In fact, other authors found that the distribution of varices is similar in patients with or without PUV [105], that PUV is more frequent in more advanced liver disease [107] and that patients with PUV bleed as frequently as non-PUV patients [108,109].

In attempt to better elucidate this issue we conducted a retrospective study on 107 consecutive cirrhotic patients without oesophageal varices ($n = 33$) or with small varices ($n = 74$) observed at our centre. They were conventionally followed-up with both endoscopy and abdominal ultrasound for 12–96 months. The preliminary results from this study show that in patients without varices PUV is uncommon (15.1%), as well as other abdominal collateral vessels (15.1%); in this subgroup PUV is observed in patients with a more advanced liver disease (Child score 9.0 ± 2.1 in PUV versus 6.2 ± 1.5, $p < 0.0001$). In patients with small varices at enrolment PUV was found in 10.8% of cases, while other abdominal collateral vessels in 8.1%.

In patients without varices, 39.4% developed small varices with a mean rate of about 5.9% per year. Patients with PUV or other abdominal collateral

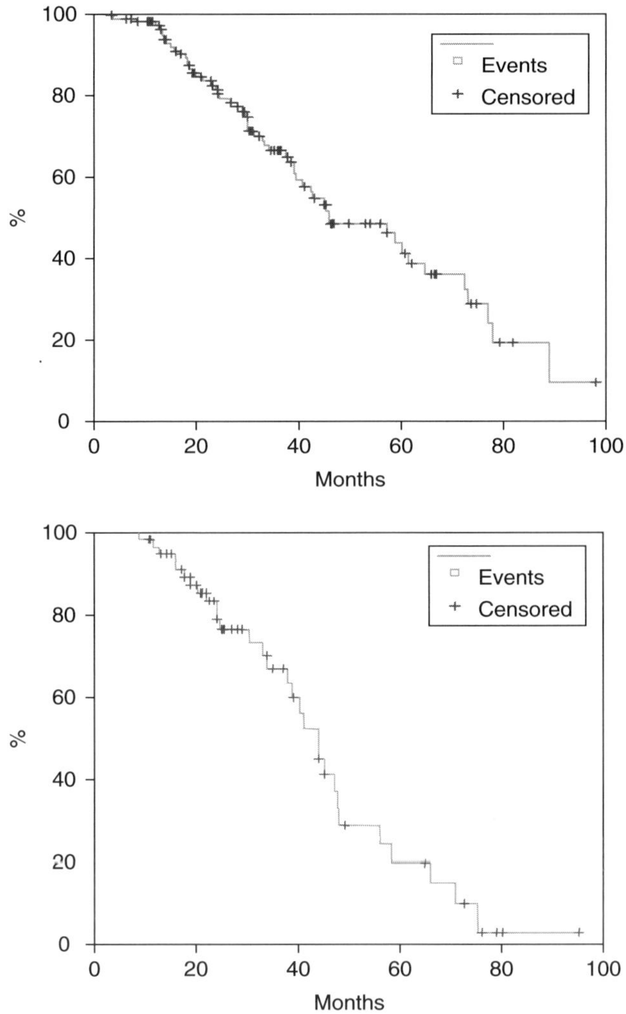

Fig. 34 Formation of new collaterals at abdominal ultrasound examination and growth of varices at endoscopy: significance of correlation $p = 0.01$.

vessels at ultrasound examination showed a trend to a greater rate of formation of varices (Fig. 33; log-rank comparison $p = 0.14$). In patients with small varices at entrance, 40.5% showed variceal enlargement with a mean rate of about 5% per year; patients with a patent PUV showed a trend to statistical significance for a greater rate of progression of varices (log-rank comparison $p = 0.09$).

During the follow-up, 43.7% of the patients developed one or more collateral abdominal vessel (Fig. 34). The formation of a new collateral vessel at abdominal ultrasound correlated with variceal appearance or growth (Pearson's coefficient of correlation 0.312, $p = 0.001$). In conclusion, our data suggest that abdominal non-variceal collaterals form in response to the worsening of portal hypertension in parallel with the dilation of varices, and they do not represent a protective factor on this complication. This observation should be re-evaluated in a study analysing a larger group of patients recruited in different centres, which is in progress.

Summary

The progressive and persistent increase of portal pressure in the course of liver cirrhosis induces the formation of a portal-systemic circulation aimed at decompressing the portal system. Oesophageal varices are the most important portal-systemic collaterals and form in the large majority of patients on long-term follow-up. Once varices have formed, they tend to enlarge and eventually rupture, exposing the patient to the risk of death.

Present knowledge about treatment in the area of pre-primary prophylaxis

Julio Vorobioff

The problem

Clinical evidence of portal hypertension (oesophageal varices/variceal bleeding, ascites, portal-systemic encephalopathy) is usually present once the portal pressure has reached a threshold value of 10–12 mmHg. For any of these circumstances, consensus regarding nomenclature, diagnostic approaches and therapeutic measures has been established [110–112].

Clinically significant portal hypertension [113], although including the presence of these complications, can also be defined only by means of portal manometry. Therefore, even when varices/variceal haemorrhage and/or ascites are absent, an increase in the portal pressure gradient to a threshold above approximately 10 mmHg also defines, by itself, the clinically significant portal hypertensive status.

Nevertheless, an important period of the natural history of chronic liver disease (in fact the longest) elapses asymptomatic and without major signs. Meanwhile, portal pressure ranges within 6–10 mmHg. This early stage of the disease, playing the hidden part of the iceberg, has recently gained the attention of portal hypertension researchers [114,115]. Then, pre-primary prophylaxis is aimed at avoiding/delaying the formation (when still non-existent) and in preventing the growth (when already formed but still small) of oesophageal varices. The different objectives of pre-primary prophylaxis and the dual definition of clinically significant portal hypertension allows to consider different patients population categories. On one side, portal hypertensive patients without significant portal hypertension (i.e. a HVPG 6–10 mmHg) and, obviously, without varices. On the other side, patients with significant portal hypertension (i.e. a HVPG > 10 mmHg) who still have not formed varices. In a third group, patients with small oesophageal varices and, by definition, with significant portal hypertension. This seemingly arbitrary division, correlating portal hypertensive status, endoscopic findings and treatment objectives is one of the most important emerging concepts derived from three recent trials [89,94,116] dealing with this new therapeutic chapter.

The screening of patients for pre-primary prophylaxis

Confronted with the evidence of oesophageal varices, variceal bleeding and/or ascites, the diagnosis of liver cirrhosis with clinically significant portal hypertension is not a difficult task. On the contrary, earlier diagnosis is not an easy one. Lack of signs and an almost symptomless course makes diagnosis at this stage a challenging exercise. Nevertheless, as most potential candidates for pre-primary prophylaxis are within this 'silent' stage, efforts must be addressed in their screening. Obviously, chronic alcohol abusers and morbid obese patients should be evaluated. Extrahepatic manifestations, not necessarily accompanying advanced stages, could help in the diagnosis of specific diseases (i.e. Wilson disease, haemochromatosis, chronic autoimmune hepatitis, PBC, PSC) and also in hepatitis C virus (HCV) chronic infection. Patient complaints, such us fatigue and/or upper abdominal discomfort and the presence of hepatosplenomegaly may also be helpful. This 'first approach' is completed by adding liver function tests and specific markers detection. However, in order to confirm diagnosis and establish the degree of portal hypertension, a second step based on histological evaluation, HVPG measurement and endoscopic examination is necessary. Complementary information obtained from Doppler ultrasound, if present, may be qualitatively helpful [113,117,118].

Performing a liver biopsy should not be a major problem. Coagulation disorders contraindicating the procedure are uncommon at this stage. However, as diagnosis can result from combining clinical, laboratory, endoscopic and manometric data, liver biopsy is not unanimously necessary. Moreover, in the three already completed pre-primary prophylaxis trials, histological evaluation was available in 95% of included patients by Calès *et al.* [116] and in 48% of those included by Merkel *et al.* [94] (C Merkel, personal communication). Diagnosis of cirrhosis was either biopsy-proven or clinically suspected and confirmed by an HVPG $>$ 10 mmHg in Groszmann *et al.* [89] study (RJ Groszmann, personal communication).

Endoscopic screening for varices of all of biopsy-proven/clinically suspected cirrhotic patients has been recommended [119]. Patients with no or small varices may represent 66–75% of cirrhotic patients screened by endoscopy [120]. Therefore, endoscopically speaking, the majority of cirrhotic patients are potential candidates for pre-primary prophylaxis. Although non-invasive screening of varices has been proposed, suggested parameters seem more accurate in predicting the existence of large varices than small ones [80,82]. Moreover, although overall interobserver agreement regarding variceal presence is near 70%, major disagreements appear when absence from presence and small from large varices are been discriminated [121,122]. Consequently, an endoscopic study, latter submitted for interobserver agreement, must be performed during the work-up for patient inclusion in pre-primary prophylaxis trials. A conceptual definition regarding small varices with red signs may be pending: should their pharmacological treatment be considered as pre-primary prophylaxis?

Pre-primary prophylaxis is a research field and, therefore, HVPG measurements should be included in every future clinical trial. Manometrically speaking, most cirrhotic patients without varices are located in an area where HVPG ranges between 6 mmHg and 10 mmHg. In other words, this is a group of portal hypertensive patients without clinically significant portal hypertension. Nevertheless, cirrhotic patients without varices are already above the threshold value of 10 mmHg; and therefore, considered as portal hypertensive patients with clinically significant portal hypertension [16,89,113]. A third group to be considered for pre-primary prophylaxis are those patients with small varices and, therefore, already established clinically significant portal hypertension. Although sharing common therapeutic aims, which look mainly endoscopic (variceal appearance/formation/growth), some characteristics within each of these three groups (i.e. different prognosis, different degree of drug responsiveness, development of other portal hypertension related complications regardless of endoscopic events) [89,94,116] will probably determine the need for tailoring pre-primary prophylaxis, according to each group. A more ambitious objective would be to establish clinical-haemodynamic correlations at this early stage, as has already been demonstrated when treating clinically significant portal hypertension [70,123].

Therapeutic aspects

Several experimental [124–131] and one clinical [132] study gave rational and enthusiastic support for clinical trials regarding prevention of formation and growth of oesophageal varices in cirrhotic patients. Therefore, three clinical studies dealing with this therapeutic aspect of portal hypertension have been performed during the last decade.

The first one, by Calès *et al.* [116], is a double-blind, randomised, multicentre trial, evaluating propranolol administration for the prevention of development of large varices in 206 cirrhotic patients, mostly alcoholics. At inclusion, oesophageal varices were absent in 79 patients and were small in 127 patients. A fixed dose (160 mg/day) of long-acting propranolol was administered to the 102 patients randomised for drug treatment and all patients were followed-up for at least 2 years. Almost one-third of the patients included in each group were lost to follow-up during the study period. After 2 years the percentage of patients with large oesophageal varices was 31% in the propranolol group versus 14% in the placebo group ($p < 0.05$), this difference being not significant at the third year (44% versus 34%, respectively). Complete abstinence from alcohol was observed in 66% of patients in both groups. New, large varices developed in 21 of the 79 (27%) patients while an increase from small to large varices was observed in 82 of the 127 (65%) patients. Bleeding episodes and death rate did not differ among both treatment groups.

An elevated patient drop-out rate and the administration of a fixed dose of propranolol may have influenced Calès *et al.*'s [116] negative results. Of note is the remarkably high abstinence rate (66%) observed among alcoholic cirrhotic patients, which accounted for 86% and 78% in propranolol and placebo groups, respectively. Alcohol abstinence has been shown to be beneficial as it not only improved liver function, but also it decreased portal pressure and variceal size, including making them disappear in some patients [133–136]. Neither such relationship nor the description of small or medium size variceal formation, a necessary step in the respective ways from both non-existent or small to large varices is mentioned by Calès *et al.* [116]. A non-stop trip from previously non-existent and/or small varices straight to large varices, suggests that development of large varices [112] is an 'all or none' phenomenon.

More recently, in a multicentre, randomised, double-blind, placebo-controlled trial, Groszmann *et al.* [89] prospectively evaluated 213 cirrhotic patients without oesophageal varices in order to investigate (1) the effects of timolol (a non-selective β-adrenergic blocker) in the prevention of the development of oesophageal varices and variceal haemorrhage and (2) the predictive value that sequential measurements of HVPG could have in the development of primary (development of varices/variceal haemorrhage), secondary (ascites/encephalopathy) and terminating events (transplant or death). Only portal hypertensive (i.e. HVPG > 6 mmHg) cirrhotics were included. HCV-related cirrhosis accounted for 53%, alcohol for 20% and alcohol + HCV for 15% of included patients, respectively. Yearly endoscopies and HVPG measurements were performed, and the median time of follow-up was 4.2 years. One hundred and eight patients received timolol and the mean dose was 10.8 mg.

The incidence of primary (*n*:84) (78 cases of varices formation and 6 of variceal haemorrhage), secondary (*n*:56) and terminating events (*n*:34) was not significantly different between drug and placebo. Simultaneously, no significant differences in HVPG were detected between both study groups. An HVPG > 10 mmHg at baseline and at year 1 after inclusion in the study was highly predictive of the development of primary, secondary and terminating events ($p < 0.0001$). A higher number of adverse events and serious adverse events (20 versus 6) were reported in the timolol group ($p < 0.01$). In summary, in cirrhotic patients without varices, non-selective β-blockers are not useful in the prevention of the development of varices/variceal haemorrhage and are associated with a higher proportion of adverse events. Moreover, an HVPG > 10 mmHg is a powerful prognostic predictor of the development of complications of portal hypertension.

What reason/s account for these 'negative' results? Cirrhotic patients without varices are probably still lacking a well-developed, collateral circulation network. Besides, but theoretically related, the systemic haemodynamic profile is more likely normal than hyperdynamic in early and compensated cirrhotics [137] (Vorobioff *et al.*, unpublished data). Therefore, it is possible that at early stages of the disease, the β-adrenergic receptor population could be quantitatively and qualitatively different than in advanced disease, resulting in low or absent responsiveness to β-blockers. This could also account for the high incidence of adverse effects observed by Groszmann *et al.* [89]. An important 'positive' result: this study demonstrates that the presence of 'clinically significant portal hypertension' [113], even (and only) manometrically defined, given that no patient had oesophageal varices at entry into the study, is by itself a prognostic indicator in cirrhotic patients.

In the third and most recent study, Merkel *et al.* [94], in a single blind, placebo-controlled clinical trial, evaluated nadolol for the prevention of growth of small varices. Of the 161 cirrhotic patients (57% alcohol-related, 39% of viral aetiology) included in the study, 83 were randomised to nadolol. Other end points were variceal haemorrhage, death, regression of varices and adverse effects resulting in withdrawal of treatment. HVPG was measured at baseline and after 2 years of treatment in 19 patients (10 assigned to nadolol and 9 to placebo). The mean daily dose of nadolol varied from 60 ± 25 mg/day to 64 ± 25 mg/day (according to the year of follow-up). Mean follow-up was 36 months.

Nine patients in the nadolol group and twenty-nine in the placebo group had growth (to F2 and F3) of oesophageal varices. The cumulative risk of growth of varices at 2, 3, 4 and 5 years of follow-up was 7% versus 31%, 13% versus 41%, 20% versus 51% and 20% versus 51% for nadolol and placebo, respectively ($p < 0.001$) (Fig. 35). Predictors of variceal growth were treatment, Child–Pugh score and aggravation of Child–Pugh score. The cumulative probability of being free of variceal bleeding was significantly higher in the nadolol group (88% at the end of follow-up) than in

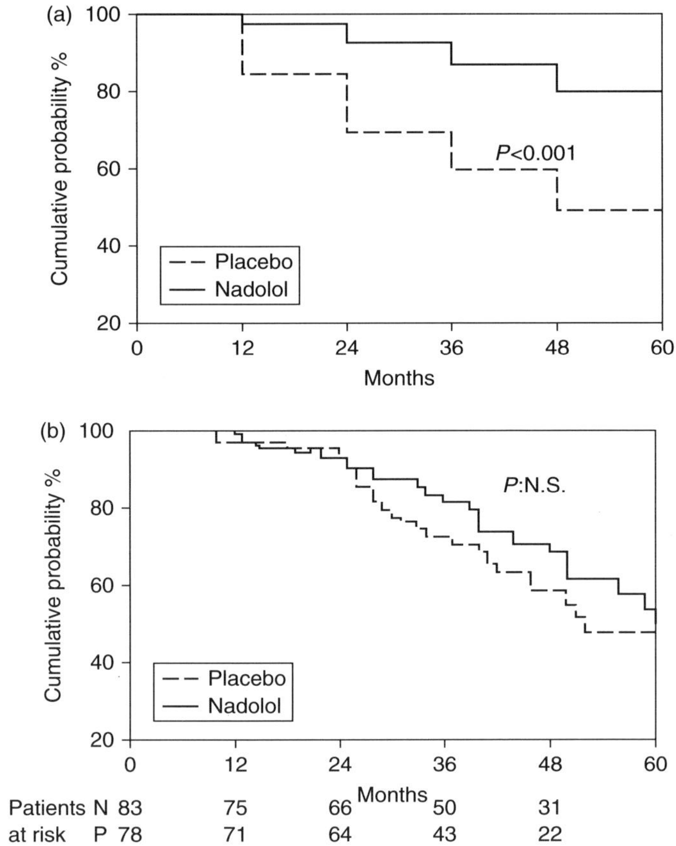

Fig. 35 Cumulative probability of remaining free of growth of varices (a) and survival (b) in the placebo-controlled clinical trial of nadolol in the prophylaxis of growth of small oesophageal varices [94] (reprinted with permission from *Gastroenterology*).

patients randomised to placebo (78%) ($p < 0.02$). But once the main end point was reached (and then all patients were pharmacologically treated) the risk of bleeding was similar for patients initially treated with drug or placebo. Regression of varices occurred in 15 patients randomised to nadolol and in 5 randomised to placebo. Among alcoholic cirrhotic patients, regression (*n*:11) was more frequent in abstainers. Non-alcoholic cirrhotic patients (*n*:9) also showed regression of varices. A high abstinence index was observed (64% and 69% for nadolol and placebo, respectively) (NS). Although the course of Child–Pugh score during follow-up was very similar in the two treatment groups, a progression of liver function impairment was observed in 19 of the 31 patients reporting incomplete abstinence or continuing alcohol abuse. HVPG decreased significantly at 2 years in the 10 patients receiving nadolol (from 12.2 ± 1.1 mmHg to 11.0 ± 1.5 mmHg) ($p < 0.009$) while it showed a slight, non-significant increase in the 9 patients receiving placebo. After 2 years, the HVPG was lower in the patients randomised to nadolol than to placebo (11.0 ± 1.5 mmHg versus 12.5 ± 1.1 mmHg, respectively) ($p < 0.03$). Survival did not differ between both treatment groups (Fig. 35). A higher number of adverse effects requiring withdrawal of treatment were observed in the nadolol group (*n*:9) than in the placebo group (*n*:1) ($p < 0.01$).

According to Merkel *et al.* [94] pharmacological treatment seems to be successful not only in preventing variceal growth but also to induce its regression (only 9 patients had variceal growth but 15 showed regression). Although no aetiology related in this study, it seems relevant that among alcoholic patients regression was more prevalent in abstainers (as was the lack of liver function impairment). Moreover, spontaneous regression (*n*:5) was also observed. Another important finding is the modest but significant decrease in HVPG induced by nadolol, implying that patients with already developed (although small) varices have a certain degree of responsiveness to β-adrenergic blockers, still not present in patients without varices [89].

Summary

The unexpected results by Groszmann *et al.* [89], far from being disappointing, constitute a captivating challenge for hepatologists. Accordingly, two clearly different stages along the natural history of hepatic cirrhosis have been delineated. On one side are patients with oesophageal varices, collateral circulation and hyperdynamic circulation, in whom non-selective β-adrenergic blockers have shown to be beneficial in both primary prophylaxis and prevention of recurrence of variceal bleeding [100]. And on the other side, is a group of patients who are already portal hypertensive (a HVPG > 6 mmHg) without oesophageal varices and who are unresponsive to β-adrenergic blockers. The challenge is to develop new and useful therapeutic tools for this stage of the disease. Both liver endothelial dysfunction [138–143] and/or the incipient collateral circulation [8] seem to be the reasonable main targets at this stage. Being effective at this time, treatment could not only delay or avoid variceal formation but also improve liver function and therefore modify the natural history of liver disease.

Not least challenging are the results of Merkel *et al.* [94]. Growth of small varices is significantly delayed by β-adrenergic blockers, but failure to prevent growth implies so in preventing bleeding. This suggests that an earlier switching point to other therapy (then prophylactic) should be considered once pre-primary prophylaxis fails. Moreover, previously described regression/disappearance of varices has been firmly established by the Italian authors. Then, bi-directional end points could be established in the pharmacological treatment of patients with small oesophageal varices.

Nevertheless, survival was not improved in any of the three studies [89,94,116], although most patients were scored as Child–Pugh A. Therefore, pre-primary prophylaxis should not be exclusively supported by drugs targeting the portal hypertensive state but also, when feasible, the specific aetiologic agent/cause of liver disease at early stages [144,145]. A wider and more accurate conceptual redefinition of pre-primary prophylaxis could then be established.

In view of recent pharmaco-economical studies suggesting the use of β-blockers in all cirrhotic patients, the discussion of this issue becomes highly pertinent.

Endoscopic screening or empiric β-blockers for prophylaxis of variceal bleeding?

Alberto Morabito and Carlo Merkel

In the most recent years we observed a rise in the number of studies dedicated to the relationships between cost and effects of health interventions. This has been due to the progressive awareness of the limitations of the resources dedicated to health, and to the fact that health costs are going to rise without control, unless a limit to the expansion of health expenses is set.

Among studies directed to define the most appropriate clinical strategies, the following types of investigations are possible:

- Cost minimisation
- cost–benefit analysis
- cost–effectiveness analysis
- cost–utility analysis
- decision analysis

The simple analyses of cost minimisation are only adequate if the effects of the strategies to be compared are the same; otherwise they are not suitable to define which treatment constitutes a rational use of resources. The cost–benefit analyses are characterised by the fact that they express both costs and benefits in monetary terms. Since frequently it is difficult for the researchers to express benefits in monetary units, the use of cost–effectiveness analysis was developed. In this kind of analysis, the incremental cost for an additional improvement in health obtained from a treatment compared to another one is assessed according to the formula:

$$C/E = \frac{[(\text{Cost}_{\text{strategy B}}) - (\text{Cost}_{\text{strategy A}})]}{[(\text{Benefit}_{\text{strategy B}}) \quad (\text{Benefit}_{\text{strategy A}})]}$$

In other words, the analysis assesses the cost for every unit of improvement of outcome (e.g. to prevent a single bleeding). In the case in which the analysis takes into account the quality of life of the patients, the analysis is termed cost–utility analysis. Decision analysis is a broader term, which includes all kinds of analyses assessing, under conditions of uncertainty, the probability of events together with the consequences of these events. Generally a decisional tree is built to represent a decisional process.

Most pharmaco-economical analyses dedicated to the problem of prophylaxis of bleeding lie in the area of cost–effectiveness analysis. In 2002, Arguedas *et al.* [146] performed a cost–effectiveness analysis comparing observation alone, endoscopic screening followed by β-blockers if large varices were seen, endoscopic screening followed by variceal ligation if large varices were seen and universal prophylaxis with β-blockers without screening. Results were separately given for patients with compensated (Child A) and decompensated (Child B-C) cirrhosis. From the analysis the authors concluded that in patients with compensated cirrhosis universal treatment with β-blockers was too costly as compared with the other strategies requiring screening. The preference between β-blockers and variceal ligation was related to the assumption of the model in terms of risk reduction and side effects of β-blockers. In patients with decompensated cirrhosis, universal prophylaxis without screening was preferable to every screening procedure. Saab *et al.* [147] made a similar analysis, comparing observation alone, universal prophylaxis without screening and endoscopic screening followed by β-blockers if large varices were seen. They did not stratify patients in compensated and decompensated cirrhosis. The main finding of their study was that the dominant strategy was universal prophylaxis without screening, although this conclusion was sensitive to changes in compliance to screening and treatment within very reasonable values. The third paper analysing this subject was published by Spiegel *et al.* in 2003 [148]. In this very detailed study they compared six strategies: observation alone, universal prophylaxis without screening, endoscopic screening followed by β-blockers if large varices were seen, endoscopic screening followed by variceal ligation if large varices were seen, endoscopic screening in high-risk patients, selected according to a prediction rule, followed by β-blockers if large varices were present and endoscopic screening in high-risk patients, followed by variceal ligation in large varices. Results were rather complex: first of all, endoscopic screening in high-risk patients was a strategy dominated by the others, that is was more costly and less effective than universal screening; furthermore, universal (or 'empiric') β-blockers given without screening was associated to a reasonable increase in cost compared to observation alone (US$12,000 for every bleeding prevented), while endoscopic screening with β-blockers or ligation if large varices were seen was extremely more costly (more than US$170,000 for every bleeding prevented). Taken together, all these pharmaco-economical studies suggest (or tend to suggest) empiric β-blockers without screening as a reasonable strategy to make a prophylaxis of first variceal bleeding in cirrhosis. Despite these promising results, a survey of the clinical management of experts in portal hypertension specifically addressing this point for this consensus conference clearly stated that this strategy should not be used in clinical practice. The reasons for this disbelief may be related to a sense of scepticism, which these analyses are prone to, but more robust reasons may play a role. Indeed, as suggested in an editorial on this topic [149], results of pharmaco-economical analyses are severely dependent on the values of many critical values introduced into the model, and on the costs, which are largely variable across countries. In addition, the effectiveness of treatment in community-based conditions is probably different, and likely to be lower. For these reasons, the authors conclude that 'it is premature to adopt the use of empiric β-blocker prophylaxis for patients with compensated or decompensated cirrhosis'. It appears that most experts in portal hypertension agree. A more formal analysis of the statistical issues related to the choice between observing without treating, treating without screening and screening with treatment in selected cases is reported in the appendix.

Appendix: evidence-based medicine and clinical decision analysis

Alberto Morabito

A treatment should never be administered if its harm is greater than its efficacy, which is generally expressed as relative risk reduction. Likewise, a diagnostic test should never be ordered if the therapeutic harm is greater than the therapeutic efficacy [150]. Intervention is always favoured if the number needed to treat to avoid one adverse outcome (NNT) is smaller than the number needed to treat to harm one individual (NNH). When faced with a choice between two therapeutic options, the action threshold above which an intervention is favoured can be expressed in terms of the harm inflicted (H) as

$$P_t = H \times \text{NNT} \quad \text{or} \quad P_t = \text{NNT}/\text{NNH}$$

If a patient's preferences are taken into account as relative value judgements (RV) of adverse events relative to that of therapeutic events, the action threshold is defined as

$$P_t = \text{NNT} \times (\text{RV}/\text{NNH})$$

In the setting of clinical decision-making, EBM summary measures derived from population studies can be effectively used to define diagnostic and therapeutic action thresholds that may help in the management of individual patients.

Popular indices of therapeutic benefit include the treatment effect, generally expressed as either the absolute change or the relative change in the rate of events, and the number of patients who need to be treated to prevent one bad outcome or attain one good outcome (NNT). Treatment effect is commonly expressed as the absolute risk difference (ARD) between event rates: $\text{ARD} = \text{Risk}_1 - \text{Risk}_2$, or as the proportional relative risk reduction (RRR) in event rates: $\text{RRR} = (\text{Risk}_1 - \text{Risk}_2)/\text{Risk}_1 = 1 - \text{Risk}_2/\text{Risk}_1$ or as the reciprocal of the difference in event rates (NNT) between the alternatives: $\text{NNT} = 1/(\text{Risk}_1 - \text{Risk}_2) = 1/\text{ARD}$.

The harmful effects of treatment can be presented in a similar way. The common way to express this is to assess the rates of adverse effects due to treatment or to calculate the NNH (the number of patients who must be treated for one individual to experience a harmful event). This can be expressed as the absolute difference between two harms (AHD) as $\text{NNH} = 1/(\text{Harm}_1 - \text{Harm}_2) = 1/\text{AHD}$.

Decision analysis

In medical literature, it has become customary to equate the term utility with a measure of strength of the patient's preference for outcome. Indeed, the outcomes expressed as morbidity or mortality can be integrated into a patient's value judgements to arrive at the optimal clinical decision. Therefore, the preferred management strategy is the one associated with the optimal expected value of utility and is not directly dictated by the value of individual strategy outcomes.

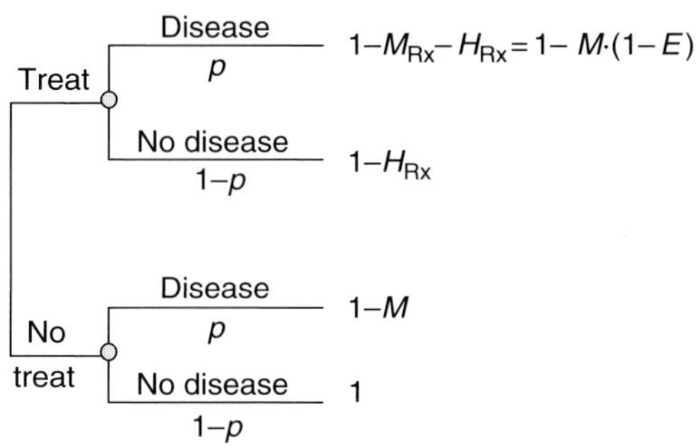

Fig. 36 Clinical setting in which an intervention is compared with no intervention.

If the net harm associated with treatment can be represented in the same units as the net benefit, the threshold probability of disease (p_t) at which the expected value of treatment is exactly the same as the expected value of no treatment can be shown by the following:

$$p_t = \frac{\text{NetHarm}}{\text{NetBenefit} + \text{NetHarm}}$$

The clinical setting in which an intervention is compared with no intervention is shown in Fig. 36.

In a clinical setting intervention, the harm associated with treatment is H and the event rate without and with treatment are M and M_{Rx}, respectively, then the absolute risk difference (ARD $= M - M_{Rx}$), and the relative risk reduction (RRR) or efficacy (E) is $(M - M_{Rx})/M$. Consequently, NNT $= 1/\text{ARD}$.

The threshold probability of disease at which the point of indifference is reached between treatment and no treatment is shown by the following:

$$p_t = H/(E \times M) = H/[M - M_{Rx}] = H/[S_{Rx} - S] = H/\text{ARD} = H \times \text{NNT}$$

If the control arm is placebo, it follows from the above equation that if the probability that the patient has the disease is less than p_t, treatment is not indicated, and if the probability is greater than p_t, treatment should be given. If we assume that a patient in the no-treatment arm is actually on placebo, as is commonly the case in randomised trials, the above relationship can be shown by the following:

$$p_t = (H_{\text{active treatment}} - H_{\text{placebo}}) \times \text{NNT} = \text{NNT}/\text{NNH}$$

A recent study randomised patients who already completed a 3-month course of warfarin to determine whether longer anticoagulation would be beneficial in the prevention of deep venous thrombosis (DVT) recurrence. The study has determined that the NNT for the prophylaxis of DVT recurrence is 4. The study concluded that a considerable risk of DVT recurrence exists beyond the typical 3-month course with warfarin and that a longer duration of anticoagulation may be necessary.

However, the optimal duration of treatment needs to be interpreted in light of not only the benefit but also the harm of warfarin treatment. Although many would argue that the NNT of 4 represents a very effective therapy, this measure alone does not provide an answer to the question of whether this treatment is better than the alternative management strategy of observation without active treatment. The crucial clinical question is: how good is one treatment strategy in comparison with another when both benefit and harm are taken into consideration? To begin to address the clinical question of whether to give warfarin or not, we note that the annual risk of major bleeding in patients given warfarin was 3.8% (compared to 0% in patients in the placebo arm), representing an NNH of 26. If we assume that the avoidance of DVT and bleeding complications represents approximately the same value to the patient, warfarin should be administered if the probability of DVT recurrence is greater than 15% (4/26).

In this study, the recurrence rate for DVT was 27.4% per year, suggesting that warfarin treatment should be continued beyond the initial 3 months of treatment in a typical patient meeting the eligibility criteria.

Now, let us consider a patient at increased risk for bleeding with continued warfarin use because of heavy alcohol intake. Although such patients were excluded from the above clinical trial, it is possible to individualise treatment by applying the above equations to the specific patient. Using published data, we may assume that the risk of bleeding in the patient under consideration is increased by at least 2.7-fold, that is, $NNH = 10\ [= 1/(0.038 \times 2.7)]$. This translates into a new action threshold of 0.4 ($NNT/NNH = 4/10$). Thus, the risk of DVT should exceed 40% per year to justify to continue warfarin. The optimal duration of warfarin could very well be only a few months for this patient. It is equally important to ask the following: what is the highest NNT at which treatment is still worth administering? As noted above, the treatment should be considered only if $NNT < NNH$. We recommend that the NNT not be used without concomitant data on treatment harm. In the example above, warfarin should not be administered if the $NNT > 26$ (or in the case of the patient at increased therapeutic harm because of heavy alcohol intake, warfarin should not be used if the $NNT > 10$). At or above this NNT, the harm of treatment would always outweigh the benefit, assuming harm and benefit are valued equivalently.

This approach enables answering a question posed by Steiner in the recent article: 'For $NNT > 1$, what is the minimal therapeutic benefit at which treatment is worth administering?' [151]. In addressing the application of population-based therapeutic measures to the care of individual patients, Steiner lamented that since we cannot be sure who will benefit from treatment, 'all you can say is that on the basis of best available evidence, everything possible is being done to prevent an adverse effect'. As shown here, treatment is worth considering if $NNT < 1/H$ or if $NNT < NNH$. On the other hand, the following question can be asked: 'How much harm is acceptable, knowing the efficacy of treatment?'

Comparison of an intervention with no intervention

The analytical solution of the tree in Fig. 36 for the treatment of a single disease involves multiplication of the outcomes of the tree by its corresponding probabilities and solving for the probability of a disease at which the point of indifference is reached for treatment and no treatment (p_t). This represents a typical clinical situation with uncertain diagnosis (e.g. whether to administer anticoagulants to a patient suspected of having pulmonary embolism or whether to administer adjuvant chemotherapy to a patient who underwent breast cancer surgery).

The threshold probability of presenting disease (p_t) at which the expected value of treatment equals the expected value of no treatment is the solution to the equation:

$$p \times (1 - M_{RX} - H) + (1 - p) \times (1 - H) = p \times (1 - M) + (1 - p) \times (1),$$

or

$$p \times ([(1 - M_{Rx} - H) - (1 - M)] + [1 - (1 - H)]) = H,$$

where $[(1 - M_{Rx} - H) - (1 - M)] = M - M_{Rx} - H$ is the net benefit from treatment in patients with disease (outcome in those treated minus outcome in those not treated) and $[1 - (1 - H)]$ is the net harm from treatment in those without disease (outcome in those treated minus outcome in those not treated). Net benefit of treatment is restricted to patients who have the disease, and net harm applies to those patients without the disease. H refers to the harm associated with treatment, and M and M_{Rx} refer to morbidity/mortality, without and with treatment, respectively. All of these parameters need to be expressed as probabilities on a scale of 0 to 1. The difference between M and M_{Rx} is equal to the absolute risk difference in event rates (ARD), ($M - M_{Rx} =$ ARD). The analytical derivation of net benefits shown here is equivalent to Glasziou and Irwig's axiomatic definition of net benefits. The solution of the tree depends on definition of benefits and harms. Our model breaks down utilities into effects of the disease (with or without treatment) and the effects of treatment. Therefore, harm [e.g. NNH $= 1/(H_1 - H_2)$] will relate only to the adverse effect of treatment, and benefit (e.g. NNT) will relate only to the effect of the disease that may or may not be treated (e.g. NNT $= 1/[M - M_{Rx}]$ or $1/[M_{Rx2} - M_{Rx1}]$) (see below and the text). Our model assumes that M_{Rx} (morbidity/mortality with treatment) and H_{Rx} (treatment related morbidity/mortality) are independent events and that the probability of the two effects occurring simultaneously is negligible and may be omitted. In most cases, the results under these assumptions do not significantly differ from the results when these assumptions are not taken into account.

From the equations above, we derive the following:

$$p_t(M - M_{Rx}) = H$$

$$p_t = H/(M - M_{Rx}) = H/(E \times M) = H/(S_{Rx} - S) = H/\text{ARD},$$

where, in those with disease, S_{RX} is the disease-specific survival in those treated and S represents disease-specific survival in those not treated.

Finally, since NNT $= 1/$ARD, we arrive at the following:

$$p_t = H \times \text{NNT}$$

Choice between withholding treatment, testing and treating without testing

The text also provides a solution for a choice between withholding treatment, treating without testing and performing a test that will determine further action. The

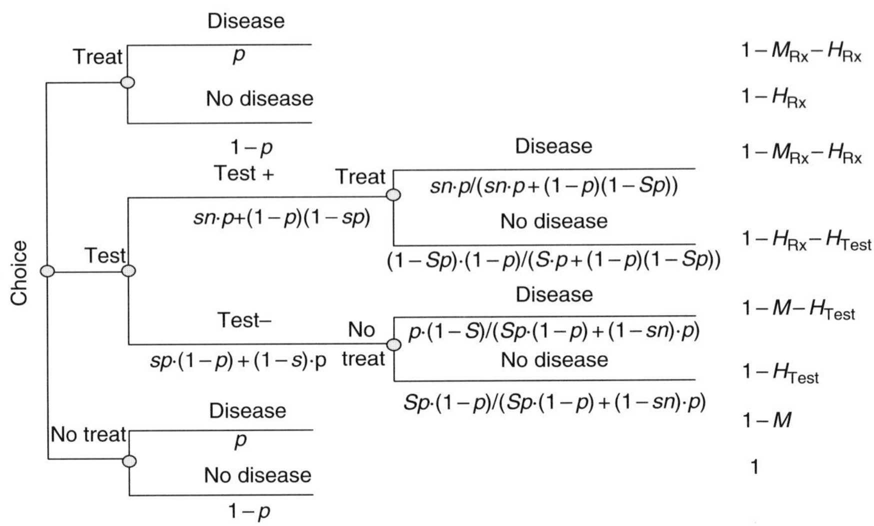

Fig. 37 Solution of the decision tree.

analytical solution of this tree provides two probabilities: the probability of a disease at which we should be indifferent between testing and withholding treatment (p_{tt}) and the probability of a disease at which we should be indifferent between testing and treatment (p_{Rx}).

The solution of the decision tree in Fig. 37 follows the same procedure illustrated earlier. Alternatively, the formulas shown in the text may be derived by simply replacing the net benefit and net harm in the original Pauker and Kassirer model [152] with the evidence-based therapeutic summary measures shown earlier.

Integration of patient's preferences within a threshold model

If we assume that a patient expresses certain value judgements toward target events (morbidity/mortality without treatment)

$$q_{\text{target}} = 1 - \text{value of experiencing target event}$$
$$= \text{value of avoiding target event}$$

and toward adverse events of the treatments

$$q_{\text{adverse event}} = 1 - \text{value of experiencing adverse event}$$
$$= \text{value of avoiding adverse event.}$$

When this definition of patient preferences is adopted in our model, we obtain the following relationships:

$$p_t = \text{NNT} \times [\text{RV} \times H] \quad \text{or} \quad \text{RV} \times \text{NNT}/\text{NNH}$$

$$E_t = \text{RV} \times H/(p \times M) \quad \text{or} \quad E_t = \text{RV} \times H/M \quad \text{if } p = 1$$

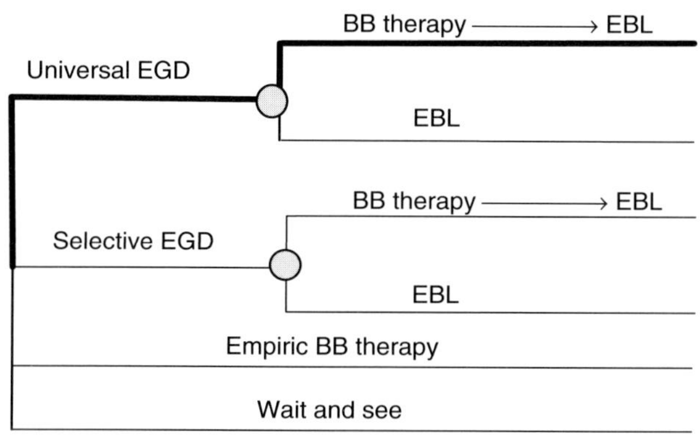

Fig. 38 Six proposed strategies for the prevention of variceal bleeding in patients with cirrhosis.

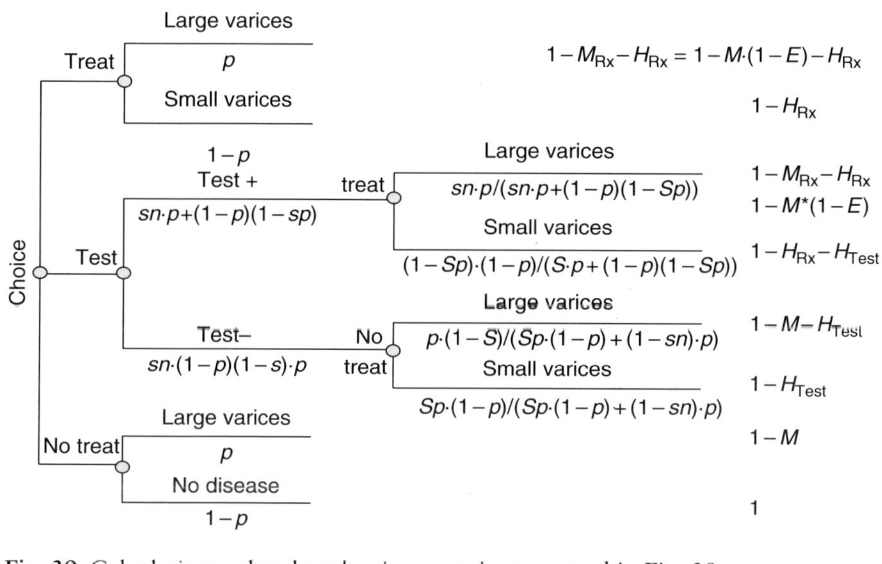

Fig. 39 Calculations related to the six strategies proposed in Fig. 38.

In the case of diagnostic certainty (i.e. $p = 1$), treatment should be administered only if NNT < NNH/RV or if efficacy of treatment is greater than E_t, as shown above.

If we apply this model to the problem of prevention of bleeding in patients with cirrhosis class A or B using the clinical probability estimates reported in the paper by Spiegel *et al.* [148], we can calculate the proportion of patients who take advantage from the treatment administered in the six branches of the tree in Figs 38 and 39.

The ratio of NNT/NNH depends on the prevalence of bleeding. Likely the cost to prevent one episode of bleeding will depend on hypothesised prevalence of the condition. The cost of intervention may enter into the modelling process as the patient's preference q_{target} with an appropriate economical evaluation of events prevented and adverse events experienced.

Conclusion

- The utilities of any strategy depend on the bleeding risk.
- The more aggressive strategies are more useful for more severe patients.
- The utilities strongly depend on the following model assumptions:
  - sensitivity and specificity of tests
  - treatment efficacy in subgroups
  - treatment harm in subgroups

REFERENCES

1 Vorobioff J, Groszmann RJ, Picabea E *et al.* Prognostic value of hepatic venous pressure gradient measurements in alcoholic cirrhosis: a 10-year prospective study. *Gastroenterology* 1996;**111**(3): 701.

2 Wiest R, Groszmann RJ. Nitric oxide and portal hypertension: its role in the regulation of intrahepatic and splanchnic vascular resistance. *Sem Liver Dis* 1999;**19**(4): 411.

3 Ignarro LJ, Cirino G, Casini A, Napoli C. Nitric oxide as a signaling molecule in the vascular system: an overview. *J Cardiovasc Pharmacol* 1999;**34**(6): 879.

4 Furchgott RF, Zawadzki JV. The obligatory role of endothelial cells in the relaxation of arterial smooth muscle by acetylcholine. *Nature* 1980;**288**(5789): 373.

5 Palmer RM, Ferrige AG, Moncada S. Nitric oxide release accounts for the biological activity of endothelium-derived relaxing factor. *Nature* 1987;**327**(6122): 524.

6 Fukumura D, Yuan F, Endo M, Jain RK. Role of nitric oxide in tumor microcirculation. Blood flow, vascular permeability, and leukocyte-endothelial interactions. *Am J Pathol* 1997;**150**(2): 713.

7 Carmeliet P. Mechanisms of angiogenesis and arteriogenesis. *Nat Med* 2000;**6**(4): 3.

8 Fernandez M, Vizzutti F, Garcia-Pagan JC, Rodes J, Bosch J. Anti-VEGF receptor-2 monoclonal antibody prevents portal-systemic collateral vessel formation in portal hypertensive mice. *Gastroenterology* 2004;**126**(3): 886.

9 Lee FY, Albillos A, Colombato LA, Groszmann RJ. The role of nitric oxide in the vascular hyporesponsiveness to methoxamine in portal hypertensive rats. *Hepatology* 1992;**16**(4): 1043.

10 Sieber CC, Groszmann RJ. Nitric oxide mediates hyporeactivity to vasopressors in mesenteric vessels of portal hypertensive rats. *Gastroenterology* 1992;**103**(1): 235.

11 Sieber CC, Groszmann RJ. In vitro hyporeactivity to methoxamine in portal hypertensive rats: reversal by nitric oxide blockade. *Am J Physiol* 1992;**262**(6 Pt 1): G996.

12 Shah V, Wiest R, Garcia-Cardena G, Cadelina G, Groszmann RJ, Sessa WC. Hsp90 regulation of endothelial nitric oxide synthase contributes to vascular control in portal hypertension. *Am J Physiol* 1999;**277**(2 Pt 1): G463.
13 Wiest R, Shah V, Sessa WC, Groszmann RJ. NO overproduction by eNOS precedes hyperdynamic splanchnic circulation in portal hypertensive rats. *Am J Physiol* 1999;**276**(4 Pt 1): G1043.
14 Tsai MH, Iwakiri Y, Cadelina G, Sessa WC, Groszmann RJ. Mesenteric vasoconstriction triggers nitric oxide overproduction in the superior mesenteric artery of portal hypertensive rats. *Gastroenterology* 2003; **125**(5): 1452.
15 Iwakiri Y, Tsai MH, McCabe TJ *et al.* The phosphorylation of endothelial nitric oxide synthase initiates excessive nitric oxide production in the early phases of portal hypertension. *Am J Physiol Heart Circ Physiol* 2002;**282**: H2084.
16 Garcia-Tsao G, Groszmann RJ, Fisher RL, Conn HO, Atterbury CE, Glickman M. Portal pressure, presence of gastroesophageal varices and variceal bleeding. *Hepatology* 1985;**5**(3): 419.
17 D'Amico G. The role of vasoactive drugs in the treatment of oesophageal varices. *Expert Opin Pharmacother* 2004;**5**(2): 349.
18 Colombato LA, Albillos A, Groszmann RJ. Temporal relationship of peripheral vasodilatation, plasma volume expansion and the hyperdynamic circulatory state in portal-hypertensive rats. *Hepatology* 1992;**15**(2): 323.
19 Mosca P, Lee FY, Kaumann AJ, Groszmann RJ. Pharmacology of portal-systemic collaterals in portal hypertensive rats: role of endothelium. *Am J Physiol* 1992;**263**(4 Pt 1): G544.
20 Sieber CC, Sumanovski LT, Stumm M, van der Kooij M, Battegay E. In vivo angiogenesis in normal and portal hypertensive rats: role of basic fibroblast growth factor and nitric oxide. *J Hepatol* 2001;**34**(5): 644.
21 Groszmann RJ, Bosch J, Grace ND *et al.* Haemodynamic events in a prospective randomised trial of propranolol versus placebo in the prevention of a first variceal haemorrhage. *Gastroenterology* 1990;**99**(5): 1401.
22 Garcia-Cardena G, Folkman J. Is there a role for nitric oxide in tumor angiogenesis? *J Natl Cancer Inst* 1998;**90**(8): 560.
23 Murohara T, Horowitz JR, Silver M *et al.* Vascular endothelial growth factor/vascular permeability factor enhances vascular permeability via nitric oxide and prostacyclin. *Circulation* 1998;**97**(1): 99.
24 Ziche M, Morbidelli L, Choudhuri R *et al.* Nitric oxide synthase lies downstream from vascular endothelial growth factor-induced but not basic fibroblast growth factor-induced angiogenesis. *J Clin Invest* 1997;**99**(11): 2625.
25 Kroll J, Waltenberger J. VEGF-A induces expression of eNOS and iNOS in endothelial cells via VEGF receptor-2 (KDR). *Biochem Biophys Res Commun* 1998;**252**(3): 743.
26 Hood JD, Meininger CJ, Ziche M, Granger HJ. VEGF upregulates ecNOS message, protein, and NO production in human endothelial cells. *Am J Physiol* 1998;**274**(3 Pt 2): H1054.
27 Papapetropoulos A, Garcia-Cardena G, Madri JA, Sessa WC. Nitric oxide production contributes to the angiogenic properties of vascular endothelial growth factor in human endothelial cells. *J Clin Invest* 1997;**100**(12): 3131.

28 Fukumura D, Gohongi T, Kadambi A *et al.* Predominant role of endothelial nitric oxide synthase in vascular endothelial growth factor-induced angiogenesis and vascular permeability. *Proc Natl Acad Sci USA* 2001; **98**(5): 2604.
29 Iwakiri Y, Cadelina G, Sessa WC, Groszmann RJ. Mice with targeted deletion of eNOS develop hyperdynamic circulation associated with portal hypertension. *Am J Physiol Gastrointest Liver Physiol* 2002; **283**(5): G1074.
30 Shah V. Cellular and molecular basis of portal hypertension. *Clin Liver Dis Portal Hypertension* 2001;**5**: 629.
31 Morales Ruiz M, Jimenez W. Neovascularization, angiogenesis and vascular remodeling in portal hypertension. In: Sanyal A, Shah V (eds). *Portal hypertension pathobiology, evaluation and treatment*, Humana Press, Totowa, New Jersey, 2005; 99–112.
32 Lee F, Colombato L, Albillos A, Groszmann R. Administration of N omega-nitro-L-arginine ameliorates portal-systemic shunting in portal-hypertensive rats. *Gastroenterology* 1993;**105**: 1464.
33 Cales P, Braillon A, Jiron M, Lebrec D. Superior portosystemic collateral circulation estimated by azygos blood flow in patients with cirrhosis. Lack of correlation with oesophageal varices and gastrointestinal bleeding. Effect of propranolol. *J Hepatol* 1985;**1**: 37.
34 Rudic R. Direct evidence for the importance of endothelium-derived nitric oxide in vascular remodeling. *J Clin Invest* 1998;**101**: 731.
35 Fernandez-Varo G, Ros J, Morales-Ruiz M *et al.* Nitric oxide synthase 3-dependent vascular remodeling and circulatory dysfunction in cirrhosis. *Am J Pathol* 2003;**162**: 1985.
36 Carmeliet P. Angiogenesis in health and disease. *Nat Med* 2003;**9**: 653.
37 Jain R. Molecular regulation of vessel maturation. *Nat Med* 2003;**9**: 685.
38 Urbich C, Dimmeler S. Endothelial progenitor cells. Characterization and role in vascular biology. *Circ Res* 2004;**95**: 343.
39 Sumanovski L, Battegay E, Stumm M, van der Kooij M, Sieber C. Increased angiogenesis in portal hypertensive rats: role of nitric oxide. *Hepatology* 1999;**29**: 1044.
40 Shah V, Lyford G, Gores G, Farrugia G. Nitric oxide in gastrointestinal health and disease. *Gastroenterology* 2004;**126**: 903.
41 Failli P, DeFranco R, Caligiuri A *et al.* Nitrovasodilators inhibit platelet-derived growth factor-induced proliferation and migration of activated human hepatic stellate cells. *Gastroenterology* 2000;**119**: 479.
42 Lee J, Decker N, Chatterjee S, Yao J, Friedman S, Shah V. Mechanisms of nitric oxide interplay with Rho GTPase family members in modulation of actin membrane dynamics in pericytes and fibroblasts. *Am J Pathol* 2005;**166**: 1861–1870.
43 Aicher A, Heeschen C, Mildner-Rihm C *et al.* Essential role of endothelial nitric oxide synthase for mobilization of stem and progenitor cells. *Nat Med* 2003;**9**: 1370.
44 Chan C, Lee F, Wang S *et al.* Effects of vasopressin on portal-systemic collaterals in portal hypertensive rats: role of nitric oxide and prostaglandin. *Hepatology* 1999;**30**: 630.

45 Papapetropoulos A, Desai K, Rudic R *et al.* Nitric oxide synthase inhibitors attenuate transforming-growth-factor-beta 1-stimulated capillary organization in vitro. *Am J Pathol* 1997;**150**: 1835.
46 Sato T. Vascular development: molecular logic for defining arteries and veins. *Curr Opin Hematol* 2003;**10**: 131.
47 Sato T. Emerging concept in angiogenesis: specification of arterial and venous endothelial cells. *Br J Pharmacol* 2003;**140**: 611.
48 Zargar SA, Javid G, Khan BA *et al.* Endoscopic ligation compared with sclerotherapy for bleeding esophageal varices in children with extrahepatic portal venous obstruction. *Hepatology* 2002;**36**: 666.
49 Davignon A, Rautaharju P, Boisselle E, Soumis F, Megelas M, Choquette A. Normal ECG standards for infants and children. *Pediatr. Cardiol.* 1979;**1**: 123.
50 Ohllson E, Rutherford R, Boitnott J. Changes in portal circulation after biliary obstruction in dogs. *Am J Surg* 1970;**120**: 16.
51 Kasai M, Okamoto A, Ohi R, Yabe K, Matsumura Y. Changes of portal vein pressure and intrahepatic blood vessels after surgery for biliary atresia. *J Pediatr Surg* 1981;**16**: 152.
52 Miyata M, Satani M, Ueda T, Okamoto E. Long-term results of hepatic portoenterostomy for biliary atresia: special reference to postoperative portal hypertension. *Surgery* 1974;**76**: 234.
53 Lilly JR, Stellin G. Variceal haemorrhage in biliary atresia. *J Pediatr Surg* 1984;**19**: 476.
54 Ohi R, Mochizuki I, Komatsu K, Kasai M. Portal hypertension after successful hepatic portoenterostomy in biliary atresia. *J Pediatr Surg* 1986;**21**: 271.
55 Stringer M, Howard E, Mowat A. Endoscopic sclerotherapy in the management of esophageal varices in 61 children with biliary atresia. *J Pediatr Surg* 1989;**24**: 438.
56 Miga D, Sokol R, MacKenzie T *et al.* Survival after first esophageal variceal haemorrhage in patients with biliary atresia. *J Pediatr* 2001;**139**: 291.
57 van Heurn LW, Saing H, Tam PK. Portoenterostomy for biliary atresia: long-term survival and prognosis after esophageal variceal bleeding. *J Pediatr Surg* 2004;**39**: 6.
58 Shneider B, Brown M, Sokol R *et al.* A multi-center analysis of outcome at 24 months of age in children with biliary atresia in the United States. *Hepatology* 2004;**40**: 201A.
59 Beath S, Pearmain G, Kelly D, McMaster P, Mayer A, Buckels J. Liver transplantation in babies and children with extrahepatic biliary atresia. *J Pediatr Surg* 1993;**28**: 1044.
60 Yonemura T, Yoshibayashi M, Uemoto S, Inomata Y, Tanaka K, Furusho K. Intrapulmonary shunting in biliary atresia before and after living-related liver transplantation. *Br J Surg* 1999;**86**: 1139.
61 Heaton ND, Davenport M, Howard ER. Incidence of haemorrhoids and anorectal varices in children with portal hypertension. *Br J Surg* 1993;**80**: 616.
62 Smith S, Wiener ES, Starzl TE, Rowe MI. Stoma-related variceal bleeding: an under-recognized complication of biliary atresia. *J Pediatr Surg* 1988;**23**: 243.
63 Schuijtvlot ET, Bax NM, Houwen RH, Hruda J. Unexpected lethal pulmonary hypertension in a 5-year-old girl successfully treated for biliary atresia. *J Pediatr Surg* 1995;**30**: 589.

64 Soh H, Hasegawa T, Sasaki T *et al.* Pulmonary hypertension associated with postoperative biliary atresia: report of two cases. *J Pediatr Surg* 1999;**34**: 1779.
65 Ling Y, Zhang J, Luo B *et al.* The role of endothelin-1 and the endothelin B receptor in the pathogenesis of hepatopulmonary syndrome in the rat. *Hepatology* 2004;**39**: 1593.
66 Shneider B. Portal hypertension. In: Suchy F, Sokol R, Balistreri W (eds). *Liver disease in children.* Philadelphia; Lippincott Williams & Wilkins, 2001; 129.
67 D'Amico G, Pagliaro L, Bosch J. The treatment of portal hypertension: a meta-analytic review. *Hepatology* 1995;**22**: 332.
68 Shneider B. Approaches to the management of paediatric portal hypertension: results of an informal survey. In: Groszmann R, Tygat N, Bosch J (eds). Portal hypertension in the 21st century. Boston; Kluwer Academic Publishers, 2004.
69 De Franchis R. Incidental esophageal varices. *Gastroenterology* 2004;**126**: 1860.
70 Feu F, Garcia-Pagan JC, Bosch J *et al.* Relation between portal pressure response to pharmacotherapy and risk of recurrent variceal haemorrhage in patients with cirrhosis. *Lancet* 1995;**346**: 1056.
71 Ozsoylu S, Kocak N, Yuce A. Propranolol therapy for portal hypertension in children. *J Paedr* 1985;**106**: 317.
72 Shashidhar H, Langhans N, Grand RJ. Propranolol in prevention of portal hypertensive haemorrhage in children: a pilot study. *J Pediatr Gastroenterol Nutr* 1999;**29**: 12.
73 de Kolster C, Rapa de Higuera M, Carvajal A, Castro J, Callegari C, Kolster J. Propranolol in children and adolescents with portal hypertension: its dosage and the clinical, cardiovascular and biochemical effects. *GEN* 1992;**46**: 199.
74 Ozsoylu S, Kocak N, Demir H, Yuce A, Gurakan F, Ozen H. Propranolol for primary and secondary prophylaxis of variceal bleeding in children with cirrhosis. *Turk J Pediatr* 2000;**42**: 31.
75 Ostman-Smith I, Wettrell G, Riesenfeld T. A cohort study of childhood hypertrophic cardiomyopathy: improved survival following high-dose beta-adrenoceptor antagonist treatment. *J Am Coll Cardiol* 1999;**34**: 1813.
76 Hoofnagle JH. Biliary Atresia Research Consortium (BARC). *Hepatology* 2004;**39**: 891.
77 Pascal J, Cales P, Desmorat H. Natural history of esophageal varices. In: Bosch J, Rodes J (eds). *Recent advances in the pathophysiology and treatment of portal hypertension*, Serono Symposia Review, Rome, 1989; 127.
78 D'Amico G. Esophageal varices: from appearance to rupture; natural history and prognostic indicators. In: Groszmann RJ, Bosch J (eds). *Portal hypertension in the 21st Century.* Boston; Kluwer Academic Publishers, 2004; 147.
79 Zaman A, Hapke R, Flora K *et al.* Factors predicting the presence of esophageal varices or gastric varices in patients with advanced liver disease. *Am J Gastroenterol* 1999;**94**: 3292.
80 Pilette C, Oberti F, Aubé C *et al.* Non-invasive diagnosis of esophageal varices in chronic liver disease. *J Hepatol* 1999;**31**: 867.
81 Ng FH, Wong SY, Loo CK *et al.* Prediction of oesophagogastric varices in patients with cirrhosis. *J Gastroenterol Hepatol* 1999;**14**: 785.
82 Schepis F, Cammà C, Niceforo D *et al.* Which patients should undergo endoscopic screening for esophageal varices detection? *Hepatology* 2001;**33**: 333.

83 Zaman A, Becker T, Lapidus J *et al.* Risk factors for the presence of varices in cirrhotic patients without a history of variceal haemorrhage. *Arch Intern Med.* 2001;**161**: 2564.

84 Riggio O, Angeloni S, Nicolini G *et al.* Endoscopic screening for esophageal varices in cirrhotic patients. *Hepatology* 2002;**35**: 501.

85 Giannini E, Botta F, Borro P *et al.* Platelet count/spleen diameter ratio: proposal and validation of a non-invasive parameter to predict the presence of oesophageal varices in patients with liver cirrhosis. *Gut* 2003; **52**: 1200.

86 Zimbwa TA, Blanshard C, Subramaniam A. Platelet count/spleen diameter ratio as a predictor of oesophageal varices in alcoholic cirrhosis. *Gut* 2004;**53**: 1055.

87 Vianna A. Anatomy of the portal venous system in portal hypertension. In: McIntyre N, Benhamou JP, Bircher J, Rizzetto M, Rodés J (eds). *Oxford textbook of clinical hepatology*, Oxford University Press, Oxford, 1991; 393–399.

88 Noda T. Angioarchitectural study of esophageal varices (with special reference to variceal rupture). *Virchows Arch* A 1984;**404**: 381.

89 Groszmann RJ, Garcia-Tsao G, Bosch J *et al.* Multicenter randomised placebo-controlled trial of non-selective beta-blockers in the prevention of the complications of portal hypertension: final results and identification of a predictive factor. AASLD, Boston. *Hepatology* 2003;**38**(4)(suppl. 1): 206A.

90 Merli M, Nicolini G, Angeloni S *et al.* Incidence and natural history of small esophageal varices in cirrhotic patients. *J Hepatol* 2003;**38**: 266.

91 Primignani M, Albè R, Preatoni P *et al.* 'De novo' development of esophageal varices in patients with a recent histologic diagnosis of liver cirrhosis. *Gastroenterology* 1998;**114**: A1324.

92 Zoli M, Merkel C, Magalotti D *et al.* Natural history of cirrhotic patients with small esophageal varices: a prospective study. *Am J Gastroenterol* 2000;**95**: 503.

93 D'Amico G, Pasta L, Madonna S *et al.* *The incidence of esophageal varices in cirrhosis.* DDW, Atlanta, 2001.

94 Merkel C, Marin R, Angeli P *et al.* A placebo-controlled clinical trial of nadolol in the prophylaxis of growth of small esophageal varices in cirrhosis. *Gastroenterology* 2004;**127**: 476.

95 Dell'Era A, Bosch J. Review article: the relevance of portal pressure and other risk factors in acute gastro-oesophageal variceal bleeding. *Aliment Pharmacol Ther* 2004;**20**(suppl. 3): 8–15; discussion 16.

96 Lee SS, Hadengue A, Moreau R *et al.* Postprandial haemodynamic responses in patients with cirrhosis. *Hepatology* 1988;**8**: 647.

97 Luca A, García-Pagán JC, Bosch J *et al.* Effects of ethanol consumption on hepatic haemodynamics in patients with alcoholic cirrhosis. *Gastroenterology* 1997;**112**: 1291.

98 García-Pagán JC, Feu F, Castells A *et al.* Circadian variations of portal pressure and variceal haemorrhage in patients with cirrhosis. *Hepatology* 1994;**19**: 595.

99 The North Italian Endoscopic Club for the Study and Treatment of Esophageal Varices. Prediction of the first variceal haemorrhage in patients with cirrhosis of the liver and esophageal varices. *N Engl J Med* 1988;**13**: 983.

100 D'Amico G, Pagliaro L, Bosch J. Pharmacological treatment of portal hypertension: An evidence-based approach. *Semin Liver Dis* 1999;**19**: 475.

101 Jensen DM. Endoscopic screening for varices in cirrhosis: findings, implications, and outcomes. *Gastroenterology* 2002;**122**: 1620.

102 Chalasani N, Imperiale TF, Ismail A *et al.* Predictors of large esophageal varices in patients with cirrhosis. *Am J Gastroenterol* 1999;**94**: 3285.

103 Thomopoulos KC, Labropoulou-Karatza C, Mimidis KP *et al.* Non-invasive predictors of the presence of large oesophageal varices in patients with cirrhosis. *Dig and Liver Dis* 2003;**35**: 473.

104 Mostbeck GH, Wittich GR, Herold C *et al.* Haemodynamic significance of the paraumbilical vein in portal hypertension: assessment with duplex US. *Radiology* 1989;**170**: 339.

105 Sacerdoti D, Bolognesi M, Bombonato G *et al.* Paraumbilical vein patency in cirrhosis: effects on hepatic haemodynamics evaluated by Doppler sonography. *Hepatology* 1995;**22**: 1689.

106 Vilgrain V, Lebrec D, Menu Y *et al.* Comparison between ultrasonographic signs and the degree of portal hypertension in patients with cirrhosis. *Gastrointest Radiol.* 1990;**15**: 218.

107 DomLand M, Gebel M, Caselitz M *et al.* Comparison of portal venous flow in cirrhotic patients with and without paraumbilical vein patency using duplex-sonography. *Ultraschall Med.* 2000;**21**: 165.

108 Morin C, Lafortune M, Pomier G *et al.* Patent paraumbilical vein: anatomic and haemodynamic variants and their clinical importance. *Radiology* 1992;**185**: 253.

109 Aagaard J, Jensen LI, Sorensen TI *et al.* Recanalized umbilical vein in portal hypertension. *AJR* 1982;**139**: 1107.

110 De Franchis R. Updating consensus in portal hypertension: report of the Baveno III consensus workshop on definitions, methodology, and therapeutic strategies in portal hypertension. *J Hepatol* 2000;**33**: 846.

111 Ferenci P, Lockwood A, Mullen K *et al.* Hepatic Encephalopathy – Definition, nomenclature, diagnosis, and quantification: final report of the working party at the 11th world congresses of gastroenterology, Vienna, 1998. *Hepatology* 2002;**35**: 716.

112 Moore KP, Wong F, Gines P *et al.* The management of ascites in cirrhosis: report of the consensus conference of the international ascites club. *Hepatology* 2003;**38**: 258.

113 D'Amico G, Garcia-Tsao G, Calès P *et al.* Diagnosis of portal hypertension: how and when. In: de Franchis R (ed). *Portal hypertension. Proceedings of the third baveno international consensus workshop on definitions, methodology and therapeutic strategies.* Oxford; Blackwell Science, 2001; 36.

114 Merkel C, Escorsell A, Sieber C *et al.* Preprimary prophylaxis: can (and should) we prevent the formation and growth of varices? In: de Franchis R (ed). *Portal hypertension. Proceedings of the third baveno international consensus workshop on definitions, methodology and therapeutic strategies.* Oxford; Blackwell Science, 2001: 97.

115 Merkel C, Bolognesi M, Gatta A. The cirrhotic patient with no varices and with small varices. In: Groszmann RJ and Bosch J (eds). *Portal hypertension in the 21st century.* Kluwer Academic Publishers, Dordrecht, 2004; 271.

116 Calès P, Oberti F, Payen JL *et al.* Lack of effect of propranolol in the prevention of large esophageal varices in patients with cirrhosis: a randomised trial. *Eur J Gastroenterol Hepatol* 1999;**11**: 741.

117 Zironi G, Gaiani S, Fenyves D *et al.* Value of measurement of mean portal flow velocity by Doppler flowmetry in the diagnosis of portal hypertension. *J Hepatol* 1992;**16**: 298.
118 Zoli M, Iervese T, Merkel C *et al.* Prognostic significance of portal haemodynamics in patients with compensated cirrhosis. *J Hepatol* 1993;**17**: 56.
119 Grace ND, Groszmann RJ, Garcia-Tsao G *et al.* Portal hypertension and variceal bleeding: an AASLD single topic symposium. *Hepatology* 1998;**28**: 868.
120 Monkewich GJ, Marcon NE. Endoscopy in the management of portal hypertension. In: Groszmann RJ and Bosch J (eds). *Portal hypertension in the 21st century.* Kluwer Academic Publishers, Dordrecht, 2004; 185.
121 Calès P, Zabotto B, Meskens J *et al.* Gastroesophageal endoscopic features in cirrhosis: observer variability, interassociations, and relationship to hepatic disfunction. *Gastroenterology* 1990;**98**: 156.
122 Bendtsen F, Skovgaard LT, Sorensen TIA *et al.* Agreement among multiple observers on endoscopic diagnosis of esophageal varices before bleeding. *Hepatology* 1990;**11**: 341.
123 Groszmann RJ, Bosch J, Grace ND *et al.* Haemodynamic events in a prospective randomised trial of propranolol versus placebo in the prevention of a first variceal haemorrhage. *Gastroenterology* 1990;**99**: 1401.
124 Genecin P, Polio J, Groszmann RJ. Sodium intake modulates portal pressure and the hyperdynamic circulation in portal hypertensive rats. *Gastroenterology* 1989;**96**: A599.
125 Colombato LA, Albillos A, Genecin P *et al.* Prevention of portal-systemic shunting in propranolol-treated and in sodium-restricted rats. *Gastroenterology* 1991;**100**: A370.
126 Sarin SK, Groszmann RJ, Mosca PG *et al.* Propranolol ameliorates the development of portal-systemic shunting in a chronic murine schistosomiasis model of portal hypertension. *J Clin Invest* 1991;**87**: 1032.
127 Lin HC, Soubrane O, Cailmail S *et al.* Early chronic administration of propranolol reduces the severity of portal hypertension and portal-systemic shunts in conscious portal vein stenosed rats. *J Hepatol* 1991;**13**: 213.
128 Lin HC, Soubrane O, Lebrec D. Prevention of portal hypertension and porto-systemic shunts by early chronic administration of clonidine in conscious portal vein-stenosed rats. *Hepatology* 1992;**14**: 325.
129 Albillos A, Colombato L, Lee FY *et al.* Octreotide ameliorates vasodilatation and Na^+ retention in portal hypertensive rats. *Gastroenterology* 1993; **104**: 575.
130 Lee FY, Colombato L, Albillos A *et al.* Administration of N(-Nitro-L-arginine ameliorates portal-systemic shunting in portal-hypertensive rats. *Gastroenterology* 1993;**105**: 1464.
131 Oberti F, Rifflet H, Maïga MY *et al.* Prevention of portal hypertension by propranolol and spironolactone in rats with bile duct ligation. *J Hepatol* 1997; **26**: 167.
132 Escorsell A, Ferayorni L, Bosch J *et al.* The portal pressure response to β blockade is greater in cirrhotic patients without varices than in those with varices. *Gastroenterology* 1997;**112**: 2012.
133 Bennet HD, Lorentzen C, Baker L. Transient esophageal varices in hepatic cirrhosis. *Arch Int Med* 1953;**92**: 507.

134 Dagradi A. The natural history of esophageal varices in patients with alcoholic liver cirrhosis. An endoscopic and clinical study. *Am J Gastroenterol* 1972;**57**: 520.

135 Calès P, Desmorat H, Vinel JP *et al.* Incidence of large esophageal varices in patients with cirrhosis: application to prophylaxis of first bleeding. *Gut* 1990;**31**: 1298.

136 Vorobioff J, Groszmann RJ, Picabea E *et al.* Prognostic value of hepatic venous pressure measurement in alcoholic cirrhosis: a ten year prospective study. *Gastroenterology* 1996;**111**: 701.

137 Braillon A, Calès P, Valla D *et al.* Influence of the degree of liver failure on systemic and splanchnic haemodynamics and on response to propranolol in patients with cirrhosis. *Gut* 1986;**27**: 1204.

138 Fiorucci S, Antonelli E, Morelli O *et al.* NCX-1000, a NO-releasing derivative of ursodeoxycholic acid, selectively delivers NO to the liver and protects against development of portal hypertension. *Proc Natl Acad Sci USA* 2001;**98**: 8897.

139 Van de CM, Omasta A, Janssens S *et al.* In vivo gene transfer of endothelial nitric oxide synthase decreases portal pressure in anaesthetised carbon tetrachloride cirrhotic rats. *Gut* 2002;**51**: 440.

140 Morales-Ruiz M, Cejudo-Martin P, Fernandez-Varo G *et al.* Tranduction of the liver with activated Akt normalizes portal pressure in cirrhotic rats. *Gastroenterology* 2003;**125**: 522.

141 Fiorucci S, Antonelli E, Brancaleone V *et al.* NCX-1000, a nitric-oxide releasing derivative of ursodeoxycholic acid, ameliorates portal hypertension and lowers norepinephrine-induced intrahepatic resistance in the isolated and perfused rat liver. *J Hepatol* 2003;**39**: 932.

142 Loureiro-Silva MR, Cadelina GW, Iwakiri Y *et al.* A liver-specific nitric oxide donor improves the intra-hepatic vascular response to both portal blood flow increase and methoxamine in cirrhotic rats. *J Hepatol* 2003;**39**: 940.

143 Zafra C, Abraldes JG, Turnes J *et al.* Simvastatin enhances hepatic nitric oxide production and decreases the hepatic vascular tone in patients with cirrhosis. *Gastroenterology* 2004;**126**: 749.

144 Burroughs AK, Groszmann RJ, Bosch J *et al.* Assessment of therapeutic benefit of antiviral therapy in chronic hepatitis C: is hepatic venous pressure a better end point? *Gut* 2002;**50**: 425.

145 Czaja AJ, Carpenter HA. Decreased fibrosis during corticosteroid therapy of autoimmune hepatitis. *J Hepatol* 2004;**40**: 646.

146 Arguedas MR, Heudebert GR, Eloubeidi MA, Abrams GA, Fallon MB. Cost-effectiveness of screening, surveillance, and primary prophylaxis strategies for esophageal varices. *Am J Gastroenterol* 2002;**97**: 2441.

147 Saab S, De Rosa V, Nieto J, Durazo F, Han S, Roth B. Costs and clinical outcomes of primary prophylaxis of variceal bleeding in patients with hepatic cirrhosis: a decision analytic model. *Am J Gastroenterol* 2003;**98**: 763.

148 Spiegel BM, Targownik L, Dulai GS, Karsan HA, Gralnek IM. Endoscopic screening for esophageal varices: is it ever cost effective? *Hepatology* 2003;**37**: 366.

149 Rubenstein JH, Inadomi JM. Empiric beta-blocker for the prophylaxis of variceal haemorrhage: cost-effective or clinically applicable? *Hepatology* 2003;**37**: 249.

150 Djulbegovic B, Hozo I, Lyman GH. Linking evidence-based medicine therapeutic summary measures to clinical decision analysis. *Med Gen Med* 2000; 2(1): E6.
151 Steiner JF. Talking about treatment: the language of populations and the language of individuals. *Ann Intern Med* 1999;**130**: 618.
152 Pauker SG, Kassirer J. The threshold approach to clinical decision making. *N Engl J Med* 1980;**302**: 1109.

Baveno IV Consensus Statements: Pre-Primary Prophylaxis

Roberto J. Groszmann, Carlo Merkel (Chairpersons), Yasuko Iwakiri, Alberto Morabito, Benjamin L. Shneider, Vijay Shah, Julio Vorobioff and Marco Zoli

Background

• Prevention of the development of complications of portal hypertension is clearly an important area for future research.
• Portal-systemic collaterals may develop before the appearance of varices, and can be diagnosed non-invasively. However, their clinical importance is uncertain. (5;D)
• Hepatic venous pressure gradient (HVPG) is predictive of varices formation. (1b;A)

Recommendations for management

• All cirrhotic patients should be screened for varices at diagnosis. (5;D)
• Despite some pharmaco-economical analysis, it is not indicated to treat cirrhotic patients with β-blockers without prior assessment of the presence of oesophageal varices. (5;D)
• There is no indication, at this time, to treat patients to prevent the formation of varices. (1b;A)

Areas requiring further study

• Basic mechanisms in the development and progression of portal hypertension.
• Natural history of low-risk varices (epidemiology and predictive factors of progression).
• Routine use of HVPG in clinical trials involved in investigating the complications of portal hypertension.
• Treatment to decrease or prevent the progression and/or prevent the development of varices.
• Biliary atresia (a very interesting entity of paediatric portal hypertension with rapid rate of progression).

Non-invasive tests

• Non-invasive tests might be useful to identify patients at risk of having or prone to develop varices (HVPG $>$ 12 mmHg), but prospective studies are required. (4;C)

LECTURE

Pulmonary Vascular Complications of Liver Disease: Implications for Diagnosis and Treatment of Portal Hypertension

Michael B. Fallon

OVERVIEW

Respiratory symptoms are common in patients who have chronic liver disease with estimates ranging as high as 50–70% of patients complaining of shortness of breath [1]. The differential diagnosis of dyspnoea is broad in these patients and there are a number of important causes to consider. Over the last 15 years, two distinct pulmonary vascular disorders have emerged as important aetiologies of pulmonary dysfunction in patients with liver disease or portal hypertension. The hepatopulmonary syndrome (HPS) occurs when intrapulmonary vasodilatation impairs arterial gas exchange and is found in as many as 15–20% of patients being evaluated for orthotopic liver transplantation (OLT) [2]. Portopulmonary hypertension (POPH) results when pulmonary arterial constriction and remodelling lead to increased pulmonary arterial pressure and is seen in as many as 6% of patients being evaluated for OLT [3]. The presence of either HPS or POPH increases morbidity and mortality in patients with liver disease. How the pathogenesis of alterations in the pulmonary vasculature relates to the mechanisms that trigger and maintain portal hypertension and whether pulmonary vascular complications influence the outcome and consequences of portal hypertension have not been carefully studied.

Recently, the results of a task force sponsored by the European Respiratory Society and conceived and led by Dr Roberto Rodriguez-Roisin have been published [4]. This group of 16 international investigators discussed and reviewed the salient clinical and pathogenetic features of both HPS and POPH. This work serves as the most comprehensive review of these disorders and as a framework for exploring whether HPS and POPH may influence the diagnosis and treatment of portal hypertension. The present review will focus on (1) the significance of HPS and POPH relative to the clinical outcome and pathogenesis of portal hypertension and (2) the diagnosis of HPS and POPH, based on the concept that recognition of these disorders will influence treatment and outcomes in portal hypertension.

HEPATOPULMONARY SYNDROME

Definition

Hepatopulmonary syndrome (HPS) is defined by a widened alveolar–arterial oxygen gradient ($AaPO_2$) on room air (> 15 mmHg) with or without hypoxaemia resulting from intrapulmonary vasodilatation in the presence of hepatic dysfunction or portal hypertension [4–6]. Early studies emphasised that the exclusion of all other causes of cardiopulmonary dysfunction were required to make the diagnosis of HPS [5]. However, it is now clear that HPS may co-exist with other cardiopulmonary abnormalities [7,8] and contribute significantly to gas exchange abnormalities in this setting. In addition, the $AaPO_2$ normally increases with age. Therefore, age correction using standard formulae for it is appropriate to avoid over-diagnosis of HPS [9].

Natural history and prognosis

The natural history of HPS is incompletely characterised. Most patients appear to develop progressive intrapulmonary vasodilatation and worsening gas exchange [10] over time and spontaneous improvement is rare [11]. A recent prospective study has evaluated the natural history of HPS in a cohort of 111 patients with cirrhosis of whom 27 (24%) had HPS [12]. The median survival among patients with HPS was significantly shorter (10.6 months) compared with patients without HPS (40.8 months). Mortality remained higher in those with HPS after adjusting for severity of underlying liver disease and after excluding patients who underwent liver transplantation during follow-up. The causes of death in patients with HPS were mainly due to complications of hepatocellular dysfunction and portal hypertension and correlated with the severity of hypoxaemia in HPS. This data raises the possibility that the presence of HPS may be an important factor that influences the progression of liver disease and the risk of complications related to portal hypertension. Finally, although speculative, even modest hypoxaemia related to HPS may worsen during sleep based on the observation that nocturnal oxygen saturation decreased in a small cohort of non-HPS cirrhotic patients [13].

Mortality after liver transplantation also appears to be higher in patients with HPS compared with those without HPS. The utility of the severity of HPS as a predictor of outcome after liver transplantation has been prospectively evaluated in a cohort of 24 patients with cirrhosis and HPS [14]. The authors found that mortality after liver transplantation was markedly increased in severe HPS, in part due to the development of unique post-operative complications recognised in HPS patients [15,16]. A preoperative PaO_2 of $\leq$ 50 mmHg alone or in combination with a macroaggregated albumin shunt fraction $\geq$ 20% were the strongest predictors of post-operative mortality. These results support that the presence of HPS may adversely affect survival in patients with cirrhosis and that the outcome of transplantation for HPS worsens as HPS progresses.

The observation that HPS increases mortality and that transplant outcomes may worsen in more severe HPS has led to the policy in some US centres of increasing priority for OLT in patients with HPS and significant hypoxaemia [17]. Since some studies have found HPS to be common in patients with well-preserved hepatic function, this approach has the potential to substantially increase the numbers of patients with relatively well-preserved hepatic function who undergo transplantation for HPS. In turn, patients without HPS would wait longer and would be expected to have a greater chance to develop complications of portal hypertension.

Pathophysiology

A fundamental question regarding pathogenesis in HPS is whether the mechanisms are similar to those involved in the systemic and splanchnic alterations of the hyperdynamic circulatory state of cirrhosis. HPS is found most commonly in the setting of cirrhosis and appears to occur across the spectrum of aetiologies of liver disease [18–20]. However, whether the presence or severity of intrapulmonary vasodilatation and HPS correlate with the severity of underlying liver disease is controversial and studies have found HPS more commonly in both less- and more-advanced cirrhosis [8,18–22]. Recently, HPS has also been recognised in patients with portal hypertension in the absence of cirrhosis (portal vein thrombosis, nodular regenerative hyperplasia, congenital hepatic fibrosis and Budd–Chiari syndrome) [23–26] and has been reported in the setting of acute and chronic hepatitis in the absence of portal hypertension [27,28]. These findings support that advanced liver disease is not required for HPS to develop and raise the possibility that unique pathophysiological events occur in patients who develop HPS.

The hallmark of HPS is microvascular dilatation occurring within the pulmonary arterial circulation. This appears to result from decreased tone in pre-capillary arterioles. In human HPS, enhanced pulmonary production of nitric oxide (NO) has been implicated as a vasodilator. Exhaled NO levels, a measure of pulmonary production, are increased in cirrhotic patients with HPS and normalise after OLT [29–31], as HPS resolves. In addition, acute inhibition of NO production or action with N^G-nitro-L-arginine methyl ester (L-NAME) or methylene blue, respectively, transiently improve HPS [32–34]. However, the mechanisms of increased endogenous NO production and its relationship to the presence of portal hypertension, the hyperdynamic circulation and the degree of liver injury, remain uncertain. In addition, whether other mediators such as haem oxygenase derived carbon monoxide (CO) [35] might contribute to intrapulmonary vasodilatation is not yet established.

Chronic common bile duct ligation (CBDL) in the rat is the only established model that reproduces the physiological features of human HPS [36,37] (Plate 2, *facing p.* 204). It is unique among rodent models of cirrhosis and/or portal hypertension in that other commonly used models such as thioacetamide-induced cirrhosis and partial portal vein ligation do not result in the development of HPS [38]. Early studies in CBDL animals focussed on the vasoconstrictor role of eicosanoids and on an increase in intravascular macrophage-like cells [39,40]. Subsequent work identified increased pulmonary vascular endothelial nitric oxide synthase (eNOS) as a major source of pulmonary NO production [41–43] and demonstrated that the administration of intravenous L-NAME improved hypoxaemia after CBDL [44]. Further studies have revealed that increased hepatic production of endothelin-1 (ET-1) with release into the circulation is an important mechanism for triggering the increase in pulmonary eNOS and the onset of vasodilatation after CBDL [42,45]. This effect appears to be driven by a shear stress mediated increase in pulmonary vascular endothelial endothelin B (ET_B) receptor expression which enhances endothelial NO production by ET-1 [46]. Accordingly, administration of a selective ET_B receptor antagonist to CBDL animals decreases pulmonary endothelial eNOS and ET_B receptor levels and significantly improves HPS [47]. Recent preliminary data supports that biliary epithelium is an important source of hepatic ET-1 production after CBDL and may explain the unique susceptibility of CBDL animals to HPS [48].

As experimental HPS progresses, there is a steady accumulation of intravascular macrophages. These cells transiently produce inducible nitric oxide synthase (iNOS) [43,44] and progressively produce haem oxygenase 1 (HO-1) [43,49]. These events contribute to further vasodilatation through production of iNOS derived NO and HO-1 derived CO. Accordingly, HO inhibition improves experimental HPS. In addition, prolonged treatment of

CBDL animals beginning at the time of ligation with norfloxacin to inhibit bacterial translocation and tumour necrosis factor-alpha (TNF-α) production, decreases macrophage accumulation and prevents the transient increase in iNOS [50], supporting that TNF-α contributes to macrophage accumulation. Further, pentoxifylline, a non-specific phosphodiesterase inhibitor that increases intracellular cAMP levels and also inhibits TNF-α production in macrophages [51], given over a similar time frame can prevent the onset or decrease the severity of HPS [52]. Both these agents initiated at the onset of liver injury influence the development of the hyperdynamic state and may modify ET_B receptor expression and endothelin related signalling events in the pulmonary microvasculature.

Findings to date in the CBDL model suggest that a sequence of events related in part to the increased vascular shear stress and to the hepatic ET-1 production may trigger the onset of experimental HPS. The observation that hepatic and plasma ET-1 levels increase within 1 week after CBDL [53] suggest that hepatic ET-1 production and release may occur with relatively modest degrees of bile duct proliferation. The finding that macrophages accumulate in the pulmonary microvasculature and may be influenced by TNF-α inhibition support that these cells may also contribute to vasodilatation. Plate 2 (*facing p.* 204) includes potential therapeutic targets for treatment in HPS based on experimental data.

Clinical features

The clinical features of HPS typically involve respiratory complaints and findings associated with chronic liver disease. The insidious onset of dyspnoea, particularly on exertion, is the most common complaint but is non-specific. Platypnoea (shortness of breath exacerbated by sitting up and improved by lying supine) and orthodeoxia (hypoxaemia exacerbated in the upright position) are classically described and result from a gravitational increase in blood flow through dilated vessels in the lung bases [54]. These findings appear to be relatively specific but are of low sensitivity [55]. Cough is not a common finding in HPS. Spider angiomata are also commonly reported in HPS but are seen frequently in cirrhotic patients without HPS. Finally, clubbing and distal cyanosis, when present in the setting of liver disease or portal hypertension should increase the suspicion for HPS [2].

Diagnosis

The diagnostic features of HPS include evidence of liver disease or portal hypertension, an elevated age-adjusted alveolar–arterial oxygen

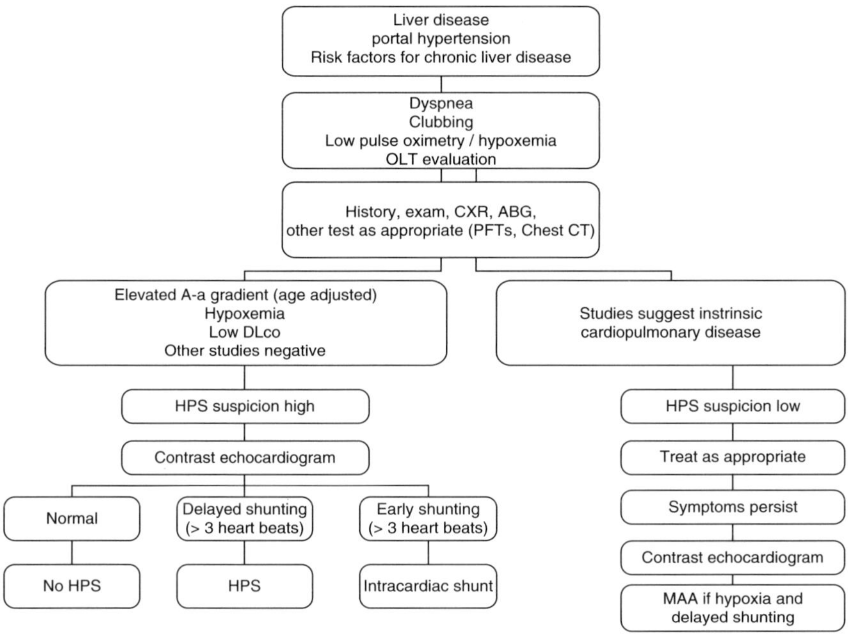

Fig. 40 Diagnosis of HPS.

gradient ($AaPO_2$), and evidence of intrapulmonary shunting. In the presence of co-existing cardiac or pulmonary disease, establishing a diagnosis of HPS can be difficult. Figure 40 presents an algorithm for the diagnosis of HPS. A logical evaluation of dyspnoea in the patient with liver disease or portal hypertension begins with a careful history and physical examination. Such an evaluation may lead the clinician to consider alternate, more common diagnoses such as COPD, CHF or myocardial ischaemia. However, if the common causes of dyspnoea can be excluded, and particularly if platypnoea or digital clubbing are present, further evaluation for HPS is warranted.

In patients with liver disease found to have dyspnoea or clubbing, or in those undergoing transplant evaluation, pulse oxymetry is a simple non-invasive screening test for hypoxaemia and a decreased SpO_2 should lead to arterial blood gas (ABG) analysis. However, caution must be exercised in interpreting a 'normal' SpO_2 as pulse oximetry may overestimate SaO_2 in nearly one-half of patients with cirrhosis [56]. Therefore, to reliably detect hypoxaemia ABG analysis should be considered when the SpO_2 values are 97% or less. In addition, if hypoxaemia or HPS is strongly suspected based on history and physical exam, ABG analysis should be performed while breathing room air regardless of pulse oximetry. In HPS, ABG reveals an elevated age-adjusted $AaPO_2$ with or without hypoxaemia. The expected room-air $AaPO_2$ at a given age can be calculated from the following equation: $AaPO_2 = 0.26 \text{ age } - 0.43$ [9].

If gas exchange abnormalities are detected, chest radiography and pulmonary function tests are performed to evaluate for the presence of other pulmonary abnormalities. Since cardiopulmonary disorders unrelated to liver disease or those related to ascites are more common than HPS, treating these abnormalities prior to further evaluation for HPS is reasonable in the absence of significant hypoxaemia (arterial oxygen pressure $PaO_2 < 70$ mmHg).

If HPS is suspected, contrast echocardiography is the preferred screening test for intrapulmonary vasodilatation [19]. Contrast echocardiography is performed by injecting agitated saline intravenously during normal transthoracic echocardiography, producing microbubbles that are visible on sonography. This bolus opacifies the right ventricle within seconds and in the absence of right-to-left shunting, bubbles are absorbed in the lungs. If an intracardiac shunt is present, contrast agent enters the left ventricle within three heartbeats (early shunting). If intrapulmonary shunting, characteristic of HPS is present, the left ventricle opacifies at least three heartbeats after the right (delayed shunting). Up to 40% of patients with cirrhosis have a positive contrast echocardiogram [19] although only a subset of these patients have sufficient vasodilatation to cause abnormal gas exchange and fulfil criteria for HPS. If a patient with liver disease or portal hypertension and hypoxaemia has a positive contrast echocardiogram in the absence of significant cardiopulmonary disease, a diagnosis of HPS has been made. A semi-quantitative scoring system for assessing intrapulmonary shunting during contrast echocardiography has been developed, although whether the degree of shunting predicts the degree of gas exchange abnormalities has not been established [57].

In hypoxaemic patients with both intrapulmonary vasodilatation and intrinsic cardiopulmonary disease, the technetium-labelled macroaggregated albumin scan (MAA scan) may be useful in defining the contribution of HPS to gas exchange abnormalities. In this test, radio-labelled aggregates of albumin measuring approximately 20 μm in diameter are infused into the venous system. Ordinarily, particles of this size become trapped in the pulmonary microvasculature and scintigraphy reveals nearly complete uptake in the lungs. In the presence of significant intrapulmonary shunting, a fraction of the macroaggregated albumin passes through the lungs and into the systemic circulation. Scintigraphy then also reveals uptake in other organs in addition to the lung, allowing the calculation of the shunt fraction. In one study, the MAA scan was positive only in patients with HPS and a $PaO_2 < 60$ mmHg and not in COPD patients with a similar degree of hypoxaemia [8]. However, the MAA scan is less sensitive than contrast echocardiogram and may be most useful in defining if HPS contributes to hypoxaemia in patients with concomitant obstructive pulmonary disease.

Pulmonary angiography is expensive and invasive and has a low sensitivity for detecting intrapulmonary vasodilatation. Therefore, it is not routinely utilised in the diagnosis of HPS. High-resolution chest computerised tomography (CT) and evaluation of pulmonary blood transit time are newer diagnostic modalities for assessing HPS [58,59]. In one study, the degree of pulmonary microvascular dilatation observed on chest CT correlated with the severity of gas exchange abnormalities in a small cohort of patients with HPS, suggesting that quantitation of intrapulmonary vasodilatation was possible. In another study, pulmonary transit time of erythrocytes, measured by echocardiographic analysis of human serum albumin–air microbubble complexes through the heart, also correlated with gas exchange abnormalities in a small group of patients with HPS. The utility of these techniques in evaluating HPS remains to be defined.

Summary

Hepatopulmonary syndrome occurs when pulmonary microvascular dilatation impairs arterial oxygenation in the setting of liver disease or portal hypertension. The syndrome is found in as many as 20% of cirrhotics and should be considered in any patient with chronic liver disease who develops dyspnoea or hypoxaemia. The presence of HPS increases mortality in the setting of cirrhosis and may influence the frequency and severity of complications of portal hypertension. The recognition in experimental models that a unique sequence of molecular alterations leads to ET-1 and TNF-α modulation of pulmonary microvascular tone may lead to the development of novel and effective medical therapies. Contrast echocardiography and standard cardiopulmonary testing are generally sufficient to make the diagnosis of HPS but further testing may be needed in patients who have both intrinsic cardiopulmonary disease and intrapulmonary vasodilatation. Treatment consists of supplemental oxygen and consideration of OLT if significant hypoxaemia is present.

PORTOPULMONARY HYPERTENSION

Definition

Portopulmonary hypertension (POPH) is defined as the presence of pulmonary arterial hypertension occurring in the setting of portal hypertension with or without liver disease. Pulmonary arterial hypertension is present when a mean pulmonary artery (PA) pressure > 25 mmHg and a pulmonary capillary wedge pressure < 15 mmHg occur in the setting of portal hypertension [4,60]. An elevated transpulmonary gradient (mean PA pressure − pulmonary capillary wedge pressure > 10 mmHg) and/or pulmonary vascular resistance (> 240 dyne/s/cm^{-5}) are additional criteria used in the definition of this syndrome, particularly when volume overload is present.

Epidemiology and outcome

Portopulmonary hypertension is found most commonly in patients with cirrhosis and portal hypertension. However, it has also been observed in disorders characterised by portal hypertension without cirrhosis supporting that portal hypertension is an important predisposing condition [3]. In an autopsy series of 17,901 specimens, pathological changes consistent with pulmonary hypertension were found in 0.73% of patients with cirrhosis compared to a prevalence of 0.13% in subjects without chronic liver disease [61]. A subsequent prospective study of 507 patients with portal hypertension who underwent right heart catheterisation revealed a 2% prevalence of POPH [62]. More recently, studies in patients referred for liver transplantation have found an even higher prevalence of this disorder with reported values ranging from 3.5% to 16% [63–66]. The prevalence and severity of POPH do not appear to correlate with the degree of hepatic synthetic dysfunction or the severity of portal hypertension [62]. Together, these findings support that POPH is a relatively common disorder in patients with cirrhosis.

An important feature of POPH, relevant to portal hypertension, is the finding that right-sided cardiac pressures are elevated. The consequences of elevated right-sided pressures in POPH on portal hypertension and varices have not been directly studied, but it is logical to assume that they would exacerbate underlying portal hypertension. In addition, β-adrenergic blockers are generally avoided to prevent worsening of right heart function. Therefore, the severity of portal hypertension may be worsened and therapeutic options altered in the setting of POPH.

Survival in POPH is also not clearly defined, particularly taking into account medical therapies and OLT. In the pre-OLT era, a mean survival of 15 months and a 58% mortality at 1 year were found in retrospective studies [62,67]. In patients not medically treated, a 5-year survival of 30% was found [68]. When evaluated, mortality appears to be equally related to complications of pulmonary hypertension and to liver disease. Therefore, the presence of POPH appears to adversely influence survival in patients with cirrhosis and may influence the course of portal hypertension.

Liver transplantation and POPH

The efficacy of liver transplantation as a treatment for POPH is controversial. Based on retrospective data and clinical experience, severe POPH (mean PA pressure > 50 mmHg) is a contraindication to transplantation due to perioperative mortality of approximately 40% and lack of reversibility of pulmonary hypertension [69,70]. Patients with mild POPH (mean PA pressure < 35 mmHg) appear to have no increase in perioperative cardiopulmonary mortality after liver transplantation, although the results of long-term follow-up and documentation of resolution of pulmonary hypertension has not been undertaken [71]. The outcome after liver transplantation in intermediate severity POPH (mean PA pressure 35–50 mmHg) and in patients who have improvement in PA pressures on long-term medical therapy is less well defined and requires further evaluation [69]. Although case reports have demonstrated successful outcomes after combination lung–liver or heart–lung–liver transplantation, limited organ availability and technical challenges limit the feasibility of such approaches for POPH [72].

Pathogenesis

The underlying mechanisms in POPH remain incompletely understood and no animal models have been developed. To date, all patients with POPH have been found to have portal hypertension, supporting that some consequence of elevated portal pressures is critical for the development of pulmonary hypertension [62]. Accordingly, two consequences of portal hypertension, the hyperdynamic circulatory state, causing increased vascular shear stress and portosystemic shunting causing altered production or metabolism of vasoactive substances have been hypothesised to contribute to vascular changes in POPH [3]. A number of specific endothelial and circulating factors (prostacyclin, thromboxane, serotonin, ET-1) as well as genetic polymorphisms in genes regulating vascular proliferative responses (serotonin, TGF-β receptor superfamily) might contribute to POPH, but have not been directly evaluated. In addition, the finding that either HPS or POPH may occur in the same clinical setting suggest that these two entities may share underlying pathogenetic mechanisms. One emerging hypothesis based on data from experimental HPS and on the recent demonstration that endothelin receptor antagonists may be useful in POPH, suggests that the degree of endothelial dysfunction or injury may determine the response to ET-1 overexpression. Specifically, vasoproliferation and inflammation may develop in the setting of greater endothelial dysfunction/injury and lead to POPH, or vasodilatation may result with less endothelial dysfunction/injury leading to HPS (Plate 3, *facing p.* 204).

Diagnosis

Since a number of patients with POPH may be asymptomatic and the diagnostic utility of various clinical features (systemic hypertension, accentuated P_2, electrocardiographic and chest radiographic abnormalities) is low [64,73], the diagnosis of POPH requires a high index of suspicion. In general, in patients not being evaluated for liver transplantation, the presence of 'compatible' symptoms and signs and/or the exclusion of other cardiopulmonary diseases signals the need for screening for POPH. In all patients being evaluated for liver transplantation, regardless of signs or symptoms, screening is warranted, because the presence of POPH may influence transplant candidacy [71].

Transthoracic Doppler echocardiography is the best non-invasive screening study to detect POPH. If combined with intravenous contrast injection, screening for HPS and POPH can be accomplished at the same time. The presence of pulmonary hypertension is suggested by an increased estimated PA systolic pressure (derived from measuring the velocity of the tricuspid regurgitant jet) pulmonary valve insufficiency, right atrial enlargement and/or right ventricular hypertrophy or dilatation. Several recent studies have evaluated the utility of estimated PA systolic pressure measurements in the diagnosis of POPH [66,73,74]. In these studies, estimated PA systolic pressures used to define an elevated value ranged from 30–50 mmHg. In each study, between 10–15% of patients had elevated estimated PA systolic pressures by echocardiography and roughly half of these patients were confirmed to have POPH on subsequent testing. In the most recent prospective study, Doppler echocardiography had positive and negative predictive values of 59% and 100% respectively in detecting POPH [66]. However, the precise methods for estimating PA systolic pressures have not been standardised between studies and may have influenced the operating characteristics of echocardiographic screening. From a practical perspective, using an estimated PA systolic pressure of $>$ 40–45 mmHg to trigger further evaluation, particularly if right atrial and/or right ventricular abnormalities are also present is likely to detect almost all patients with POPH. The false positive rate for echocardiography most commonly results from elevated pulmonary venous pressures due to the hyperdynamic circulatory state and volume overload in cirrhosis [66].

Patients with suggestive echocardiographic findings should undergo right heart catheterisation to confirm elevated mean PA pressure and to exclude pulmonary venous hypertension. Direct measurement of PA pressures, pulmonary capillary wedge pressure, cardiac output and calculation of systemic and pulmonary vascular resistance are included. Vasodilator responsiveness with a number of agents, most frequently NO and/or epoprostenol, is often undertaken in those with confirmed POPH in an effort to predict a favourable response to long-term vasodilator therapy [3]. However, the utility of vasodilator testing in the management of POPH has not been studied.

Summary

Portopulmonary hypertension results when pulmonary arterial hypertension develops in the setting of portal hypertension. This process occurs in up to 6% of patients being evaluated for OLT. Mortality appears to be increased in patients with POPH, and its presence may specifically influence the treatment and outcomes related to portal hypertension. The use of OLT in moderate to severe POPH is controversial as perioperative mortality is significantly increased. The pathogenesis of POPH is not well understood, although pulmonary endothelial dysfunction/injury may play a key role. Echocardiography is the best screening test for POPH and should be performed in all patients undergoing OLT evaluation because a significant number of patients with POPH are asymptomatic.

REFERENCES

1 Sood G, Fallon MB, Niwas S *et al* Utility of a dyspnea-fatigue index for screening liver transplant candidates for hepatopulmonary syndrome. *Hepatology* 1998;**28**: 2319 (abstract).
2 Fallon M, Abrams G. Pulmonary dysfunction in chronic liver disease. *Hepatology* 2000;**32**: 859–865.
3 Budhiraja R, Hassoun PM. Portopulmonary hypertension: a tale of two circulations. *Chest* 2003;**123**: 562–576.
4 Rodriguez-Roisin R, Krowka MJ, Herve P, Fallon MB, on behalf of the ERS Task Force Pulmonary-Hepatic Vascular Disorders Scientific Committee ERS Task Force PHD Scientific Committee. Pulmonary-hepatic vascular disorders (PHD). *Eur Respir J* 2004;**24**: 861–880.
5 Rodriguez-Roison R, Agusti AG, Roca J. The hepatopulmonary syndrome: new name, old complexities. *Thorax* 1992;**47**: 897–902.
6 Lange PA, Stoller JK. The hepatopulmonary syndrome. *Ann Intern Med* 1995;**122**: 521–529.
7 Martinez G, Barbera J, Navasa M, Roca J, Visa J, Rodriguez-Roisin R. Hepatopulmonary syndrome associated with cardiorespiratory disease. *J Hepatol* 1999;**30**: 882–889.

8 Abrams G, Nanda N, Dubovsky E, Krowka M, Fallon M. Use of macroaggregated albumin lung perfusion scan to diagnose hepatopulmonary syndrome: a new approach. *Gastroenterology* 1998;**114**: 752–758.
9 Harris E, Kenyon A, Nisbet H, Seelye E, Whitlock R. The normal alveolar-arterial oxygen-tension gradient in man. *Clin Sci Mol Med* 1974;**46**: 89–104.
10 Krowka MJ, Dickson ER, Cortese DA. Hepatopulmonary syndrome. Clinical observations and lack of therapeutic response to somatostatin analogue. *Chest* 1993;**104**: 515–521.
11 Saunders KB, Fernando SSD, Dalton HR, Joseph A. Spontaneous improvement in a patient with the hepatopulmonary syndrome assessed by serial exercise tests. *Thorax* 1994;**49**: 725–727.
12 Schenk P, Schoniger-Hekele M, Fuhrmann V, Madl C, Silberhumer G, Muller C. Prognostic significance of the hepatopulmonary syndrome in patients with cirrhosis. *Gastroenterology* 2003;**125**: 1042–1052.
13 Javaheri S, Almoosa KF, Saleh K, Mendenhall CL. Hypocapnia is not a predictor of central sleep apnea in patients with cirrhosis. *Am J Respir Crit Care Med* 2005;**171**: 908–911.
14 Arguedas M, Abrams GA, Krowka MJ, Fallon MB. Prospective evaluation of outcomes and predictors of mortality in patients with hepatopulmonary syndrome undergoing liver transplantation. *Hepatology* 2003;**37**: 192–197.
15 Kaspar MD, Ramsay MA, Shuey CB, Jr, Levy MF, Klintmalm GG. Severe pulmonary hypertension and amelioration of hepatopulmonary syndrome after liver transplantation. *Liver Transpl Surg* 1998;**4**: 177–179.
16 Martinez-Palli G, Barbera JA, Taura P, Cirera I, Visa J, Rodriguez-Roisin R. Severe portopulmonary hypertension after liver transplantation in a patient with preexisting hepatopulmonary syndrome. *J Hepatol* 1999;**31**: 1075–1079.
17 http://www.unos.org.
18 Martinez G, Barbera J, Visa J *et al.* Hepatopulmonary syndrome in candidates for liver transplantation. *J Hepatol* 2001;**34**: 756–758.
19 Abrams GA, Jaffe CC, Hoffer PB, Binder HJ, Fallon MB. Diagnostic utility of contrast echocardiography and lung perfusion scan in patients with hepatopulmonary syndrome. *Gastroenterology* 1995;**109**: 1283–1288.
20 Schenk P, Fuhrmann V, Madl C *et al.* Hepatopulmonary syndrome: prevalence and predictive value of various cut offs for arterial oxygenation and their clinical consequences. *Gut* 2002;**51**: 853–859.
21 Krowka M, Wiseman G, Burnett O *et al.* Hepatopulmonary syndrome: a prospective study of relationships between severity of liver disease, PaO_2 response to 100% oxygen, and brain uptake after 99mTc MAA lung scanning. *Chest* 2000;**118**: 615–624.
22 Whyte M, Hughes J, Peters A, Ussov W, Patel S, Burroughs A. Analysis of intrapulmonary right to left shunt in hepatopulmonary syndrome. *J Hepatol* 1998;**29**: 85–93.
23 Dimand RJ, Heyman MB, Bass NM *et al.* Hepatopulmonary syndrome: response to hepatic transplantation. *Hepatology* 1991;**141** (Pt. 2): 55A (Abstract).
24 Abrams G, Fallon M. The hepatopulmonary syndrome. *Clin Liver Dis* 1997;**1**: 185–200.

25 Binay K, Sen S, Biswas PK, Sanyal R, Jumdar DM, Biswas J. Hepatopulmonary syndrome in inferior vena cava obstruction responding to cavoplasty. *Gastroenterology* 2000;**118**: 192–196.
26 Gupta D, Vijaya DR, Gupta R *et al*. Prevalence of hepatopulmonary syndrome in cirrhosis and extrahepatic portal venous obstruction. *Am J Gastroenterol* 2001;**96**: 3395–3399.
27 Regev A, Yeshurun M, Rodriguez M *et al*. Transient hepatopulmonary syndrome in a patient with acute hepatitis A. *J Viral Hep* 2001;**8**: 83–86.
28 Teuber G, Teupe C, Dietrich C, Caspary W, Buhl R, Zeuzem S. Pulmonary dysfunction in non-cirrhotic patients with chronic viral hepatitis. *Eur J Intern Med* 2002;**13**: 311–318.
29 Rolla G, Brussino L, Colagrande P *et al*. Exhaled nitric oxide and oxygenation abnormalities in hepatic cirrhosis. *Hepatology* 1997;**26**: 842–847.
30 Rolla G, Brussino L, Colagrande P. Exhaled nitric oxide and impaired oxygenation in cirrhotic patients before and after liver transplantation. *Ann Intern Med* 1998;**129**: 375–378.
31 Cremona G, Higenbottam TW, Mayoral V *et al*. Elevated exhaled nitric oxide in patients with hepatopulmonary syndrome. *Eur Respir J* 1995;**8**: 1883–1885.
32 Rolla G, Bucca C, Brussino L. Methylene blue in the hepatopulmonary syndrome. *N Eng J Med* 1994;**331**: 1098.
33 Brussino L, Bucca C, Morello M, Scappaticci E, Mauro M, Rolla G. Effect on dyspnoea and hypoxaemia of inhaled NG-nitro-L-arginine methyl ester in hepatopulmonary syndrome. *Lancet* 2003;**362**: 43–44.
34 Schenk P, Madl C, Rezale-Majd S, Lehr S, Muller C. Methylene blue improves the hepatopulmonary syndrome. *Ann Int Med* 2000;**133**: 701–706.
35 Arguedas MR, Drake BB, Kapoor A, Fallon MB. Carboxyhemoglobin levels in cirrhotic patients with and without hepatopulmonary syndrome. *Gastroenterology* 2005;**128**: 328–333.
36 Chang SW, Ohara N. Pulmonary circulatory dysfunction in rats with biliary cirrhosis. An animal model of the hepatopulmonary syndrome. *Am Rev Respir Dis* 1992;**145**: 798–805.
37 Fallon MB, Abrams GA, McGrath JW, Hou Z, Luo B. Common bile duct ligation in the rat: a model of intrapulmonary vasodilatation and hepatopulmonary syndrome. *Am J Physiol* 1997;**272**: G779–G784.
38 Luo B, Liu L, Tang L, Zhang J, Ling Y, Fallon MB. ET-1 and TNF-{alpha} in HPS: analysis in prehepatic portal hypertension and biliary and nonbiliary cirrhosis in rats. *Am J Physiol Gastrointest Liver Physiol* 2004;**286**: G294–G303.
39 Chang SW, Ohara N. Increased pulmonary vascular permeability in rats with biliary cirrhosis: role of thomboxane A_2. *Am J Physiol* 1992;**264**: L245–L252.
40 Chang SW, Ohara N. Chronic biliary obstruction induces pulmonary intravascular phagocytosis and endotoxin sensitivity in rats. *J Clin Invest* 1994;**94**: 2009–2019.
41 Fallon MB, Abrams GA, Luo B, Hou Z, Dai J, Ku DD. The role of endothelial nitric oxide synthase in the pathogenesis of a rat model of hepatopulmonary syndrome. *Gastroenterology* 1997;**113**: 606–614.
42 Luo B, Abrams GA, Fallon MB. Endothelin-1 in the rat bile duct ligation model of hepatopulmonary syndrome: correlation with pulmonary dysfunction. *J Hepatol* 1998;**29**: 571–578.

43 Zhang J, Ling Y, Luo B *et al.* Analysis of pulmonary heme oxygenase-1 and nitric oxide synthase alterations in experimental hepatopulmonary syndrome. *Gastroenterology* 2003;**125**: 1441–1451.
44 Nunes H, Lebrec D, Mazmanian M *et al.* Role of nitric oxide in hepatopulmonary syndrome in cirrhotic rats. *Am J Respir Crit Care Med* 2001;**164**: 879–885.
45 Zhang M, Luo B, Chen SJ, Abrams GA, Fallon MB. Endothelin-1 stimulation of endothelial nitric oxide synthase in the pathogenesis of hepatopulmonary syndrome. *Am J Physiol* 1999;**277**: G944–G952.
46 Luo B, Liu L, Tang L *et al.* Increased pulmonary vascular endothelin B receptor expression and responsiveness to endothelin-1 in cirrhotic and portal hypertensive rats: a potential mechanism in experimental hepatopulmonary syndrome. *J Hepatol* 2003;**38**: 556–563.
47 Ling Y, Zhang J, Luo B *et al.* The role of endothelin-1 and the endothelin B receptor in the pathogenesis of experimental hepatopulmonary syndrome. *Hepatology* 2004;**39**: 1593–1602.
48 Luo B, Tang L, Zhang J *et al.* Biliary epithelial derived endothelin-1: an endocrine mediator of experimental hepatopulmonary syndrome. *Hepatology* 2004;**40**: 214A.
49 Carter EP, Hartsfield CL, Miyazono M, Jakkula M, Morris KG Jr, McMurtry IF. Regulation of heme oxygenase-1 by nitric oxide during hepatopulmonary syndrome. *Am J Physiol – Lung Cell Mol Physiol* 2002;**283**: L346–L353.
50 Rabiller A, Nunes H, Lebrec D *et al.* Prevention of gram-negative translocation reduces the severity of hepatopulmonary syndrome. *Am J Respir Crit Care Med* 2002;**166**: 514–517.
51 Ward A, Clissold S. Pentoxifylline. A review of its pharmacodynamic and pharmacokinetic properties, and its therapeutic efficacy. *Drugs* 1987;**34**: 50–97.
52 Sztrymf B, Rabiller A, Nunes H *et al.* Prevention of hepatopulmonary syndrome by pentoxifylline in cirrhotic rats. *Eur Respir J* 2004;**23**: 752–758.
53 Luo B, Tang L, Wang Z *et al.* Cholangiocyte endothelin-1 and transforming growth factor-beta1 production in rat experimental hepatopulmonary syndrome. *Gastroenterology* 2005;**129**: 682–695.
54 Gomez F, Martinez-Palli G, Barbera J, Roca J, Navasa M, Rodriguez-Roisin R. Gas exchange mechanism of orthodeoxia in hepatopulmonary syndrome. *Hepatology* 2004;**40**: 660–666.
55 Martinez GP, Barbera JA, Visa J *et al.* Hepatopulmonary syndrome in candidates for liver transplantation. *J Hepatol* 2001;**34**: 651–657.
56 Abrams GA, Sanders MK, Fallon MB. Utility of pulse oximetry in the detection of arterial hypoxemia in liver transplant candidates. *Liver Transpl* 2002;**8**: 391–396.
57 Vedrinne JM, Duperret S, Bizollon T *et al.* Comparison of transesophageal and transthoracic contrast echocardiography for detection of an intrapulmonary shunt in liver disease. *Chest* 1997;**111**: 1236–1240.
58 Katsuta Y, Honma H, Zhang X *et al.* Pulmonary blood transit time and impaired arterial oxygenation in patients with chronic liver disease. *J Gastroenterol* 2005;**40**: 57–63.
59 Lee KN, Lee HJ, Shin WW *et al.* Hypoxemia and liver cirrhosis (hepatopulmonary syndrome) in eight patients: comparison of the central and peripheral pulmonary vasculature. *Radiology* 1999;**211**: 549–553.

60 Rich S, Dantzker D, Ayres S *et al.* Primary pulmonary hypertension: a national prospective study. *Ann Int Med* 1987;**107**: 216–223.
61 McDonnell P, Toye P, Hutchins G. Primary pulmonary hypertension and cirrhosis: are they related? *Am Rev Respir Dis* 1983;**127**: 437–441.
62 Hadengue A, Benhayoun M, Lebrec D, Benhamou J. Pulmonary hypertension complicating portal hypertension: prevalence and relation to splanchnic hemodynamics. *Gastroenterology* 1991;**100**: 520–528.
63 Benjaminov FS, Prentice M, Sniderman KW, Siu S, Liu P, Wong F. Portopulmonary hypertension in decompensated cirrhosis with refractory ascites. *Gut* 2003;**52**: 1355–1362.
64 Kuo P, Plotkin J, Johnson L *et al.* Distinctive clinical features of portopulmonary hypertension. *Chest* 1997;**112**: 980–986.
65 Plevak D, Krowka M, Rettke S, Dunn W, Southorn P. Successful liver transplantation in patients with mild to moderate pulmonary hypertension. *Transplant Proc* 1993;**25**: 1840.
66 Colle I, Moreau R, Godinho E *et al.* Portopulmonary hypertension in candidates for liver transplantation: diagnosis at evaluation comparing Doppler echocardiography with cardiac catheterization and incidence on the waiting list. *Hepatology* 2003;**37**: 401–409.
67 Robalino B, Moodie D. Association between primary pulmonary hypertension and portal hypertension: analysis of its pathophysiology and clinical, laboratory and hemodynamic manifestations. *J Am Coll Cardiol* 1991;**17**: 492–498.
68 Swanson K, McGoon M, Krowka MJ. Survival in portopulmonary hypertension. *Am J Respir Crit Care Med* 2003;**167**: A683.
69 Mandell M, Groves B. Pulmonary hypertension in chronic liver disease. *Clin Chest Med* 1996;**17**: 17–33.
70 Krowka M. Hepatopulmonary syndromes. *Gut* 2000;**46**: 1–4.
71 Krowka M, Plevak D, Findlay J, Rosen C, Wiesner R, Krom R. Pulmonary hemodynamics and perioperative cardiopulmonary-related mortality in patients with portopulmonary hypertension undergoing liver transplantation. *Liver Transpl* 2000;**6**: 443–450.
72 Wallwork J, Calne R, Williams R. Tranplantation of liver, heart and lungs for primary biliary cirrhosis and primary pulmonary hypertension. *Lancet* 1987;**2**: 182–185.
73 Pilatis N, Jacobs L, Rerkpattanapipat P *et al.* Clinical predictors of pulmonary hypertension in patients undergoing liver transplant evaluation. *Liver Transpl* 2000;**6**: 85–91.
74 Torregrosa M, Genesca J, Gonzalez A *et al.* Role of Doppler echocardiography in the assessment of portopulmonary hypertension in liver transplantation candidates. *Transplantation* 2001;**71**: 572–574.

SESSION 4

Primary Prophylaxis for Variceal Bleeding

Norman D. Grace, Juan Carlos Garcia-Pagan, Mario Angelico, Richard Moreau, Agustin Albillos, Michael Schepke, Thomas D. Boyer and Naga Chalasani

INTRODUCTION

Over the past two decades, considerable progress has been made in the primary prophylaxis of variceal bleeding. With the widespread use of non-selective β-blockers, and more recently, variceal ligation, the risk of first variceal haemorrhage has been reduced by 50% to about 15% for large oesophageal varices [1]. The morbidity for a variceal haemorrhage has been dramatically reduced to 15% [2–4]. Nevertheless, variceal haemorrhage remains a very serious complication of cirrhosis and portal hypertension.

Five years ago, the Baveno III and Reston consensus conferences reached several conclusions relative to primary prophylaxis for oesophageal varices [5,6]. They recommended that all patients with cirrhosis and large varices (greater than 5 mm in diameter) who were compliant and had no contraindications to treatment, be offered non-selective β-blockers. Measurements of the hepatic venous pressure gradient (HVPG) at baseline and 3 months were felt to be helpful in assessing efficacy of treatment but not mandatory because of the relatively low risk of bleeding in patients not reaching the desired end points of a 20% reduction in HVPG or an HVPG below 12 mmHg. Concerns were expressed about the use of long acting nitrates as monotherapy for patients intolerant of or having contraindications to non-selective β-blockers. Studies supporting the use of endoscopic variceal ligation for high-risk patients were encouraging but it was felt that more data were needed before this technique could be generally recommended as an alternative to non-selective β-blockers. Finally, there was insufficient data to support the use of combination therapy, either pharmacological or combined with endoscopic therapy.

It was felt that patients with small varices should be monitored but data was insufficient to support initiating treatment at that stage. There was no benefit derived from follow-up endoscopy to monitor β-blocker therapy. Studies to evaluate the use of β-blockers in patients with gastric varices were needed. In the intervening five years, considerable progress has been achieved in some areas whereas little new information is available in others. This charge for Baveno IV is to evaluate new data generated over the last 5 years and to revise the prior recommendations as indicated.

Prophylaxis in patients with small oesophageal varices

M. Angelico

At the Baveno III conference it was agreed that the risk of bleeding in patients with small oesophageal varices is low. Also recognised was the low reproducibility in the diagnosis of small varices. In addition, it was noted that small varices may regress in alcoholic cirrhotics who are long-term abstainers. Based on these considerations and the limited and contradictory data on prophylactic treatment, it was concluded that there was no indication to treat patients with small varices and that more data were needed before a conclusion could be drawn about the usefulness of prophylaxis in these patients.

New data

A recent paper by Merli *et al.* [7] reported in a group of 93 patients with small varices prospectively followed with yearly upper endoscopy exams showed that the probability of variceal growth from small to medium or large is 12% at 1 year and 31% at 3 years. Independent predictors of variceal growth were alcoholic aetiology, Child–Pugh B or C score and presence of red wale marks at first examination. The authors confirmed that the risk of bleeding from small oesophageal varices is low (12% after 2 years) and is predicted by the presence of red wale markings.

In agreement with this finding, approximately one-third of the panel of experts in the current survey have indicated that they usually treat only patients with small varices who display red signs. In contrast, a small number of experts (13%) reported that they treat all patients with small varices whereas more than half do not treat these patients at all. However, the experts continue to use different methods to classify variceal size, making it quite difficult to compare different studies.

Theoretically, the end point of treating patients with small oesophageal varices is two-fold: first to avoid or delay the progression of small to large varices; second, to reduce the bleeding risk. Since small varices have a low rate of bleeding and bleeding occurs more frequently when varices are medium or large sized, one may assume that decreasing the rate of progression of small varices to larger sizes will ultimately result in a reduced bleeding rate. However, this assumption has not been demonstrated until recently [8].

To date, few data have been generated on the prophylactic treatment of patients with small varices. These include only the following: (1) one randomised study on prophylactic sclerotherapy versus no treatment which resulted in a disappointingly greater number of bleedings in the treated arms [9]; (2) the treated and untreated arms of previous randomised trials on the use of non-selective β-blockers, isosorbide mononitrate (ISMN) or their combination (Table 30) [10–15]; (3) two more recent randomised controlled trials (RCTs) specifically aimed at addressing this issue [8,16].

Previous trials reporting on the pharmacological prophylaxis of oesophageal varices which comprised a sizeable number of patients with small varices have included collectively a total of 179 patients in the treated arms and 177 untreated controls [10–15]. Yet, a number of problems make it difficult to evaluate the combined analysis of these studies. First, different treatment modalities have been used in the various studies and there is a wide variation in the methods used to classify variceal size and to define small varices; second, individual patient data are seldom reported; most importantly, there are a limited number of patients in individual trials who had small varices. In addition, the number of bleeding episodes in this subgroup is remarkably small (usually no more than two patients in each study). The small sample size does not achieve enough statistical power to make firm conclusions and also precludes the possibility of performing an adequate meta-analysis of the data.

Table 30 Previous RCTs reporting data on primary prophylaxis in patients with small varices.

	Treated with BB and/or IMN	Treated with placebo	Definition of small varices	Mean follow-up
Conn *et al.* 1991 USA, Spain	26 (prop) 2 (8%) bled	29 2 (7%) bled	Up to 3 mm	17 months
PROVA, 1991 Denmark, Norway	27 (prop) Bleeds unknw	28 Bleeds unknw	Grade 1	15 months
Merkel, 2000 Italy	2 (nad + IMN) Bleeds unknw	4 Bleeds unknw	F1 with red weal marks	55 months
Angelico, 1997 Italy	14 (prop) Bleeds unknw	13 (IMN) Bleeds unknw	F1	46 months
Garcia-Pagan, 2001 Spain	28 (IMN) Bleeds unknw	32 Bleeds unknw	≤ 5 mm	24 months
Garcia-Pagan, 2003 Spain	82 (prop) 2 (1.6%) bled	71 (prop + IMN) 1 (0.7%) bled	≤ 5 mm	24 months

The only two available studies specifically addressing the issue give more precise information; yet their results are divergent. Calés *et al.* [16] performed a double-blind trial including 206 cirrhotic patients, 80% of whom were of alcoholic aetiology, who were randomised to receive either 160 mg of propranolol or placebo. Patients were included in the study if they had no varices ($n = 79$) or varices less than 5 mm ($n = 127$) and if the Child–Pugh score was less than 13. Almost two-thirds of potential candidates were excluded from this study, mostly due to expected poor compliance, previous use of β-blockers or other vasoactive drugs. The 2-year results showed that the progression from small to large varices occurred in 31% of patients treated with propranolol and in only 14% of those receiving placebo, the difference being statistically significant ($p < 0.05$). Only three and four patients respectively in the two groups eventually bled during this period and nine and ten, respectively, died. Extending the follow-up to 3 years showed the same unfavourable trend in the propranolol treated group. These data strongly discouraged the prophylactic use of propranolol in this setting. It is interesting to note that the progression rate of varices from small to medium/large sized in the placebo arm in this study was close to that observed by Merli *et al.* [7] in their prospective evaluation of untreated patients.

Opposite results were recently obtained by Merkel *et al.* [8], who included 161 cirrhotics with small varices in a single-blinded RTC, where patients were randomised to receive nadolol or placebo. Patients were included if they had F1 varices according to Beppu *et al.* [17], and if the Child–Pugh score was < 12. In contrast to Calés' paper, a smaller though consistent proportion of these patients were of alcoholic aetiology. The cumulative risk of variceal growth up to 5 years was significantly lower ($p < 0.005$) in patients receiving nadolol, than in those receiving placebo, with a bleeding risk at the end of follow-up of 12% in the nadolol group compared to 22% in the placebo group. Notably, only two patients in the placebo group bled before variceal progression from small to large size. The cumulative probability of dying from hepatic causes did not differ between the two groups (50% versus 47%, respectively). These encouraging results are in clear contrast with those of Calés, for unexplained reasons. Differences between the two studies are shown in Table 31. The aetiology of the patients enrolled differed, as there were more alcoholics and less alcohol abstainers in the Calés' study [16]. In addition, the type of β-blocker also differed, as well as the mean daily dose (which in the French study was more than twice that in the Italian study). Finally, Calés' patients were more often males, were slightly younger and less compliant to treatment than those in the Merkel study [8]. Thus, it seems possible that a greater adherence to treatment combined with the use of

Table 31 Differences between Cales' and Merkel's study.

	Cales *et al.*	Merkel *et al.*
Number of patients	206	161
Males	66%	51%
Patients with small varices	62% (< 5 mm)	100% (F1)
Lost to follow-up	33%	13%
Mean age	52	56
Child–Pugh score	6.8	6.9
Alcoholic aetiology	80%	57%
Abstinence from alcohol	66%	81%
Type β-blocker	Propranolol	Nadolol
Daily β-blocker dose (mg)	160	62

a low-to-medium dose of a non-selective β-blocker may be necessary to delay the progression of variceal size, and that achievement of this result depends critically on abstinence from alcohol. An indirect argument in favour of the usefulness of prophylactic β-blockade in this setting is given by the observation of Escorsell *et al.* [18] who showed that the response to a single dose of β-blockers is considerably greater in compensated cirrhotics without varices than in those with varices, particularly in those with an HVPG > 11 mmHg. Unfortunately, there are no data available on this issue in patients with small varices after prolonged administration of β-blockers.

Based on these data we conclude that prophylactic treatment with non-selective β-blockers can be considered in patients with small oesophageal varices with the primary intent to reduce variceal growth, thus delaying bleeding, which is an uncommon event in the presence of small varices. Yet, more data are required before this suggestion can be accepted as a formal recommendation. Further data are also required to explore whether the benefit of non-selective β-blockade is restricted to patients with small varices with specific HVPG values (e.g. > 10–12 mmHg) or to those with good liver function or applies also to patients with decompensated liver disease.

Gastric varices

Almost all the experts involved in the current survey stated that they usually perform some sort of treatment in patients with gastric varices. Of these, 55% declare that they treat prophylactically only patients with evidence of large gastric varices. This indication, however, is not currently supported by any evidence, but is based only on common sense. For example, one reason to treat these patients prophylactically with β-blockers is that most patients with gastric varices also have oesophageal varices. Another reason is that there is often a direct connection between gastric and oesophageal varices. A third reason is that patients to be treated could be selected on the basis of HVPG measurements.

However, based on the currently available data no recommendation about prophylaxis of gastric varices can be made until results of RCTs become available.

Is there a rationale outside research to monitor HVPG in primary prophylaxis?

R. Moreau

Four studies performed in patients with cirrhosis have monitored HVPG in the context of primary prophylaxis [19–22]. The pioneer study by Groszmann *et al.* was a double-blind randomised trial comparing propranolol to placebo in 102 patients with cirrhosis [19]. In this study, there was no pre-specified haemodynamic end point but HVPG was measured at different time points during a follow-up (1 year). Thirteen patients had an initial bleeding episode. Interestingly, all bleeders had an HVPG of more than 12 mmHg. A study by Merkel *et al.* enrolled 49 patients treated with nadolol alone or nadolol plus isosorbide-5-mononitrate (ISMN) [20]. Patients were followed-up for 5 years. This was the first study to use the concept of haemodynamic responder defined by a decrease in HVPG below the value of 12 mmHg or of at least 20% from the baseline value. There were 30 haemodynamic responders (61%) and 9 first bleeders (18%). The proportion of bleeders was 80% in haemodynamic non-responders and only 20% in haemodynamic responders [20]. Two other studies [21,22] used the same haemodynamic end points as that used in the Merkel's study. A study by Bureau *et al.* enrolled 20 patients treated with propranolol alone or propranolol plus ISMN [21]. Follow-up lasted 28 months. There were 14 haemodynamic responders (70%) and 2 first bleeders (10%). The proportion of bleeders was 100% in haemodynamic non-responders and 0% in responders [21]. Finally, a study by Turnes *et al.* enrolled 91 patients treated with propranolol alone or propranolol plus ISMN [22]. Patients were followed for up to 8 years. There were 25 haemodynamic responders (35%) and 16 first bleeders (23%). The proportion of bleeders was 87.5% in haemodynamic non-responders and 12.5% in responders [22]. In summary, when the results of the four studies are pooled, it appears that among 100 patients with cirrhosis and oesophageal varices, there are 45 haemodynamic non-responders and 15 first bleeders. Among these first bleeders there are 13 haemodynamic non-responders. In other words, the proportion of bleeders was 29% in haemodynamic non-responders and only 2% in responders. It is important to note that the mean frequency of first bleeding measured in patients treated with endoscopic band ligation is only 14%, a figure that is lower than the 29% incidence of bleeding in haemodynamic non-responders. Further studies are needed in this field.

From a clinical viewpoint, it would be useful to have non-invasive methods able to predict the severity of portal hypertension, for example in patients with compensated hepatitis C-related virus (HCV)-induced cirrhosis. Before commenting on this, it should be kept in mind that, in the cirrhotic liver, morphological changes (including fibrosis) play an important role in the increase in the intrahepatic vascular resistance and thus in the pathogenesis of portal hypertension [23]. It is reasonable to speculate that the degree of liver fibrosis and that of portal hypertension are positively correlated. Therefore, surrogate markers assessing the degree of liver fibrosis might also be used as surrogate markers of the degree of portal hypertension. Fibrotest which takes into account changes in five biological variables (α2-macroglobulin, total bilirubin, gamma-GT, haptoglobin and apolipoprotein A1) has been proposed to assess liver fibrosis in HCV-positive patients [24]. Fibrotest and HVPG have been measured in 95 patients with histologically proven cirrhosis due to alcohol, HCV or other causes [25]. Fibrotest was significantly lower in patients with HVPG $\leq$ 12 mmHg than in those with HVPG $>$ 12 mmHg [25]. These findings suggest that, in patients with cirrhosis, markers of fibrosis may be useful to predict the degree of portal hypertension. Markers other than Fibrotest have been proposed to assess liver fibrosis in HCV-positive patients. These include other biomarkers [26–31] and the FibroScan [32]. It would be interesting to evaluate the performance of all these markers of fibrosis in predicting the degree of portal hypertension.

Pharmacological alternatives to β-blockers in primary prophylaxis

A. Albillos

Alternatives to β-blockers for primary prophylaxis against variceal bleeding are required in two possible settings: (1) to treat patients with contraindication or intolerance to β-blockers or (2) to reduce the residual risk of bleeding in a patient on β-blockers.

Prophylaxis for first variceal bleeding using β-blockers is not feasible in 20% of cirrhotic patients because of contraindications or intolerance to these agents [1,14]. The administration of ISMN alone reduces portal pressure by 7.5% [33] and has been proposed as a pharmacological alternative to β-blockers. However, a double-blind RCT comparing ISMN and placebo in patients with contraindication or intolerance to β-blockers has indicated that ISMN is ineffective at preventing first variceal bleeding [14]. In this study, there was a trend towards a higher 1-year actuarial probability of first bleeding in patients on ISMN compared to those on placebo (29% versus 16%, respectively). The number of patients bleeding while on ISMN is in keeping with the results of a meta-analysis comparing the use of ISMN and β-blockers for the primary prophylaxis of variceal bleeding (Table 32) [13,34,35]. In this meta-analysis, the bleeding rate was found to be significantly lower in patients on β-blockers (16%) than in those on ISMN (27%) (RR: 0.63, 95% CI: 0.40–0.98); the two groups show no difference in mortality. Thus, the available evidence does not support ISMN monotherapy for primary prophylaxis, even in patients with contraindication or intolerance to β-blockers.

Table 32 RCTs of β-blockers compared with isosorbide-5-mononitrate for primary prophylaxis of variceal bleeding.

		Bleeding		Mortality	
Author, year	Patients	BB	ISMN	BB	ISMN
Angelico, 1997	118	23%	28%	39%	49%
Borroni, 2002	52*	8%	37%	32%	26%
Lui, 2002	128	14%	23%	17%	29%
Total	298	16%	27%	28%	36%
RR (95% CI)		0.63 (0.40–0.98)		0.78 (0.57–1.08)	

BB, β-blockers; ISMN, Isosorbide-5-mononitrate; RR, relative risk; CI, confidence interval

* Only patients with ascites

The residual risk of first bleeding in patients with varices of any size on β-blockers is 10%, and increases to 15% if only patients with large varices are considered [1]. Adding to β-blockers, drugs such as vasodilators or diuretics can improve the HVPG drop achieved and increase the proportion of patients with a clinically significant reduction in HVPG (to $\leq$ 12 mmHg or $>$ 20% responders). β-blockers provide a significant HVPG reduction in about 60% of patients without previous variceal bleeding [20]. Addition of ISMN enhances the fall in HVPG produced by β-blockers alone, and increases the rate of responders by about one-third [36,37]. Based on this rationale, the efficacy of β-blockers + ISMN and of β-blockers alone was compared in three RCTs totalling 552 patients [12,15,38]. Meta-analysis of these studies revealed a non-significantly lower bleeding rate and greater occurrence of side effects in the combination therapy group, along with similar mortality (Table 33). The bleeding rate in the combination therapy group was also similar to that for β-blockers alone, when only patients with large varices in the trial by Garcia-Pagán *et al.* were analysed (20% versus 17%, respectively) [15]. Thus, contrary to the secondary prophylaxis setting in which ISMN improves the efficacy of β-blockers [39], the available evidence does not support the use of β-blockers + ISMN for primary prophylaxis. A plausible explanation for these findings could depend on two facts: (1) contrary to patients with previous bleeding, most of those without episodes of previous bleeding respond to β-blockers [19,20], and (2) the addition of ISMN to the treatment regime further reduces HVPG in non-responders to β-blockers, but not in responders [37].

Spironolactone and a low-sodium diet lower portal pressure in patients with cirrhosis by diminishing the increased plasma volume and splanchnic blood flow [40]. Hence, in a trial comparing the efficacy of nadolol and

Table 33 RCTs of β-blockers compared with β-blockers plus isosorbide-5-mononitrate for primary prophylaxis of variceal bleeding.

		Bleeding		Mortality		Side effects	
Author, year	Patients	BB	BB + ISMN	BB	BB + ISMN	BB	BB + ISMN
Pietrosi, 1999	57	37%	17%	18%	10%		
Merkel, 2000	146	22%	11%	40%	35%	5.4%	11%
Garcia-Pagán, 2000	349	8.6%	8.6%	6.3%	8.0%	5.7%	13%
Total	552	15%	10%	17%	15%	5.6%	12%
RR (95% CI)		1.50 (0.95–2.36)		1.10 (0.77–1.58)		0.86 (0.58–1.27)	

BB, β-blockers; ISMN, Isosorbide-5-mononitrate; RR, relative risk; CI, confidence interval spironolactone with that of nadolol alone for the primary prophylaxis of variceal bleeding [41], similar HVPG reductions (−16 ± 12% versus −11 ± 14%), bleeding rates (17% versus 14%) and 2-year mortality rates (2% versus 6%) were achieved.

Other drugs and combinations have been tested. Of these, the most promising is carvedilol, a non-selective β-blocker with intrinsic anti-α1-adrenergic activity, and as such, its haemodynamic effects mimic those of the β-blockers + prazosin combination [37], but it has not yet been tested in RCTs with clinical end points. Table 34 describes the three studies that have addressed the haemodynamic effects of this drug [42–44]. When compared with propranolol in a randomised trial performed on patients without previous bleeding, carvedilol achieved a greater rate of responders in terms of a target reduction in HVPG (54% versus 23%, $p < 0.05$) [44]. In this study, mean arterial pressure decreased by 11% despite careful titration of the carvedilol dose against the degree of β-1 blockade, which was associated with increases in plasma volume and diuretic dose in about one-third of the patients. Thus, it would be worthwhile testing carvedilol in an RCT limited to patients with compensated cirrhosis, and titrating the drug against the heart rate response.

Angiotensin-II (AT-II) receptor blockers are another class of drugs that have been studied in recent years for the treatment of portal hypertension. A first non-randomised trial reported a dramatic portal pressure lowering effect of long-term administration of losartan in cirrhotic patients [45]. These results were not confirmed in three randomised trials comparing losartan or irbesartan (another AT-II receptor blocker) with propranolol or placebo [46–48]. Losartan and irbesartan caused null or slight decreases in portal pressure in the three trials, but caused marked arterial hypotension and renal function impairment. In a fourth trial, including a large number of alcoholic patients, the lowering effect on portal pressure by losartan

Table 34 Studies that have evaluated the haemodynamic effects of carvedilol in patients with cirrhosis and portal hypertension.

Author, year	Dose	HVPG reduction	HVPG responders	MAP reduction
Stanley, 1997	25 mg (fixed)	−16 ± 3%	4/13 (40%)	−8.8 ± 3%
Tripathy, 2002	12.5 mg (fixed)	−24 ± 3%	8/9 (80%)	−4.4 ± 2%
Bañares, 2002	31 ± 4 mg (titrated)	−19 ± 2%	14/26 (54%)	−11 ± 1%*

HVPG, hepatic venous pressure gradient; MAP, mean arterial pressure
* Significant increases in plasma volume and in the dose of diuretics

was similar to that shown by propranolol [49]. In view of all these data, AT-II receptor blockers are not recommended for the treatment of portal hypertension.

Current research into the pharmacological treatment of portal hypertension focuses on drugs that reduce the vascular resistance of the cirrhotic liver by restoring the low capacity of the hepatic microcirculation to release nitric oxide – such as simvastatin – or by selectively donating nitric oxide to the liver microvessels. The role of these new agents in the prophylaxis of first variceal bleeding is yet to be established.

Statins have the potential to increase intrahepatic nitric oxide bioavailability in cirrhosis, since they are known to up-regulate endothelial nitric oxide synthase (eNOS) expression, to increase eNOS activity at a post-translational level and to decrease superoxide production. A single oral dose of simvastatin given to cirrhotic patients was observed to reduce hepatic vascular resistance without modifying the HVPG, to attenuate the postprandial increase in HVPG and to increase the hepatosplanchnic output of nitric oxide products [50].

Highly selective hepatic nitric oxide donors could be used as single drugs at doses high enough to effectively reduce portal pressure without lowering arterial pressure. For the time being, these drugs have been developed only in the experimental setting. NCX-1000 is a stable compound obtained by adding a nitric oxide releasing moiety to ursodeoxycholic acid [51]. Two recently published studies have tested the haemodynamic effects of the long-term administration of NCX-1000 in rats with established cirrhosis and portal hypertension [52,53]. One study uses the CCl_4 cirrhotic rat model (considered as the model that best mimics the disease in humans), and the other uses the bile duct ligated model. In both studies, NCX-1000 attenuated the hyper-response to α1-adrenergic stimulation of the perfused cirrhotic rat liver. In bile duct ligated rats, NCX-1000 markedly reduced baseline portal pressure [52], while in CCl_4 cirrhotic rats the compound failed to modify portal pressure, and only blunted the portal pressure increase induced by blood volume expansion [53]. The published results are promising, but preliminary. They show that it is possible to selectively deliver nitric oxide to the liver and modify hepatic, but not systemic haemodynamics.

Prevention of the first bleeding episode: endoscopic band ligation versus no treatment

M. Schepke

Especially due to its lower complication rate, endoscopic banding ligation (EBL) has replaced sclerotherapy for the elective endoscopic treatment of bleeding oesophageal varices.

With respect to the prevention of a first bleeding episode, band ligation has been compared to non-active treatment in six trials published during the late 1990s [54–59]. Three of these trials have been published as full papers [54–56] and three only in abstract form [4–6]. Data from five of these trials [54–58] have been included in a meta-analysis published in 2001 [60]. Since unselective β-blockers (i.e. propranolol, nadolol) effectively reduce the risk of first bleeding [61], nowadays primary prevention trials without an effective treatment in the control group are considered to be unethical. Thus, with respect to patients without contraindications to β-blockers, it is unlikely that additional data on that issue will be available in the near future. One more recent trial compared band ligation with non-active treatment for primary prophylaxis in patients with contraindications or intolerance to β-blockers [62].

Data derived from a total of 601 patients were included into the meta-analysis of five trials comparing EBL to non-active treatment [60]. This meta-analysis demonstrated that ligation significantly reduced the risk of first bleeding by 64% (relative risk, RR [95% CI]: 0.36 [0.26–0.5], number needed to treat, NNT [95% CI]: 4 [3–6]), the bleeding related mortality by 80% (RR [95% CI]: 0.20 [0.11–0.39], NNT [95% CI]: 7 [5–11]), and also had a significant beneficial effect on the overall mortality (RR [95% CI]: 0.55 [0.43–0.71], NNT [95% CI]: 5 [4–9]). There was no statistically significant heterogeneity among these five trials, neither was there a significant difference between the results from full published papers and those published only in abstract form. Recalculation of the meta-analysis after inclusion of the sixth trial [59] did not substantially alter the results [60]. Thus, it can be concluded that endoscopic band ligation is effective for the primary prevention of variceal bleeding in patients with high-risk varices.

Although there was no significant heterogeneity, some important details of the three fully published trials should be discussed: in all three studies varices could successfully be eradicated (Sarin *et al.* [54] and Lay *et al.* [55] 100% and Lo *et al.* [56] 86%, respectively). On average, this required between 2.9 [56] and 3.6 [55] therapeutic endoscopies. The trial showing the greatest difference of bleeding incidence between the treatment arm (EBL) and control group, published by Lay and co-workers [55], only included highly selected patients with a very high baseline bleeding risk (Beppu score < -0.38). Conceivably, the bleeding incidence in the control group reached 60% in that study (EBL: 19%) which is much higher than in most trials on primary prophylaxis of variceal bleeding published to date. The trial by Lo *et al.* [56] included patients with F2 and F3 varices and red colour signs. This study has by far the longest follow-up period among the three fully published trials and reports a bleeding incidence of 35% in the control group and of 22% in the ligation arm. Interestingly, a statistically significant benefit of EBL could be shown only for the subgroup of patients belonging to the Child–Pugh class B.

Major complications of EBL have not been reported in the study by Lay *et al.* [55]. In the trial by Sarin *et al.* [54] which recruited 68 patients, three ligation-induced bleeding episodes and one oesophageal perforation occurred. In the third trial (Lo *et al.*, $n = 127$) [56], EBL-induced bleeding was observed in three patients, one patient developed aspiration pneumonia. It should, however, be noted that all of these three studies utilised single-band ligation devices which were usually used in combination with an overtube. At present, however, modern multiband ligation devices are used almost exclusively and therefore, the risk of oesophageal perforation, and possibly also the risk of aspiration pneumonia is presumably lower.

A very recent study by Triantos *et al.* specifically addressed the issue of prophylactic band ligation in patients who cannot be treated with unselective β-blockers due to contraindications or intolerance [62]. These investigators randomised 52 patients with all size varices (40% of patients had large varices) to receive either endoscopic ligation ($n = 25$) or non-active treatment ($n = 27$). After a follow-up period of 19 months, three patients in the EBL group and two patients in the control group bled from varices, respectively. Two additional patients in the EBL arm bled from portal hypertensive gastropathy. Seven patients in the EBL group and eleven patients in the control group died during follow-up. Thus, probably due to the small number of patients with high baseline bleeding risk, this trial failed to show a beneficial effect of prophylactic band ligation in patients who cannot tolerate β-blockers.

In summary, the meta-analysis of five statistically homogeneous RCTs showed that endoscopic band ligation is an effective treatment for the primary prevention of variceal bleeding in patients with high-risk varices.

In those patients, when compared to non-active treatment, it reduces the bleeding incidence and also the bleeding related mortality and overall mortality [60]. However, in a small percentage of patients this treatment may be associated with serious complications (i.e. bleeding from ligation ulcers).

β-blockers versus variceal band ligation (VBL)

T.D. Boyer

Gastrooesophageal varices are present in approximately 50% of patients with cirrhosis and bleeding from varices is one of the complications of portal hypertension that leads to significant morbidity and mortality. Although survival has improved over the past two decades in patients who have bled from varices, still 15% to 20% of patients die within the first 3 months of the index bleed [63,64]. Given the persistently high rates of morbidity and mortality following a variceal bleed, most feel primary prophylaxis is warranted for this group of patients.

Most experts agree that β-blockers are the preferred therapy for prevention of the first bleed from oesophageal varices [5]. Unfortunately, either many patients have a contraindication to the use of β-blockers or they are intolerant of the drugs thus limiting their usefulness [15]. Endoscopic therapy has been proposed as an excellent way to prevent bleeding in patients with varices. Although sclerotherapy was effective in some studies, the high incidence of side effects, cost and lack of uniformity of the results in the different studies limited enthusiasm for this approach [1,65]. The advent of VBL and demonstration that it is superior to sclerotherapy [66], has again raised the issue of whether endoscopic therapy is better than pharmacological therapy in the prevention of the initial bleed from varices.

A meta-analysis of studies published before 2001 suggested that VBL was superior to β-blocker therapy [67]. In a recently published second meta-analysis of eight trials (five published as full papers), there was a significant reduction in the risk of the first bleed with VBL as compared to β-blocker therapy with no difference in survival between the two groups [68]. Since the last meta-analysis two more studies comparing VBL to β-blockers have been published as complete reports bringing the total number of the complete published papers to seven [69–75]. A meta-analysis of all seven trials is shown in Fig. 41. The studies were relatively uniform as to size of varices and use of β-blockers. In all but one study [71] the goal was to reduce the heart rate by more than 25% or to 50 beats/min. Obvious differences in these studies are the number of patients enrolled (62–152), length of follow-up (11 to 34 months), percentage of patients with Child's C cirrhosis (13% to 33%), numbers of patients with alcoholic cirrhosis (10–70%) and length of time between banding sessions (1 to 6 weeks) (Table 35). Two of the six studies showed a significantly reduced risk of bleeding in those receiving

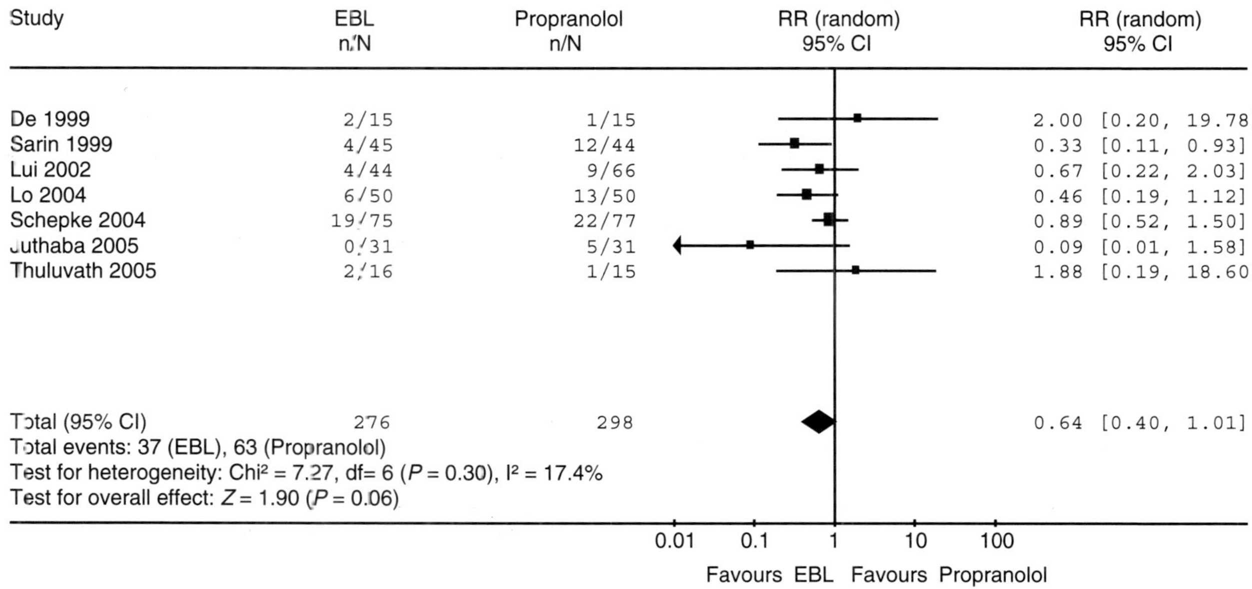

Fig. 41 EBL versus β-blockers in primary prophylaxis. Bleeding (full published papers).

Table 35 Complete studies comparing variceal band ligation to β-blockers in primary prophylaxis of variceal bleeding.

Ref #	Number patients	% CP-C	% ETOH	Size varices	VBL repeat EGD	β-blockers % decrease pulse	F/U months	VB B versus L %	Mortality B versus L %
15	30	18	17	M–L	Q6W	≥ 25%	17.6	7 13	NS
13	100	16	20	M–L	Q3–4W	≥ 25%	21.8	18 10	22 24
11	152	13	49–53	L	QW	≥ 25%	34	29 25	43 45
14	89	33	22	M–L	QW	≥ 25%	13–14	27 9*	11 11
10	62	23–26	10–13	M–L	Q4–5W	≥ 25%	11–18	13 0*	13 0*
12	110	33	65–70	M–L	QW	160 mg#	19.7	14 7	25 23
16	31	19	19	M–L	Q2–3W	≥ 25%	27	7 12	20 37

B, β-blocker versus L, variceal band ligation; CP-C, Child's Pugh class C; NS, not stated; ETOH, cirrhosis due to alcohol; VB, cumulative rate of variceal bleeding; W, weeks

VBL [69,73] and in one, mortality was less in those receiving VBL as compared to β-blockers [69]. In the other studies no significant differences in the primary end points of variceal bleeding or death were observed. Severe side effects of treatment were more common in those receiving β-blockers. However, two deaths from bleeding following treatment with VBL have been reported [68,70]. Lastly, impact of treatment on quality of life and cost cannot be determined from these trials.

In the study of Sarin *et al.* [73] cumulative rate of variceal bleeding was 9% in those who received VBL whereas 27% bled in the β-blocker group, the latter being much higher than expected [1]. In the report of Jutabha *et al.* [69] the rate of variceal bleeding with β-blockers was 13% (about the expected rate) but the rate of bleeding with VBL was 0%, much below the rates observed in previous studies (Table 35) [66].

There are a number of concerns about the results of the only two studies [69,74] that found an advantage for VBL as compared to β-blockers. First, bleeding rates with β-blockers were unusually high in one [73] and bleeding rates with VBL were too low in the second [69]. Both studies enrolled small numbers of patients and had short periods of follow-up relative to most of the other published series (Fig. 42). One study [69] was terminated early by the investigators because of significant differences in both rates of bleeding and mortality between the VBL and β-blocker treated patients. In well-designed clinical trials, the investigators are blinded to the results of the study and a Data Safety Monitoring Board follows the results of the trial, thus preventing either premature stopping of the study or prolonging a study that has shown no or a significant difference between the groups of subjects. In the report of Jutabha *et al.* [69] there was no Data Safety Monitoring Board and the decision to stop was made by the investigators. With early termination

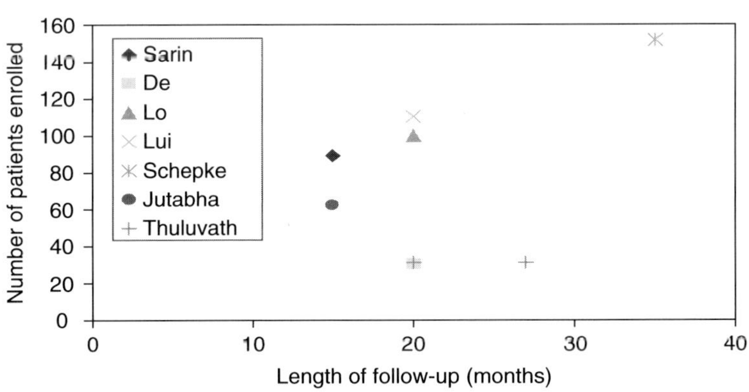

Fig. 42 Relationship between number of patients and length of follow-up.

and a short period of follow-up the number of patients enrolled was small as were the number of end points, four episodes of variceal bleeding and four deaths, leading this author to be concerned about the value of the statistical difference found by the investigators. Using a Chi-Square analysis with Yates' correction, the difference in failure rate between the two groups was found to be marginally significant ($p = 0.03$) and the difference in rates of variceal bleeding and death not to be significant ($p = 0.12$). If there was one episode of variceal bleeding or death in the band-ligation group, then statistical significance would not be achieved by any test ($p = 0.35$).

The other concern about all of the studies is the power analysis (or lack thereof) that was used to determine sample size. The power analysis performed for one study [69] estimated that a total 104 patients would be required to achieve a statistically significant difference between the two groups with expected rates of bleeding in the VBL group of 4% and 19% in those receiving β-blockers. This is an overly optimistic estimate of the risk of variceal bleeding following VBL as in the previously published studies the lowest risk observed with VBL was 7% with an average risk of at least 10%. If a 10% failure rate for VBL and 24% for β-blocker therapy had been used, then approximately 200 patients in each group would be required to achieve a statistically significant difference. In support of this suggestion is that in the study with the largest number of patients and longest follow-up, the risk of bleeding with either therapy was virtually the same [70].

If β-blockers and VBL are equivalent therapies, then is it possible to improve on the effectiveness of either? Recently Sarin and colleagues performed an RCT comparing VBL with and without β-blockers in the primary prevention of variceal bleeding [76]. The actuarial probability of bleeding at 20 months in the VBL plus β-blockers versus VBL alone groups was 7% versus 11% respectively (difference not significant). The addition of sclerotherapy to VBL also does not appear to improve efficacy [77]. It may be possible to improve the efficacy of β-blocker therapy by monitoring the response of the HVPG. The risk of bleeding in patients whose HVPG falls to below 12 mmHg or by at least 20% with β-blocker therapy is significantly less than in those who fail to achieve this response [20]. Thus, it is possible that monitoring β-blocker therapy by measuring the patients' HVPG before and after treatment and using VBL in those who fail to respond may be an effective way to prevent variceal bleeding. However, controlled trials are needed before we embrace this approach.

Markov models for primary prophylaxis

N. Chalasani

Markov models are simulation techniques that predict outcomes of a disease state and the costs of various treatment strategies over a time horizon, and these models take transition probabilities into account. With this technique, information about the natural history of a disease and its response to therapeutic manoeuvres can be obtained. This is particularly useful for diseases involving several stages and several treatment possibilities that require very large clinical trials for appropriate subgroup analyses. Some advantages of Markov models include the following: (1) they compare strategies where clinical trials are not possible (e.g. a clinical trial of endoscopic variceal band ligation (EVL) versus placebo in patients with high-risk varices will not be possible due to ethical reasons); (2) they provide data on the cost-effectiveness of various treatment strategies (most RCTs do not provide cost-effectiveness data) and (3) they have the ability to do sensitivity analyses and to combine data. Although the Markov models are attractive, they carry several disadvantages such as the following: (1) they are not clinical trials and thus the results should not be viewed as confirmatory; (2) their results depend on the strategies constructed and the probabilities and assumptions taken into account and (3) their acceptability will depend on whether or not a strategy has been proven in clinical trials (e.g. interferon for HCV infection versus haemodynamic monitoring (HDM) for primary prophylaxis).

As patients with cirrhosis and varices have various disease stages and as there are different treatment options available to prevent the first variceal bleeding, Markov technique has been applied to assess the cost-effectiveness of different treatment strategies. Table 36 depicts various published studies that employed Markov modelling for primary prophylaxis [65,78–83].

Noteworthy is the study by Spiegel and colleagues which compared five strategies for primary prophylaxis to 'do nothing' strategy over a 36-month time horizon [81]. These strategies included (1) screening upper endoscopy followed by β-blockers for those with high-risk oesophageal varices, (2) screening upper endoscopy followed by prophylactic banding for those with high-risk oesophageal varices, (3) selective endoscopy (endoscopy is offered based on clinical prediction rules) followed by β-blockers for those with high-risk oesophageal varices, (4) selective endoscopy (endoscopy is offered based on clinical prediction rules) followed by β-blockers for those with high-risk oesophageal varices and (5) universal β-blocker therapy to all cirrhotics.

Table 36 Summary of published decision analyses of various strategies for primary prophylaxis.

First author	Journal and year published	Target population	Strategies compared	Conclusions
Teran	*Gastro* 1996	Cirrhotic patients with any oesophageal varices	• Propranolol • Prophylactic sclerotherapy • Prophylactic shunt surgery	Propranolol is the cost-effective prophylactic therapy for preventing variceal bleeding Sclerotherapy was less cost-effective and had no effect on QALE Shunt surgery decreased life expectancy and was not cost-effective
Aoki	*GIE* 2000	Cirrhotic with high-risk oesophageal varices	• Watchful waiting • BB • Variceal ligation	Variceal ligation is more effective than BB in preventing variceal bleeding. But, 23% of patients with high-risk oesophageal varices benefit from BB more than from variceal ligation
Arguedas	*AJG* 2002	Patients with cirrhosis	• No screening for varices and no prophylaxis • Screening for varices and BB for eligible patients • Screening for varices and ligation for eligible patients • BB for all	Results depended on whether or not patients had decompensated cirrhosis *For those with compensated cirrhosis*: Screening for varices followed by BB for eligible patients is the most cost-effective strategy *For those with decompensate cirrhosis*: Universal BB therapy is the most cost-effective strategy
Saab	*AJG* 2003	Patients with cirrhosis	• No screening for varices and no prophylaxis • Screening for varices and BB for eligible patients • BB for all	Universal BB was the most cost-effective strategy but some assumptions were questionable. These include no regression in the severity of liver disease or size of varices and 100% compliance to BB

Spiegel	*Hepatology* 2003	Patients with cirrhosis	• Do nothing • Universal EGD for varices and BB for eligible patients • Universal EGD for varices and ligation for eligible patients • Selective EGD for varices and BB for eligible patients • Selective EGD for varices and ligation for eligible patients • BB for all	Universal BB therapy is the most cost-effective strategy for preventing variceal bleeding Screening endoscopy adds significant cost with marginal increase in effectiveness
Hickens	*APT* 2003	Cirrhotics with high-risk oesophageal varices	• BB versus single HDM at 4 weeks after starting BB. If HVPG > 12 mmHg, BB are discontinued and patients receive ligation • BB versus HDM before and 4 weeks after starting BB. Haemodynamic non-responders discontinue BB but receive ligation	HDM monitoring was not cost-effective in this study. Compared to no HDM, single HDM had incremental cost of $108,185 per each VB prevented. Compared to no HDM, two HDM strategy had incremental cost of $202,796 per VB prevented
Imperiale	*AJG* 2003	Cirrhotics with high-risk oesophageal varices	• No HDM (BB followed by ligation for those who are intolerant) • HDM-1: BB followed by nitrates for those who are non-responders • HDM-2: BB followed by ligation for those who are non-responders	Both HDM-1 and HDM-2 are more cost-effective than a strategy of no HDM

BB, β-blockers; HDM, Haemodynamic monitoring

Compared to 'do nothing strategy', empiric β-blockers to all cirrhotics cost an incremental US $12,408 per additional variceal bleeding prevented. Compared to empiric β-blockers, all other strategies were substantially more expensive and less effective. This study concluded that empiric β-blockers to all cirrhotics without subjecting them to screening endoscopy is the most effective form of therapy for primary prophylaxis against variceal bleeding, as the use of screening endoscopy to guide therapy adds significant costs with only marginal increase in effectiveness.

Two recent studies that examined the cost-effectiveness of HDM in providing the primary prophylaxis have arrived at different conclusions [82,83]. In the study by Hickens and colleagues, two different strategies of HDM were compared to current standard of providing β-blocker therapy without HDM [82]. In the first strategy, β-blocker therapy alone was compared to single HDM 4 weeks after initiating the β-blocker therapy. Patients who are intolerant to β-blockers and those in the HDM group with HVPG $>$ 12 mmHg at 4 weeks underwent variceal ligation to eradicate the varices. In the second strategy, β-blocker therapy alone was compared to HDM prior to and 4 weeks after initiating the β-blocker therapy. Patients who are intolerant to β-blockers and the haemodynamic non-responders ($\leq$ 20% drop in HVPG or HVPG $>$ 12 mmHg at 4 weeks) underwent variceal ligation to eradicate the varices. The total expected costs, variceal bleeding episodes and deaths were calculated over a 1-year time horizon. Compared to β-blocker therapy alone, the incremental cost per variceal bleeding episode prevented and death averted were, respectively, US $108,185 and US $355,100 (one HDM strategy) and US $202,796 and US $719,300 (for two HDM strategics) indicating that HDM to guide primary prophylaxis is an expensive strategy for reducing variceal bleeding or death. The results in these analyses were sensitive to the time horizon of the analysis, the probability of bleeding while receiving β-blockers and the cost of HDM. In another study, Imperiale and colleagues constructed a Markov model to compare HDM with no HDM in cirrhotic patients with moderate-to-large oesophageal varices [83]. Patients intolerant to β-blocker therapy would undergo endoscopic variceal ligation; those with an inadequate haemodynamic response (HDR) to β-blocker therapy could have nitrates added before ligation was considered. Only direct costs were considered during the 5-year time horizon. In the base-case analysis, either HDM was cost saving (US $2,523 per life year gained) or cost-effective (incremental cost-effectiveness ratio of US $5,200 per life year saved) compared with no HDM, depending on whether nitrates are added to β-blocker therapy. HDM reduced variceal bleeding by nearly 60% and had a small effect on all-cause mortality. In sensitivity analysis, HDM was sensitive to time horizon, as it was not cost-effective for a time horizon of less than

22 months, and was not cost saving prior to 49 months. The difference in the results of these two decision analyses is likely due to the time horizon of analyses (1 year for Hickens *et al.* versus 5 years for Imperiale *et al.*) and due to the assumed cost of each HDM (US $4,000 [range 0–US $20,000] for Hickens *et al.* versus US $450 [range US $300–US $900] for Imperiale *et al.*). Further clinical studies as well as decision analyses are needed to clarify the utility of HDM in providing primary prophylaxis for those with high-risk oesophageal varices.

REFERENCES

1 D'Amico G, Pagliaro L, Bosch J. Pharmacological treatment of portal hypertension: an evidence-based approach. *Sem Liv Dis* 1999;**19**: 475–505.

2 Chalasani N, Kahi C, Francois F *et al.* Improved patient survival after acute variceal bleeding: a multicenter, cohort study. *Am J Gastroenterol* 2003;**98**: 653–659.

3 Carbonell N, Pauwels A, Serfaty L, Fourdan O, Levy VG, Poupon R. Improved survival after variceal bleeding in patients with cirrhosis over the past two decades. *Hepatology* 2004;**40**: 652–659.

4 D'Amico G, De Franchis R. Cooperative Study Group. Upper digestive bleeding in cirrhosis. Post-therapeutic outcome and prognostic indicators. *Hepatology* 2003;**38**: 599–612.

5 Garcia-Pagan JC, Grace ND. Primary prophylaxis. In: de Franchis R (ed). *Portal hypertension III*. Oxford, UK; Blackwell Science Ltd., 2001; 127–131

6 Grace ND, Groszmann RJ, Garcia-Tsao G *et al.* Portal hypertension and variceal bleeding: an AASLD single topic symposium. *Hepatology* 1998;**28**: 868–880

7 Merli M, Nicolini G, Angeloni S *et al.* Incidence and natural history of small esophageal varices in cirrhotic patients. *J Hepatol* 2003;**38**: 266–272

8 Merkel C, Marin R, Angeli P *et al.* A placebo controlled trial of nadolol in the prophylaxis of growth of small esophageal varices in cirrhosis. *Gastroenterology* 2004;**127**: 476–484

9 Strauss E, Gomes Ribeiro M, Albano A *et al.* Long-term follow-up of a randomised controlled trial of prophylactic sclerotherapy of small esophageal varices in cirrhosis. *J Gastroenterol Hepatol* 1999;**14**: 225–230

10 Conn HO, Grace ND, Bosch J *et al.* Propranolol in the prevention of the first haemorrhage from esophageal varices: a multicenter randomised clinical trial. *Hepatology* 1991;**13**: 902–912

11 Prova, Study Group. Prophylaxis of first haemorrhage from esophageal varices by sclerotherapy, propranolol or both in cirrhotic patients: a randomised multicenter trial. *Hepatology* 1991;**14**: 1016–1024

12 Merkel C, Marin R, Sacerdoti D *et al.* Long-term results of a clinical trial of nadolol with and without isosorbide mononitrate for primary prophylaxis of variceal bleeding in cirrhosis. *Hepatology* 2000;**31**: 324–329

13 Angelico M, Carli L, Piat C *et al.* Effects of isosorbide-5-mononitrate compared to propranolol on first bleeding and long-term survival in cirrhosis. *Gastroenterology* 1997;**113**: 1632–1639

14 Garcia-Pagan JC, Villanueva C, Vila MC *et al.* Isosorbide mononitrate in the prevention of first bleed in patients who cannot receive beta-blockers. *Gastroenterology* 2001;**121**: 908–914
15 Garcia-Pagan JC, Morillas R, Banares R *et al.* Propranolol versus propranolol plus isosorbide-5-mononitrate in the prevention of a first variceal bleed: a double blind RCT. *Hepatology* 2003;**37**: 1260–1266
16 Cales P, Oberti F, Payen JL *et al.* Lack of effect of propranolol in the prevention of large esophageal varices in patients with cirrhosis: a randomised trial. *Eur J Gastroenterol Hepatol* 1999;**11**: 741–745
17 Beppu K, Inokuchi K, Koyanagi N *et al.* Prediction of variceal hemorrhage by esophageal endoscopy. *Gastrointest Endosc* 1981;**27**: 213–218
18 Escorsell A, Ferayorni L, Bosch J *et al.* The portal pressure response to beta-blockade is greater in patients without varices than in those with varices. *Gastroenterology* 1997;**112**: 2012–2016
19 Groszmann RJ, Bosch J, Grace ND *et al.* Haemodynamic events in a prospective randomised trial of propranolol versus placebo in the prevention of a first variceal haemorrhage. *Gastroenterology* 1990;**99**: 1401–1407.
20 Merkel C, Bolognesi M, Sacerdoti D *et al.* The haemodynamic response to medical treatment of portal hypertension as a predictor of clinical effectiveness in the primary prophylaxis of variceal bleeding in cirrhosis. *Hepatology* 2000;**32**: 930–934.
21 Bureau C, Peron JM, Alric L *et al.* 'A La Carte' treatment of portal hypertension: adapting medical therapy to haemodynamic response for the prevention of bleeding. *Hepatology* 2002;**36**: 1361–1366.
22 Turnes J, Garcia-Pagan JC, Abraldes JG *et al.* Pharmacological reduction of portal pressure and long term risk of first variceal bleeding in patients with cirrhosis. *Hepatology* 2003;**38**(suppl. 1): 219A.
23 Lebrec D, Moreau R. Pathophysiology of portal hypertension. *Hepatogastroenterology* 1999;**46**: 1426–1428.
24 Imbert-Bismut F, Ratziu V, Pieroni L, Charlotte F, Benhamou Y, Poynard T for the MULTIVIRC Group. Biochemical markers of liver fibrosis in patients with hepatitis C virus infection: a prospective study. *Lancet* 2001;**357**: 1069–1075.
25 Thabut D, Imbert-Bismuth F, Cazals-Hatem D *et al.* Diagnostic value of fibrosis biochemical markers (Fibrotest-Fibrosure) for the prediction of portal hypertension in patients with or without cirrhosis. *Hepatology* 2004;**40**(suppl. 1): 202A–203A.
26 Leroy V, Monier F, Bottari S *et al.* Circulating matrix metalloproteinases 1, 2, 9 and their inhibitors TIMP-1 and TIMP-2 as serum markers of liver fibrosis in patients with chronic hepatitis C: comparison with PIIINP and hyaluronic acid. *Am J Gastroenterol* 2004;**92**: 271–279.
27 Forns X, Ampurdanuès S, Llovet JM *et al.* Identification of chronic hepatitis C patients without hepatic fibrosis by a simple predictive model. *Hepatology* 2002;**36**: 986–992.
28 Rosenberg WMC, Voelker M, Thiel R *et al.* Serum markers detect the presence of liver fibrosis; a cohort study. *Gastroenterology* 2004;**127**: 1704–1713.
29 Wai CT, Greenson JK, Fontana RJ *et al.* A simple noninvasive index can predict both significant fibrosis and cirrhosis in patients with chronic hepatitis C. *Hepatology* 2003;**38**: 518–526.

30 Patel K, Gordon SC, Jacobson I *et al.* Evaluation of a panel of non-invasive serum markers to differentiate mild from moderate-to-advanced liver fibrosis in chronic hepatitis C patients. *J Hepatol* 2004;**41**: 935–942.

31 Collewaert N, Van Vlierberghe H, Van Hecke A, Laroy W, Delanghe J, Contreras R. Noninvasive diagnosis of liver cirrhosis using DNA sequencer-based total serum protein glycomics. *Nat Med* 2004;**10**: 429–434.

32 Castera L, Vergniol J, Foucher J *et al.* Prospective comparison of transient elastography, Fibrotest, APRI, and liver biopsy for the assessment of fibrosis in chronic hepatitis C. *Gastroenterology* 2005;**128**: 343–350.

33 Garcia-Pagan JC, Feu F, Navasa M *et al.* Long-term haemodynamic effects of isosorbide-5-mononitrate in patients with cirrhosis and portal hypertension. *J Hepatol* 1990;**11**: 189–195.

34 Borroni G, Salerno F, Cazzaniga M *et al.* Nadolol is superior to isosorbide mononitrate for the prevention of the first variceal bleeding in cirrhotic patients with ascites. *J Hepatol* 2002;**37**: 315–321.

35 Lui HF, Stanley AJ, Forrest EH *et al.* Primary prophylaxis of variceal haemorrhage: a randomised controlled trial comparing band ligation, propranolol, and isosorbide mononitrate. *Gastroenterology* 2002;**123**: 735–744.

36 Garcia-Pagan JC, Feu F, Bosch J, Rodes J. Propranolol compared with propranolol plus isosorbide-5-mononitrate for portal hypertension in cirrhosis. A randomised controlled study. *Ann Intern Med* 1991;**114**: 869–873.

37 Albillos A, Garcia-Pagan JC, Iborra J *et al.* Propranolol plus prazosin compared with propranolol plus isosorbide-5-mononitrate in the treatment of portal hypertension. *Gastroenterology* 1998;**115**: 116–123.

38 Pietrosi G, D'Amico G, Pasta L *et al.* Isosorbide mononitrate with nadolol compared to nadolol alone for primary prophylaxis of variceal bleeding in cirrhosis. A double-blind placebo-controlled randomised trial. *J Hepatol* 1999;**30**(suppl. 1): 66.

39 Gournay J, Masliah C, Martin T, Perrin D, Galmiche JP. Isosorbide mononitrate and propranolol compared with propranolol alone for the prevention of variceal rebleeding. *Hepatology* 2000;**31**: 1239–1245.

40 Garcia-Pagan JC, Salmeron JM, Feu F *et al.* Effects of low-sodium diet and spironolactone on portal pressure in patients with compensated cirrhosis. *Hepatology* 1994;**19**: 1095–1099.

41 Abecasis R, Kravetz D, Fassio E *et al.* Nadolol plus spironolactone in the prophylaxis of first variceal bleed in nonascitic cirrhotic patients: a preliminary study. *Hepatology* 2003;**37**: 359–365.

42 Stanley AJ, Therapondos G, Helmy A, Hayes PC. Acute and chronic haemodynamic and renal effects of carvedilol in patients with cirrhosis. *J Hepatol* 1999;**30**: 479–484.

43 Tripathi D, Therapondos G, Lui HF, Stanley AJ, Hayes PC. Haemodynamic effects of acute and chronic administration of low-dose carvedilol, a vasodilating beta-blocker, in patients with cirrhosis and portal hypertension. *Aliment Pharmacol Ther* 2002;**16**: 373–380.

44 Bañares R, Moitinho E, Matilla A *et al.* Randomised comparison of long-term carvedilol and propranolol administration in the treatment of portal hypertension in cirrhosis. *Hepatology* 2002;**36**: 1367–1373.

45 Schneider AW, Friedrich J, Klein CP. Effect of losartan, an angiotensin II receptor antagonist, on portal pressure in cirrhosis. *Hepatology* 1999;**29**: 334–339.
46 Gonzalez-Abraldes J, Albillos A, Banares R *et al.* Randomised comparison of long-term losartan versus propranolol in lowering portal pressure in cirrhosis. *Gastroenterology* 2001;**121**: 382–388.
47 Schepke M, Werner E, Biecker E *et al.* Haemodynamic effects of the angiotensin II receptor antagonist irbesartan in patients with cirrhosis and portal hypertension. *Gastroenterology* 2001;**121**: 389–395.
48 Venon WD, Baronio M, Leone N *et al.* Effects of long-term irbesartan in reducing portal pressure in cirrhotic patients: comparison with propranolol in a randomised controlled study. *J Hepatol* 2003;**38**: 455–460.
49 De BK, Bandyopadhyay K, Das TK *et al.* Portal pressure response to losartan compared with propranolol in patients with cirrhosis. *Am J Gastroenterol* 2003;**98**: 1371–1376.
50 Zafra C, Abraldes JG, Turnes J *et al.* Simvastatin enhances hepatic nitric oxide production and decreases the hepatic vascular tone in patients with cirrhosis. *Gastroenterology* 2004;**126**: 749–755.
51 Fiorucci S, Antonelli E, Morelli O *et al.* NCX-1000, a NO-releasing derivative of ursodeoxicholic acid, selectively delivers NO to the liver and protects against development of portal hypertension. *Proc Natl Acad Sci USA* 2001;**98**: 8897–8902.
52 Fiorucci S, Antonelli E, Brancaleone V *et al.* NCX-1000, a nitric oxide-releasing derivative of ursodeoxycholic acid, ameliorates portal hypertension and lowers norepinephrine-induced intrahepatic resistance in the isolated and perfused rat liver. *J Hepatol* 2003;**39**: 932–939.
53 Loureiro-Silva MR, Cadelina GW, Iwakiri Y, Groszmann RJ. A liver specific nitric oxide donor improves the intra-hepatic vascular response to both portal blood flow increase and methoxamine in cirrhotic rats. *J Hepatol* 2003;**39**: 940–946.
54 Sarin S, Guptan, R, Jain A, Sundaram K. A randomised controlled trial of endoscopic variceal band ligation for primary prophylaxis of variceal bleeding. *Eur J Gastroenterol Hepatol* 1996;**4**: 337–342.
55 Lay C, Tsai J, Teg C *et al.* Endoscopic variceal ligation in prophylaxis of first variceal bleeding in cirrhotic patients with high-risk esophageal varices. *Hepatology* 1997;**25**: 1346–1350.
56 Lo G, Lai K, Cheng J, Lin C, Hsu P, Chiang H. Prophylactic banding ligation of high risk esophageal varices in patients with cirrhosis: a prospective randomised trial. *J Hepatol* 1999;**31**: 451–456.
57 Gameel K, Wahid I, Saleh S, Sallam M, Abdel-Fattah S. Prophylactic endoscopic variceal band ligation (EVL) versus sclerotherapy (ES) for the prevention of variceal bleeding in high risk varices: a prospective randomised controlled trial (abstract). *Hepatology* 1996;**27**: A361.
58 Chen C, Chen C, Chang T. Prophylactic endoscopic variceal ligation (EVL) for esophageal varices (abstract). *Gastroenterology* 1998;**114**: A1224.
59 Omar M, Attia M, Mostafa IM. Prophylactic band ligation to prevent first bleeding from large esophageal varices (abstract). *Gastrointest Endosc* 2000;**51**: AB122.

60 Imperiale T, Chalasani N. A meta-analysis of endoscopic variceal ligation for primary prophylaxis of esophageal variceal bleeding. *Hepatology* 2001;**33**: 802–807.

61 Poynard T, Cales P, Pasta L *et al.* Beta adrenergic antagonists in the prevention of first gastrointestinal bleeding in patients with cirrhosis and esophageal varices. *N Engl J Med* 1991;**324**: 1532–1538.

62 Triantos C, Vlachogiannakos J, Anastasios A *et al.* Primary prophylaxis of variceal bleeding in cirrhotics unable to take beta-blockers: a randomised trial of ligation. *Aliment Pharmacol Ther* 2005;**21**: 1435–1443.

63 Chalasani N, Kahi C, Francois F *et al.* Improved patient survival after acute variceal bleeding: a multicenter, cohort study. *Am J Gastroenterol* 2003;**98**: 653–659.

64 Carbonell N, Pauwels A, Serfaty L, Fourdan O, Levy VG, Poupon R. Improved survival after variceal bleeding in patients with cirrhosis over the past two decades. *Hepatology* 2004;**40**: 652–659.

65 Teran J, Imperiale T, Mullen K, Tavill A, McCullough A. Primary prophylaxis of variceal bleeding in cirrhosis: a cost-effectiveness analysis. *Gastroenterology* 1997;**112**: 473–482.

66 Laine L, Cook D. Endoscopic ligation compared with sclerotherapy for treatment of esophageal variceal bleeding. A meta-analysis. [see comment]. *Ann Intern Med* 1995;**123**: 280–287.

67 Imperiale (1–3) T, Chalasani (2) N. A meta-analysis of endoscopic variceal ligation for primary prophylaxis of esophageal variceal bleeding. *Hepatology* 2001;**33**: 802–807.

68 Khuroo MS, Khuroo NS, Farahat KLC, Khuroo YS, Sofi AA, Dahab ST. Meta-analysis: endoscopic variceal ligation for primary prophylaxis of esophageal variceal bleeding. *Alim Pharmacol Ther* 2005;**21**: 347–361.

69 Jutabha R, Jensen DM, Martin P, Savides T, Han S-H, Gornbein J. Randomised study comparing banding and propranolol to prevent initial variceal haemorrhage in cirrhotics with high risk esophageal varices. *Gastroenterology* 2005;**128**: 870–881.

70 Schepke M, Kleber G, Nurnberg D *et al.* German Study Group for the Primary Prophylaxis of Variceal Bleeding. Ligation versus propranolol for the primary prophylaxis of variceal bleeding in cirrhosis. *Hepatology* 2004;**40**: 65–72.

71 Lui HF, Stanley AJ, Forrest EH *et al.* Primary prophylaxis of variceal haemorrhage: a randomised controlled trial comparing band ligation, propranolol, and isosorbide mononitrate. [see comment]. *Gastroenterology* 2002;**123**: 735–744.

72 Lo GH, Chen WC, Chen MH *et al.* Endoscopic ligation vs. nadolol in the prevention of first variceal bleeding in patients with cirrhosis. *Gastrointestinal Endosc* 2004;**59**: 333–338.

73 Sarin SK, Lamba GS, Kumar M, Misra A, Murthy NS. Comparison of endoscopic ligation and propranolol for the primary prevention of variceal bleeding. [see comment]. *N Engl J Med* 1999;**340**: 988–993.

74 De BK, Ghoshal UC, Das T, Santra A, Biswas PK. Endoscopic variceal ligation for primary prophylaxis of oesophageal variceal bleed: preliminary report of a randomised controlled trial. *J Gastroenterol Hepatol* 1999;**14**: 220–224.

75 Thuluvath PJ, Maheshwari A, Jagannath S, Arepaliy A. A randomised controlled trial of +/− blockers versus endoscopic band ligation for primary

prophylaxis: a large sample size is required to show a difference in bleeding rates. *Dig Dis Sci* 2005;**50**: 407–410.
76 Sarin SK WMAS. Endoscopic variceal ligation plus propranolol versus endoscopic variceal ligation alone in primary prophylaxis of variceal bleeding. *Am J Gastroenterol* 2005;**100**: 797–804.
77 Singh P, Pooran N, Indaram A, Bank S. Combined ligation and sclerotherapy versus ligation alone for secondary prophylaxis of esophageal variceal bleeding: a meta-analysis. *Am J Gastroenterol* 2002;**97**: 623–629.
78 Aoki N, Kajiyama T, Beck JR, Cone RW, Soma K, Fukui T. Decision analyses of prophylactic treatment for patients with high-risk varices. *Gastrointest Endosc* 2000;**52**: 707–714.
79 Arguedas MR, Heudebert GR, Eloubedi MA, Abrams GA, Fallon MB. Cost-effectiveness of screening, surveillance and primary prophylaxis strategies for esophageal varices. *Am J Gastroenterol* 2002;**97**: 2441–2452.
80 Saab SM, DeRosa V, Nieto J, Durazo F, Han S, Roth B. Costs and clinical outcomes for primary prophylaxis of varices; bleeding in patients with hepatic cirrhosis: a decision analytic model. *Am J Gastroenterol* 2003;**98**: 763–770.
81 Spiegel BMR, Targowik L, Dulai GS, Karsan HA, Gralnek IM. Endoscopic screening for esophageal varices: is it ever cost effective? *Hepatology* 2003;**37**: 366–377.
82 Hickens BL, Shahara AI, Abrams GA, Eloubedi M, Fallon MB, Arguedas MR. Hepatic venous pressure gradient measurements to assess response to primary prophylaxis in patients with cirrhosis: a decision analytical study. *Aliment Pharmacol Ther* 2003;**17**: 145–153.
83 Imperiale TF, Chalasani N, Klein R. Cost-effectiveness analysis of measuring haemodynamic response to primary pharmacoprophylaxis of variceal bleeding. *Am J Gastroenterol* 2003;**98**: 2742–2750.

Baveno IV Consensus Statements: Prevention of the First Bleeding Episode

Norman D. Grace, Juan Carlos Garcia-Pagàn (Chairpersons), Agustin Albillos, Mario Angelico, Thomas D. Boyer, Naga Chalasani and Michael Schepke

Use of HVPG measurements

• Hepatic venous pressure gradient (HVPG) monitoring identifies patients with cirrhosis who will benefit from non-selective β-blocker therapy in primary prophylaxis. (1b;A)
• 'A La Carte' treatment using HVPG response in primary prophylaxis needs to be evaluated, especially in high-risk patients. Until then, routine use of HVPG cannot be recommended. (5;D)

Patients with small varices

• Patients with small varices could be treated with non-selective β-blockers to prevent progression of varices and bleeding, but further studies, especially as relates to prevention of bleeding, are required before a formal recommendation on their use can be made. (5;D)
• Patients with small varices with red weal signs or of Child C class have an increased risk of bleeding and may benefit from treatment. (5;D)

Pharmacological treatments

• Non-selective β-blockers reduce the risk of first variceal bleeding. (1a;A)
• Isosorbide mononitrate (ISMN) administered alone must not be used. (1a;A)
• There is not enough data to recommend the use of the combination of β-blockers plus ISMN or spironolactone plus β-blockers for primary prophylaxis. (1b;A)
• Other pharmacological agents able to reduce portal pressure must be adequately tested before their clinical use. (5;D)

Endoscopic treatment

• Prophylactic endoscopic band ligation (EBL) is useful in preventing variceal bleeding in patients with medium and large oesophageal varices. (1a;A)

• EBL is more effective than non-selective β-blockers in preventing first variceal bleeding but does not improve survival. However the long-term benefits of EBL are uncertain because of the short duration of follow-up. (1a;A)
• EBL should be offered to patients with medium/large varices and with contraindications or intolerance to β-blockers. (5;D)

Gastric varices

• In the absence of specific data on prophylactic studies, randomised controlled trials (RCTs) should be performed in patients with gastric varices.

Cost-effectiveness analysis

• Markov models are not a substitute for well-designed clinical trials. However, well-designed Markov models are complementary to clinical studies and should be pursued for exploratory purposes and to establish the cost-effectiveness of various strategies. Markov models may fill in a void where clinical trials are simply not feasible.

Areas requiring further study (5;D)

• Comparison of EBL and β-blockers with respect to cost-effectiveness and quality of life to determine the treatment of choice.
• Studies to clarify whether the use of EBL + β-blockers is better than each treatment alone.

LECTURE

Hepatorenal Syndrome: Current Concepts

Andrés Cárdenas and Pere Ginés

INTRODUCTION

Renal failure commonly complicates the clinical course of patients with advanced cirrhosis. Although there are several causes of renal failure in the setting of advanced liver disease, renal dysfunction in cirrhosis most commonly occurs in the absence of histological abnormalities in the kidney. This type of renal dysfunction is known as hepatorenal syndrome (HRS), a unique form of functional renal failure that develops in patients with cirrhosis. Although HRS occurs predominantly in advanced cirrhosis, it may also develop in other chronic liver diseases associated with severe liver failure and portal hypertension, such as alcoholic hepatitis, or in acute liver failure [1–4].

Hepatorenal syndrome occurs in less than 10% of hospitalised patients with cirrhosis and ascites. The probability of developing HRS in patients with cirrhosis and ascites is near 20% at 1 year and increases to 40% at 5 years [5]. Patients with ascites and marked sodium and solute-free water retention with dilutional hyponatraemia as well as those with marked arterial hypotension have a high risk of developing HRS [5]. Two types of HRS are observed in clinical practice [1]. Type 1 HRS is characterised by an acute and severe renal failure with a very poor prognosis while type 2 HRS is less severe and progressive compared to type 1; these patients usually do not respond well to diuretics and have a better prognosis compared with those with type 1 HRS.

There are several mechanisms that play a contributory role in pathogenesis of HRS, including extrarenal and intrarenal factors, abnormalities in systemic haemodynamics, and the diseased liver causing portal hypertension and hepatic failure. This review will describe the pathogenesis, clinical features, diagnostic approach and current treatment of HRS in cirrhosis.

Table 37 Vasoactive factors involved in the regulation of renal perfusion in cirrhosis and the pathogenesis of hepatorenal syndrome.

Vasodilators
Prostacyclin
Prostaglandin E2
Nitric oxide
Atrial natriuretic peptide
Kallikrein-kinin system
Vasoconstrictors
Angiotensin II
Norepinephrine
Neuropeptide Y
Endothelin-1
Adenosine
Thromboxane A2
Cysteinyl leukotrienes
F2-isoprostanes

Pathophysiology

The pathophysiological hallmark of HRS is severe vasoconstriction of the renal circulation [6,7]. The underlying mechanisms are complex and include interactions between changes in the systemic arterial circulation, increased portal pressure, activation of vasoconstrictor factors and suppression of vasodilator factors acting on the renal circulation (Table 37). A common pathway for these derangements is the development of an intense splanchnic arterial vasodilation, mainly due to an increased production of local vasodilators substances (mainly nitric oxide), which causes arterial underfilling and triggers an important compensatory response by activating vasoconstrictor and antinatriuretic systems such as the renin–angiotensin–aldosterone system (RAAS), the sympathetic nervous system (SNS) and arginine vasopressin (AVP) accounting for sodium and solute-free water retention as well as renal vasoconstriction [7–10] (Fig. 43).

In early or moderately advanced stages of cirrhosis, renal blood flow is kept within normal limits due to the effect of local vasodilators that antagonise the renal vascular effect of the systemic vasoconstrictors. When there is stimulation of the endogenous vasoconstrictors, there is also activation of renal vasodilators (prostaglandins, nitric oxide and natriuretic peptides) in order to maintain renal perfusion and glomerular filtration rate (GFR) [11]. Although the renal production of prostaglandins and circulating levels of natriuretic peptides are increased in patients with cirrhosis and ascites without HRS, with disease progression circulating vasoconstrictors

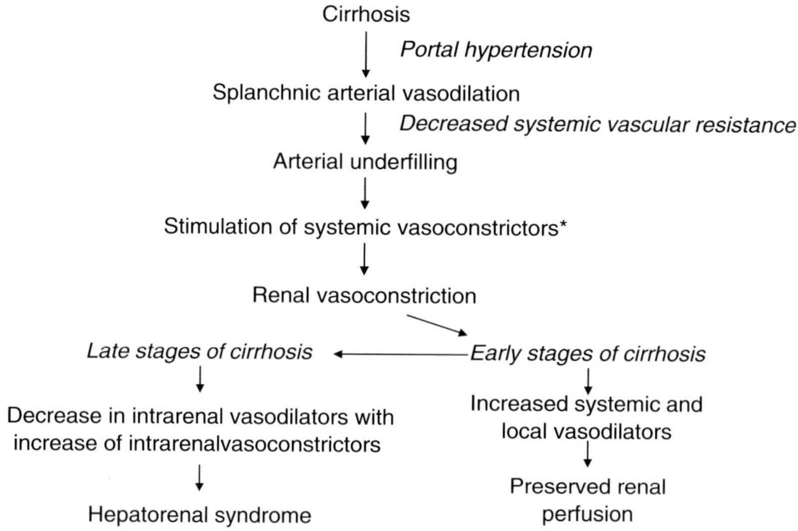

Fig. 43 Pathogenesis of hepatorenal syndrome as proposed by the peripheral arterial vasodilation theory. * Renin-angiotensin-aldosterone system (RAAS), sympathetic nervous system (SNS), endothelin and arginine vasopressin (AVP).

overcome the effect of renal vasodilators, leading to severe renal vasoconstriction and reduction in GFR [12]. In some patients a precipitating cause of circulatory dysfunction such as spontaneous bacterial peritonitis (SBP) leads to worsening of renal vasoconstriction [13]. Once vasoconstriction develops, intrarenal mechanisms probably perpetuate HRS due to the development of intrarenal vicious cycles in which hypoperfusion leads to an imbalance in intrarenal vasoactive systems that in turn cause more vasoconstriction.

Clinical and laboratory findings

Although there are no specific clinical findings in HRS, the majority of patients have features of advanced liver disease with jaundice, prolonged prothrombin time, thrombocytopenia, hepatic encephalopathy, hypoalbuminaemia and ascites. In addition, patients have a low arterial blood pressure and reduced systemic vascular resistance as well as tachycardia and increased cardiac output. Some patients may also have cirrhotic cardiomyopathy, a condition characterised mainly by diastolic dysfunction which may contribute to haemodynamic changes occurring in HRS, particularly when precipitated by SBP [14,15]. Renal failure in HRS is frequently associated with oliguria (urine volume < 500 ml/24 h), although some patients

Table 38 Clinical types of hepatorenal syndrome.

Type 1. Rapid and progressive impairment of renal function as defined by a doubling of the initial serum creatinine to a level higher than 2.5 mg/dL or a 50% reduction of the initial 24-h creatinine clearance to a level lower than 20 mL/min in less than 2 weeks.
Type 2. Impairment in renal function (serum creatinine > 1.5 mg/dL) that does not meet the criteria of type 1.

may have preserved urine volume, intense urinary sodium retention (urine sodium < 10 meq/L) and spontaneous dilutional hyponatraemia (serum sodium < 130 meq/L).

As described earlier, there are two types of HRS [1] (Table 38). Type 1 HRS is characterised by a rapid and progressive impairment of renal function as defined by a doubling of the initial serum creatinine to a level higher than 2.5 mg/dL in less than 2 weeks. Serum creatinine levels in HRS are usually lower than values observed in patients with acute renal failure without liver disease, due to a reduced muscle mass and low endogenous production of creatinine in cirrhosis [16]. Nonetheless, there are no other reliable non-invasive methods of assessing renal function in cirrhosis and therefore the diagnosis of HRS is still based on the level of serum creatinine. In contrast to type 1 HRS, type 2 HRS is characterised by a more subtle course with serum creatinine levels around 1.5–2.5 mg/dL [1]. The main clinical consequence of type 2 HRS is diuretic-resistant ascites. As expected, survival is longer in this group of patients than in those with type 1 HRS, but is shorter than that of patients with ascites without renal failure.

In some patients, type 1 HRS develops spontaneously without any identifiable precipitating factor, whereas in others it can occur in close association with systemic bacterial infections in particular SBP, acute alcoholic hepatitis and large-volume paracentesis without albumin infusion. SBP precipitates type 1 HRS in approximately 30% of cases despite appropriate treatment and resolution of the infection [13]. This proportion is reduced to 10% when albumin infusion is given in association with antibiotic therapy (see later). Large-volume paracentesis (> 5 L) without albumin expansion may precipitate type 1 HRS in up to 20% of cases [17]. This complication is one of the reasons why intravenous albumin should be administered after large-volume paracentesis in patients with cirrhosis and ascites. Renal failure occurs in approximately 10% of cirrhotic patients with gastrointestinal bleeding [18]. The development of renal failure occurs mainly in patients who develop hypovolaemic shock, and in most cases is associated with ischaemic hepatitis, which suggests that renal failure in patients with gastrointestinal

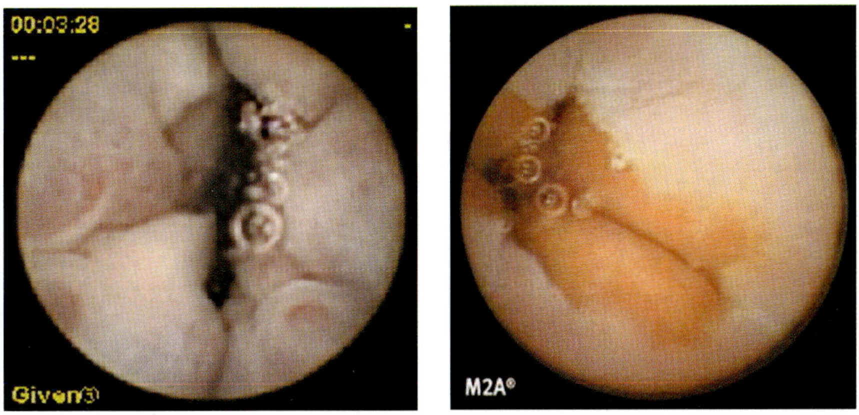

Plate 1 Appearance of oesophageal varices (left panel) in comparison with normal GE junction (right panel) on PillCam Eso® endoscopy.

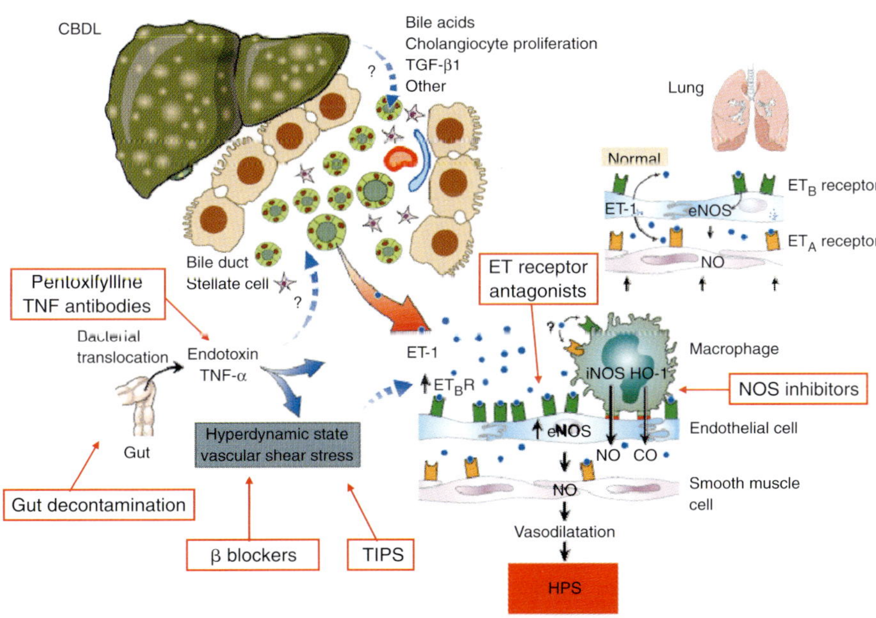

Plate 2 Potential mechanisms and treatments in experimental HPS.

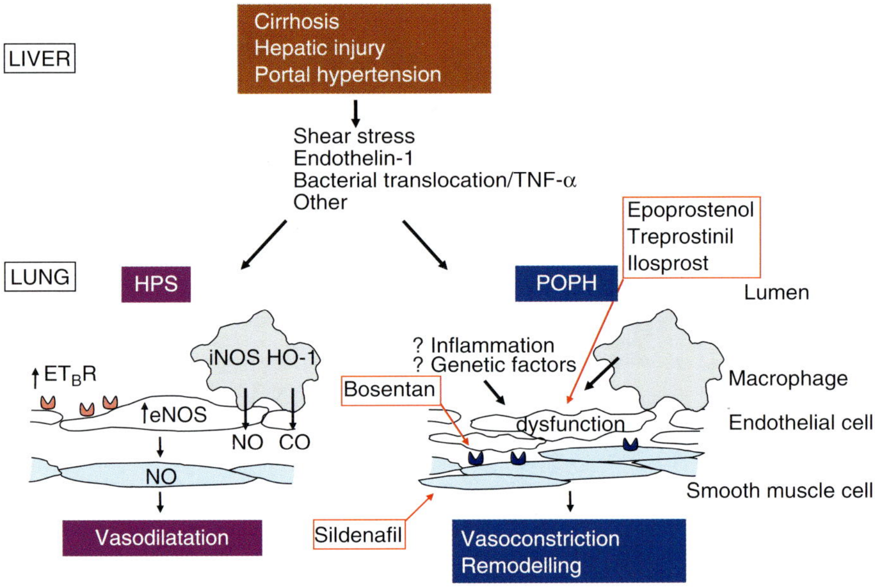

Plate 3 Potential pathogenesis of POPH in relation to HPS.

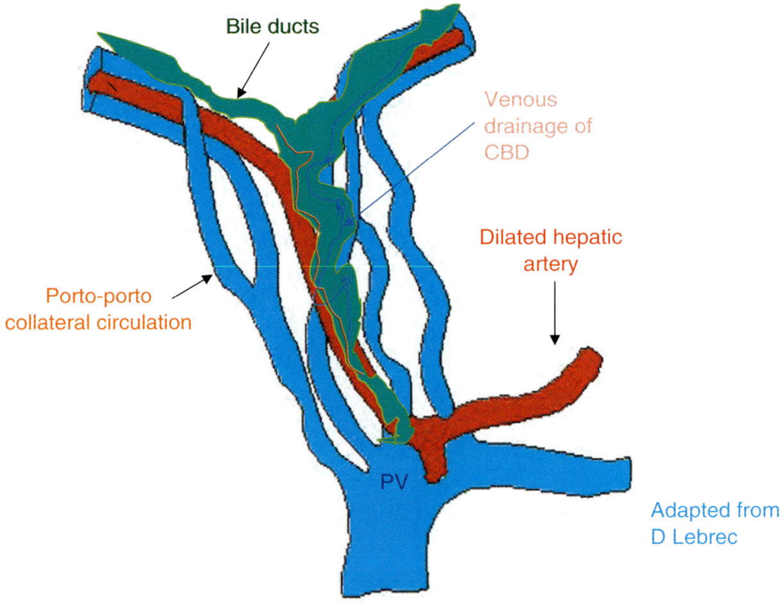

Plate 4 Schematic diagram of a portal cavernoma along with biliary duct anomalies.

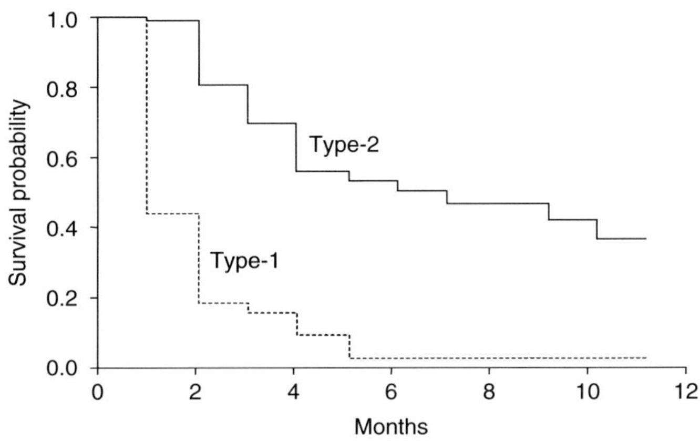

Fig. 44 Survival of patients with cirrhosis and type 1 and 2 hepatorenal syndrome. (From Ginés P *et al.* Hepatorenal syndrome. *Lancet* 2003;**362**: 1819–1827, with permission.)

bleeding is probably related to the development of acute tubular necrosis and not HRS [18].

Prognosis

Hepatorenal syndrome carries the worst prognosis of all the complications of cirrhosis. Without treatment, the median survival time of patients with type 1 HRS is less than 2 weeks and practically all patients die within 8–10 weeks after the onset of renal failure [5,19]. On the other hand patients with type 2 HRS have a longer median survival time of approximately 6 months (Fig. 44) [5,19].

Diagnosis

The diagnosis of HRS is one of exclusion that depends mainly on the level of serum creatinine. Unfortunately serum creatinine does not provide an exact estimation of GFR in cirrhosis, since its level is lower than expected due to a low endogenous production of creatinine which frequently occurs in advanced cirrhosis [16]. Creatinine clearance usually overestimates GFR and in addition is difficult to perform because it depends on the adequate collection of urine volume over 24 h, which in many cases is inadequate, especially in oliguric patients unless they have bladder catheterisation [16,20]. Since the use inulin clearance for estimation of GFR is expensive and cumbersome, the serum creatinine concentration is currently used to estimate GFR in cirrhosis. In fact the diagnosis of HRS is made when serum creatinine is greater

Table 39 Diagnostic criteria of hepatorenal syndrome.

Major criteria*
1 Low glomerular filtration rate, as indicated by serum creatinine greater than 1.5 mg/dL.
2 Exclusion of shock, ongoing bacterial infection, volume depletion and use of nephrotoxic drugs.
3 No improvement in renal function despite stopping diuretics and volume repletion with 1.5 L of saline.
4 No proteinuria or ultrasonographic evidence of obstructive uropathy or parenchymal renal disease.

Minor criteria
1 Urine volume lower than 500 mL/day.
2 Urine sodium lower than 10 meq/L.
3 Urine osmolality greater than plasma osmolality.
4 Urine red blood cells less than 50 per high power field.
5 Serum sodium concentration lower than 130 meq/L.

* Only major criteria are necessary for the diagnosis of hepatorenal syndrome

than 1.5 mg/dL [1], and there are no identifiable causes of renal failure (see below).

Due to the lack of specific diagnostic tests to distinguish between HRS and other causes of renal failure that may occur in cirrhosis, the diagnosis of HRS is based on several criteria described in Table 39 [1]. Serum creatinine should be assessed without diuretic therapy for at least 5 days. Other criteria include the absence of clinical conditions that predispose to the development of acute renal failure (i.e. volume depletion, shock, bacterial infections or nephrotoxic drugs), no improvement of renal function following diuretic withdrawal and plasma expansion, no proteinuria and a normal renal ultrasound. Most cases of HRS have urine sodium below 10 meq/L and urine osmolality above plasma osmolality because of a preserved tubular function. Nevertheless, a minority of patients may have higher urine sodium and low urine osmolality, similar to values found in acute tubular necrosis [1,21]. Conversely, some cirrhotic patients with acute tubular necrosis may have low urine sodium and high urine osmolality. For these reasons, urinary indices are not considered major criteria for diagnosis of HRS [1,19].

As indicated above, causes of renal failure common in cirrhosis such as prerenal failure secondary to volume depletion, acute tubular necrosis, drug-induced nephrotoxicity (mainly from non-steroidal anti-inflammatory agents or aminoglycosides) and glomerulonephritis should be excluded before the diagnosis of HRS is made. Causes that may predispose to prerenal failure such as volume depletion due to vomiting or diarrhoea, or renal fluid losses due to excessive diuretic therapy are common in cirrhotic patients and should be sought after. In prerenal failure due to volume depletion, renal function improves after the intravenous administration of fluids, whereas no improvement occurs in patients with HRS. Shock before the development of renal failure in a cirrhotic patient precludes the diagnosis of HRS, and usually indicates acute tubular necrosis. In regard to bacterial infections, the diagnosis of HRS should be made if renal failure persists after complete resolution of the infection. Proteinuria (> 500 mg/dL) and/or ultrasonographic abnormalities in the kidneys are indicative of parenchymal renal disease.

Management

General measures

Type 1 HRS develops in the setting of advanced liver disease in most cases but in some others it occurs in the setting of acute liver failure. In either it is recommended that patients be hospitalised and closely monitored in an intensive care setting, if possible. Central line access with central venous pressure measurement is helpful in assessing volume status, particularly when intravenous fluid challenge of a plasma expander is administered to rule out renal failure due to intravascular volume depletion. Adequate measures to ensure proper nutrition are very important since these patients are frequently malnourished. In patients with dilutional hyponatraemia, fluid restriction of 1 L/day is recommended [22]. Since the majority of patients have ascites, diagnostic paracentesis must be performed to rule out SBP. Diuretics must be stopped as they can cause worsening of renal failure and severe hyper kalaemia (in the case of spironolactone). In patients with tense ascites, a therapeutic tap associated with albumin infusion (6–8 g/L tapped) may aid in providing comfort. The most important aspect of management is to assess the patient for candidacy for liver transplantation. In order to better prepare patients for liver transplantation, renal function must be reversed, if possible, in order to obtain a better outcome after transplantation. Available therapies for type 1 HRS include the use splanchnic vasoconstrictors and transjugular portosystemic shunts (TIPS) [23,24] (Fig. 45). Patients with type 2 HRS are less sick and for the most part have refractory ascites that can be managed on outpatient basis with large-volume paracentesis and albumin expansion [2].

Vasoconstrictor therapy

A variety of pharmacological interventions has been used to treat HRS. The use of renal vasodilators such as dopamine and prostaglandin analogues was

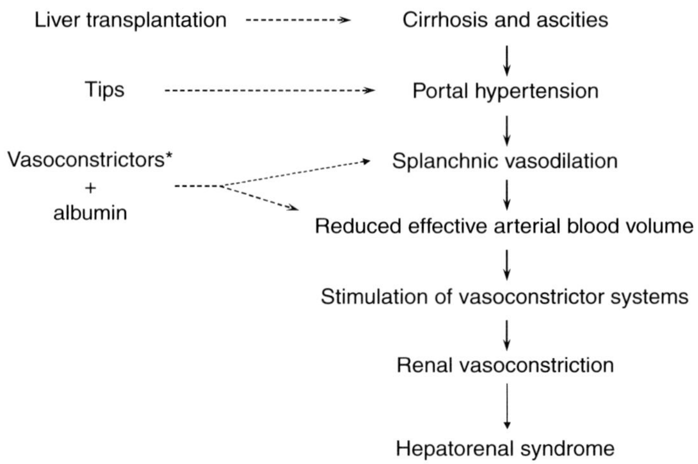

Fig. 45 Proposed therapies for hepatorenal syndrome in relation to the pathophysiological events leading to its development. TIPS: transjugular intrahepatic portosystemic shunt. Vasoconstrictors*: terlipressin, midodrine, octreotide and noradrenaline.

abandoned due to side effects and lack of benefits [25]. Other drugs such as endothelin blockers (BQ123) and N-acetylcysteine are promising, but information available is extremely limited [26,27]. Systemic vasoconstrictors with plasma expansion are the best therapy at present, because several uncontrolled studies have confirmed a beneficial role in HRS [28–39]. Vasoconstrictors with plasma expansion are used because the initial event in the pathogenesis of HRS is arterial splanchnic vasodilation causing a decrease in effective arterial blood volume with activation of endogenous vasoconstrictors systems; this approach suppresses these systems and reverses renal vasoconstriction with improvement of renal function [28].

Vasoconstrictors used for HRS include vasopressin analogues (ornipressin and terlipressin), somatostatin analogues (octreotide) and α-adrenergic agonists (midodrine and noradrenaline). In most studies vasoconstrictors were given in combination with albumin, with the aim of improving the efficacy of treatment. Vasopressin analogues have a marked vasoconstrictor effect in the splanchnic circulation and have been used for several years in the management of acute variceal bleeding in cirrhotic patients. Ornipressin, although effective in HRS, caused significant ischaemic side effects and was abandoned [28]. The most studied vasopressin analogue in HRS is terlipressin. The administration of terlipressin and albumin is associated with a significant improvement of GFR and reduction of serum creatinine below 1.5 mg/dL in approximately 40–90% of patients with type 1 HRS [23,30–36]

Table 40 Treatment of patients with type 1 hepatorenal syndrome with terlipressin. Data on response rate, side effects and survival in different series of patients.

Author/year (ref)	Response* (%)	Recurrence† (%)	Side effects‡ (%)	Median survival (days)
Uriz *et al.* 2000 [30]	7/9 (77)	0/7 (0)	1/9 (11)	39
Mulkay *et al.* 2001 [33]	11/12 (92)	6/11 (55)	0/12 (0)	42
Moreau *et al.* 2002 [31]	53/91 (58)	NR	18/99 (18)	43
Colle *et al.* 2002 [35]	11/18 (61)	7/11 (64)	0/18 (0)	24
Halimi *et al.* 2002 [34]	13/18 (72)	NR	4/18 (22)	NR
Ortega *et al.* 2002 [32]	14/21 (66)	2/12 (17)	1/21 (5)	40
Solanki *et al.* 2003 [36]	5/12 (42)	NR	3/12 (25)	NR

* The definition of response varies between studies

† Recurrence of hepatorenal syndrome after treatment withdrawal in responder patients, definition of recurrence also varies between studies

‡ Most patients presented self-limited abdominal cramps and/or diarrhoea during the administration of the first doses of terlipressin, which were not counted as severe side effects; NR, not reported

Source: Modified from Gines P *et al. Aliment Pharmacol Ther.* Sep 2004; 20(suppl. 3): 57–62

(Table 40). In most cases improvement in urine volume occurs within the first 24 h, but significant improvement in GFR happens over several days. Although one of the initial concerns about using terlipressin was the development of ischaemia (heart and/or extremities), the occurrence of this complication has been reported infrequently. There is a low incidence of ischaemic side effects ($\sim$ 10%), as demonstrated by several studies [30–36]. Patients with Child–Pugh scores greater than 13 and those who do not receive albumin expansion did not seem to respond well to this treatment [31,32]. Reversal of HRS occurs over several days but despite reduction of serum creatinine to normal or near-normal levels, GFR remains below normal values in most patients who respond [30,32]. Recurrence of HRS after stopping treatment is variable (Table 40) and a repeat course of terlipressin with albumin is usually effective [30,32].

A drawback of terlipressin is that it is not available in many countries, including the United States, and therefore α-adrenergic agonists are a reasonable alternative given that they are widely available. Administration of midodrine in association with octreotide (an inhibitor of the release of glucagon and other vasodilator peptides) and albumin also improves renal function in cirrhotic patients with HRS although information about this therapeutic approach is limited to only two studies with a total of 17 patients [37,38]. In a recent study of 14 patients with type 1 HRS treated with midodrine, octreotide and albumin, 10 had a good response (serum creatinine remained stable at < 1.5 mg/dL for 3 days) and were subsequently treated with TIPS if not contraindicated by INR > 2.0, serum bilirubin > 5 mg/dL and a Child–Pugh score > 12 [38]. Five patients underwent TIPS with excellent outcome and one of them received living donor liver transplantation. Interestingly, renal function continued to improve and completely normalised in these five patients. Of the five who responded to vasoconstrictors and albumin but did not get TIPS, two underwent successful liver transplantation, but three died as a consequence of liver failure, sepsis and arrhythmia. There was improved survival in all responders, but the real impact of TIPS in improving survival is difficult to assess, given the low number of patients treated. The findings of this study indicate that reversal of HRS achieved by pharmacological treatment is further enhanced by TIPS placement in appropriate candidates, leading to complete normalisation of renal function. Finally, the administration of noradrenaline in association with intravenous albumin resulted in a significant improvement of renal function in a small group of 12 cirrhotic patients with type 1 HRS [39].

One of the primary goals of pharmacological therapy is that of successfully reversing renal failure, so that suitable liver transplant candidates can undergo transplantation without renal failure, which is a well-known risk factor of poor outcome after transplantation. A recent study revealed that patients treated successfully with vasopressin analogues and albumin before liver transplantation had a post-transplantation outcome and survival similar to that of patients transplanted without HRS [40]. This study supports the concept that HRS should be treated before liver transplantation because improvements in renal function are probably associated with better outcomes. In three studies, patients who responded to therapy of HRS (decrease of creatinine to < 1.5 mg/dL) with terlipressin and albumin and octreotide, midodrine and albumin had an increased survival compared to those who did not respond to this therapy [31,32,38]. The recommended doses and duration of vasoconstrictor therapy are summarised in Table 41.

Transjugular intrahepatic portosystemic shunt (TIPS)

Transjugular intrahepatic portosystemic shunt is a non-surgical method of portal decompression used as an alternative therapy for cirrhotic patients bleeding from oesophageal or gastric varices who are refractory to endoscopic and medical treatment. TIPS reduces portal pressure and returns some of the volume of blood pooled in the splanchnic circulation to the systemic circulation. This event suppresses RAAS and SNS activity and reduces the

Table 41 Recommendations for using vasoconstrictors in type 1 hepatorenal syndrome.

1 Goal of treatment: reduction of serum creatinine below 1.5 mg/dL.
2 Recommended drugs and doses:
(a) Terlipressin 0.5 mg intravenously every 4 h; can increase dose in a stepwise fashion (i.e. every 2–3 days) to 1 mg/4 h and then up to 2 mg/4 h in cases showing no decrease in creatinine [30–36].
(b) Midodrine 2.5–7.5 mg orally three times daily with an increase to 12.5 mg three times daily if needed and octreotide 100 μg subcutaneously three times daily with an increase to 200 μg three times daily if needed [37,38].
(c) Noradrenaline 0.5–3 mg/h continuous intravenous infusion [39].
3 Concomitant intravenous albumin infusion (1 g/kg on the first day, followed by 20–50 g/day)* should be considered in all patients.
4 Avoid in patients with cardiac diseases, peripheral vascular disease and/or cerebrovascular disease due to the potential risk of ischaemic events.
5 Duration of therapy: 1–2 weeks

* This dose of albumin has been arbitrarily proposed. It is not known if smaller doses of albumin or use of other plasma expanders are beneficial in HRS

vasoconstriction in the renal circulation [38,41]. Small uncontrolled studies indicate that TIPS may improve renal function and GFR as well as reduce the activity of RAAS and SNS in cirrhotics with type 1 HRS [24,38,42]. Improvement in renal function after TIPS placement alone is generally slow with success in approximately 60% of patients [24,42]. One problem with the studies assessing TIPS for type 1 HRS is that patients included were highly selected and those with advanced Child–Pugh score > 12 were excluded due to the risk of worsening liver failure and/or hepatic encephalopathy.

In patients with type 2 HRS, TIPS improves renal function, prevents the development of type 1 HRS and reduces ascites formation [24,43–46]. However, despite these beneficial effects, survival is not significantly improved [43].

Dialysis

Small uncontrolled studies using haemodialysis and peritoneal dialysis suggest that both are ineffective, mainly due to a high incidence of severe side effects, including arterial hypotension, coagulopathy, gastrointestinal bleeding and increased mortality. Continuous arterovenous or venovenous haemofiltration have also been used but their efficacy remains to be determined. Although haemodialysis is not routinely recommended in HRS, it may be a reasonable option in suitable liver transplant candidates as a bridge to transplantation when there is no response to vasoconstrictors or TIPS or patients develop severe volume overload, metabolic acidosis or refractory hyperkalaemia.

The beneficial effect of an extracorporeal albumin dialysis system (MARS) was reported in 13 patients with Child C cirrhosis and type 1 HRS [47]. This system is a modified dialysis method that enables the selective removal of albumin-bound substances that accumulate in liver failure by the use of an albumin containing dialysate. In this study, five patients were treated with haemodialysis and standard medical therapy (low-dose dopamine and albumin) and eight patients were treated with the same plus MARS. The authors reported a significant decrease in bilirubin and creatinine, an improvement in serum sodium, urine volume, mean arterial blood pressure and decreased mortality in the MARS group. The procedure was well tolerated in all patients. Unfortunately, no other systemic haemodynamics parameters such as cardiac output or peripheral vascular resistance were assessed. In addition there were no measurements of renal functions such as renal blood flow and GFR. A shortcoming of this study is that improvement in serum values of bilirubin, creatinine and sodium could represent the effect of the dialysis and not a significant change in hepatic and renal function. Although promising, these results require further evaluation in order to consider dialysis as a therapy, or more importantly as a bridge to liver transplantation in patients with HRS.

Liver transplantation

Liver transplantation is the best treatment for suitable candidates with HRS, as it offers a cure to both the diseased liver and the circulatory and renal dysfunction. Unfortunately transplantation for type 1 HRS is limited by the fact that a significant proportion of patients die before the operation because they have a short survival and there is a prolonged waiting time in most centres. Priority for liver transplantation in the United States is based on the Model for End-stage Liver Disease (MELD) score which includes three variables; bilirubin, serum creatinine and international normalised ratio (INR) [48]. A recent study showed that patients with type 1 HRS with a MELD score equal to or greater than 20 showed an extremely poor outcome with a median survival of 1 month and those with type 2 HRS and a score lower than 20 showed a slightly better outcome with a median survival of 11 months. The majority of patients with type 1 HRS will have a high MELD score and hence a higher possibility of getting a liver transplant. Other countries have different allocation systems that give higher priority to patients with type 1 HRS. Regardless of the system used for organ allocation, patients with type 1 HRS need to be appropriately treated before transplantation. As mentioned previously, patients with HRS treated with vasopressin analogues and albumin before transplantation have a good outcome, similar to that of non-HRS patients [40].

Because cyclosporin and tacrolimus treatment may contribute to renal impairment post-operatively, other drugs such as azathioprine, steroids, IL-2 receptor antagonists or anti-lymphocyte agents should preferably be used in patients transplanted with renal failure until diuresis and improvement of renal function is observed, usually in 2–4 days after transplantation.

Prevention

HRS can be prevented in two clinical settings. First, in patients with SBP, a condition which entails high risk of development of HRS, the administration of albumin (1.5 g/kg at diagnosis of infection and 1 g/kg 48 h later) prevents the circulatory dysfunction and subsequent development of HRS [49]. Since it appears that SBP may trigger HRS by decreasing effective arterial blood volume, the rationale for albumin administration is to prevent arterial underfilling and subsequent activation of vasoconstrictor systems during the infection [49]. The incidence of HRS in patients with SBP receiving albumin together with antibiotic therapy is of 10% compared with an incidence of 33% in patients not receiving albumin [49]. Most importantly, hospital mortality was lower in patients receiving albumin (10%) versus those not receiving plasma expansion (29%) [49]. Second, in patients with acute alcoholic hepatitis, the administration of pentoxifylline, an inhibitor of tumour necrosis factor (400 mg t.i.d. orally for 28 days) reduces the incidence of HRS and mortality (8% and 24%, respectively) with respect to a control group (35% and 46%, respectively) [3]. Although there are no follow-up studies confirming these results, these two approaches are widely used in the clinical setting due to the high efficacy reported in the two studies and lack of alternative treatments.

REFERENCES

1 Arroyo V, Ginès P, Gerbes A *et al.* Definition and diagnostic criteria of refractory ascites and hepatorenal syndrome in cirrhosis. *Hepatology* 1996;**23**: 164–176.

2 Ginès P, Cárdenas A, Arroyo V, Rodés J. Management of cirrhosis and ascites. *N Engl J Med* 2004;**350**: 1646–1654.

3 Akriviadis E, Botla R, Briggs W *et al.* Pentoxifylline improves short-term survival in severe acute alcoholic hepatitis. a double-blind, placebo-controlled trial. *Gastroenterology* 2000;**119**: 1637–1648.

4 Moore K. Renal failure in acute liver failure. *Eur J Gastroenterol Hepatol* 1999;**11**: 967–975.

5 Ginès A, Escorsell A, Ginès P *et al.* Incidence, predictive factors, and prognosis of hepatorenal syndrome in cirrhosis. *Gastroenterology* 1993;**105**: 229–236.
6 Epstein M, Berk DP, Hollenberg NK *et al.* Renal failure in the patient with cirrhosis. The role of active vasoconstriction. *Am J Med* 1970;**49**: 175–185.
7 Schrier RW, Arroyo V, Bernardi M *et al.* Peripheral arterial vasodilation hypothesis: a proposal for the initiation of renal sodium and water retention in cirrhosis. *Hepatology* 1988;**8**: 1151–1157.
8 Martin PY, Ginès P, Schrier RW. Role of nitric oxide as mediator of hemodynamic abnormalities and sodium and water retention in cirrhosis. *N Engl J Med* 1998;**339**: 533–541.
9 Dudley FJ, Esler MD. The sympathetic nervous system in cirrhosis. In: Ginès P, Arroyo V, Rodés J, Schrier RW (eds). *Ascites and renal dysfunction in liver disease.* 2nd edn, Oxford; Blackwell Publishing, 2005; 54–72.
10 Arroyo V, Clària J, Saló J *et al.* Antidiuretic hormone and the pathogenesis of water retention in cirrhosis with ascites. *Semin Liver Dis* 1994;**14**: 44–58.
11 Ippolito S, Moore K. Arachidonic acid metabolites and the kidney in cirrhosis. In: Ginès P, Arroyo V, Rodés J, Schrier RW (eds). *Ascites and renal dysfunction in liver disease.* 2nd edn, Oxford; Blackwell Publishing, 2005; 84–104.
12 Cárdenas A. Hepatorenal syndrome: a dreaded complication of end-stage liver disease. *Am J Gastroenterol* 2005;**100**: 1–8.
13 Follo A, Llovet JM, Navasa M *et al.* Renal impairment after spontaneous bacterial peritonitis in cirrhosis: incidence, clinical course, predictive factors and prognosis. *Hepatology* 1994;**20**: 1495–1501.
14 Ruiz-del-Arbol L, Urman J, Fernandez J *et al.* Systemic, renal, and hepatic hemodynamic derangement in cirrhotic patients with spontaneous bacterial peritonitis. *Hepatology* 2003;**38**: 1210–1218.
15 Lee SS. Cardiac dysfunction in spontaneous bacterial peritonitis: a manifestation of cirrhotic cardiomyopathy? *Hepatology* 2003;**38**: 1089–1091.
16 Caregaro L, Menon F, Angeli P *et al.* Limitations of serum creatinine level and creatinine clearance as filtration markers in cirrhosis. *Arch Intern Med* 1994;**154**: 201–205.
17 Gines P, Guevara M, Delas Heras D, Arroyo V. Review article: albumin for circulatory support in patients with cirrhosis. *Aliment Pharmacol Ther* 2002; **16**(suppl. 5): 24–31.
18 Cárdenas A, Ginès P, Uriz J *et al.* Renal failure after upper gastrointestinal bleeding in cirrhosis. Incidence, clinical course, predictive factors and short-term prognosis. *Hepatology* 2001;**34**: 671–676.
19 Ginès P, Guevara M, Arroyo V, Rodes J. Hepatorenal syndrome. *Lancet* 2003;**362**: 1819–1827.
20 Roy L, Legault L, Pomier-Layrargues G. Glomerular filtration rate measurement in cirrhotic patients with renal failure. *Clin Nephrol* 1998;**50**: 342–346.
21 Dudley FJ, Kanel GC, Wood JL *et al.* Hepatorenal syndrome without sodium retention. *Hepatology* 1986;**6**: 248–259.
22 Cárdenas A, Ginès P. Pathogenesis and treatment of dilutional hyponatremia in cirrhosis. In: Arroyo V, Forns X, Garcia-Pagan JC, Rodes J (eds). *Progress in the treatment of liver diseases.* Ars Medica, Barcelona, 2003; 31–42.

23 Alessandria C, Venon WD, Marzano A *et al.* Renal failure in cirrhotic patients: role of terlipressin in clinical approach to hepatorenal syndrome type 2. *Eur J Gastroenterol Hepatol* 2002;**14**: 1363–1368.
24 Brensing KA, Textor J, Perz J *et al.* Long-term outcome after transjugular intrahepatic portosystemic stent-shunt in non-transplant cirrhotics with hepatorenal syndrome: a phase II study. *Gut* 2000;**47**: 288–295.
25 Arroyo V, Terra C, Torre A *et al.* Hepatorenal syndrome in cirrhosis: clinical features, diagnosis and management. In: Ginès P, Arroyo V, Rodés J, Schrier RW (eds). *Ascites and renal dysfunction in liver disease.* 2nd edn, Oxford; Blackwell Publishing, 2005; 341–359.
26 Soper CP, Latif AB, Bending MR. Amelioration of hepatorenal syndrome with selective endothelin-A antagonist. *Lancet* 1996;**347**: 1842–1843.
27 Holt S, Goodier D, Marley R *et al.* Improvement in renal function in hepatorenal syndrome with N-acetylcysteine. *Lancet* 1999;**353**: 294–295.
28 Guevara M, Gines P, Fernandez-Esparrach G *et al.* Reversibility of hepatorenal syndrome by prolonged administration of ornipressin and plasma volume expansion. *Hepatology* 1998;**27**: 35–41.
29 Gulberg V, Bilzer M, Gerbes AL. Long-term therapy and retreatment of hepatorenal syndrome type 1 with ornipressin and dopamine. *Hepatology* 1999;**30**: 870–875.
30 Uriz J, Gines P, Cárdenas A *et al.* Terlipressin plus albumin infusion: an effective and safe therapy of hepatorenal syndrome. *J Hepatol* 2000;**33**: 43–48.
31 Moreau R, Durand F, Poynard T *et al.* Terlipressin in patients with cirrhosis and type 1 hepatorenal syndrome: a retrospective multicenter study. *Gastroenterology* 2002;**122**: 923–930.
32 Ortega R, Ginès P, Uriz J *et al.* Terlipressin therapy with and without albumin for patients with hepatorenal syndrome. Results of a prospective, non-randomized study. *Hepatology* 2002;**36**: 941–948.
33 Mulkay JP, Louis H, Donckier V *et al.* Long-term terlipressin administration improves renal function in cirrhotic patients with type 1 hepatorenal syndrome: a pilot study. *Acta Gastroenterol Belg* 2001;**64**: 15–19.
34 Halimi C, Bonnard P, Bernard B *et al.* Effect of terlipressin (Glypressin) on hepatorenal syndrome in cirrhotic patients: results of a multicentre pilot study. *Eur J Gastroenterol Hepatol* 2002;**14**: 153–158.
35 Colle I, Durand F, Pessione F *et al.* Clinical course, predictive factors and prognosis in patients with cirrhosis and type 1 hepatorenal syndrome treated with terlipressin: a retrospective analysis. *J Gastroenterol Hepatol* 2002;**17**: 882–888.
36 Solanki P, Chawla A, Garg R *et al.* Beneficial effects of terlipressin in hepatorenal syndrome: a prospective, randomized placebo-controlled clinical trial. *J Gastroenterol Hepatol* 2003;**18**: 152–156.
37 Angeli P, Volpin R, Gerunda G *et al.* Reversal of type 1 hepatorenal syndrome with the administration of midodrine and octreotide. *Hepatology* 1999;**29**: 1690–1697.
38 Wong F, Pantea L, Sniderman K. Midodrine, octreotide, albumin, and TIPS in selected patients with cirrhosis and type 1 hepatorenal syndrome. *Hepatology* 2004;**40**: 55–64.

39 Duvoux C, Zanditenas D, Hezode C *et al.* Effects of noradrenaline and albumin in patients with type 1 hepatorenal syndrome: a pilot study. *Hepatology* 2002;**36**: 374–380.

40 Restuccia T, Ortega R, Guevara M *et al.* Effects of treatment of hepatorenal syndrome before transplantation on posttransplantation outcome. A case-control study. *J Hepatol* 2004;**40**: 140–146.

41 Boyer TD. Transjugular intrahepatic portosystemic shunt: current status. *Gastroenterology* 2003;**124**: 1700–1710.

42 Guevara M, Gines P, Bandi JC *et al.* Transjugular intrahepatic portosystemic shunt in hepatorenal syndrome: effects on renal function and vasoactive systems. *Hepatology* 1998;**28**: 416–422.

43 Ginès P, Uriz J, Calahorra B *et al.* Transjugular intrahepatic portosystemic shunting versus paracentesis plus albumin for refractory ascites in cirrhosis. *Gastroenterology* 2002;**123**: 1839–1847.

44 Ochs A, Rössle M, Haag K *et al.* The transjugular intrahepatic portosystemic stent shunt procedure for refractory ascites. *N Engl J Med* 1995;**332**: 1192–1197.

45 Rossle M, Ochs A, Gulberg V *et al.* A comparison of paracentesis and transjugular intrahepatic portosystemic shunting in patients with ascites. *N Engl J Med* 2000;**8**;**342**: 1701–1707.

46 Sanyal AJ, Genning C, Reddy RK *et al.* Nastra Group. The North American Study of Treatment for Refractory Ascites (NASTRA). *Gastroenterology* 2003;**124**: 634–641.

47 Mitzer SR, Stange J, Klammt S *et al.* Improvement of hepatorenal syndrome with extracorporeal albumin dialysis MARS: results of a prospective, randomized, controlled clinical trial. *Liver Transpl* 2000;**6**: 277–286.

48 Kamath PS, Wiesner RH, Malinchoc M *et al.* A model to predict survival in patients with end-stage liver disease. *Hepatology* 2001;**33**: 464–470.

49 Sort P, Navasa M, Arroyo V *et al.* Effect of intravenous albumin on renal impairment and mortality in patients with cirrhosis and spontaneous bacterial peritonitis. *N Engl J Med* 1999;5: 403–409.

SESSION 5

Treatment of the Acute Bleeding Episode

Loren Laine, Ramón Planas, Frederik Nevens, Rafael Bañares, David Patch and Jaime Bosch

PRESENTATION AND DIAGNOSIS

Ruptured oesophageal varices cause approximately 70% of all upper gastrointestinal bleeding episodes in cirrhosis [1]. Although overall survival has improved in recent years [2], mortality is still closely related to failure to control haemorrhage or early rebleeding, which occurs in as many as 40% of patients within the first 5 days after the initial bleeding episode [1,3]. Ideally, all variceal bleeders should be managed in an intensive care setting by a team of experienced medical staff, including well-trained nurses, hepatologists, endoscopists, surgeons and interventional radiologists. The management of variceal bleeding requires simultaneous and coordinated attention to (1) correct hypovolaemia; (2) prevent and treat complications associated with bleeding and (3) control of active bleeding and prevention of early rebleeding. The first two goals, which are independent of the cause of the haemorrhage, demand immediate management. By contrast, specific therapy to stop bleeding is usually given when the patient has had the initial resuscitation and following diagnostic endoscopy, with the important exception of pharmacological therapy that can be started earlier in the course of the bleeding episode, on arrival to the hospital or even during transfer to the hospital.

Patients usually present with haematemesis or melaena. Specific features to be noted in the history are those of prolonged alcohol excess, ingestion of NSAIDs or aspirin, previous variceal bleeding, previously diagnosed liver diseases, past abdominal sepsis or history of umbilical vein catheterisation. The physical examination should emphasise determining whether the patient is haemodynamically stable, and must also include a search for signs of chronic liver disease. The severity of blood loss is roughly estimated by the haemodynamic status. The initial examination and investigations need to include an assessment of the presence of renal dysfunction, the presence of infection, disease in other systems and the severity of liver disease. A recent study has shown that measurements of hepatic venous pressure gradient (HVPG) within 48 h of admission for acute variceal bleeding provide useful prognostic information on the outcome of the bleeding episode and long-term survival [4]. In that study, an initial HVPG of $\geq$ 20 mmHg was associated with a significant greater risk of failure to control bleeding, early rebleeding, longer hospital stay, greater transfusion requirements and lower probability of survival. If confirmed, such high-risk patients might benefit from early aggressive therapy. The presence of portal vein thrombosis and/or hepatocellular carcinoma needs to be established early on, by ultrasound imaging.

The gold standard for the diagnosis of varices is endoscopy, which should be performed as soon as resuscitation is adequate, and preferably within 12 h of admission [5], especially in patients with clinically significant bleeding or in patients with features suggesting cirrhosis. In mild bleeds, causing neither haemodynamic change nor requiring blood volume restitution, endoscopy could be done electively, but within 24 h. A diagnosis of bleeding varices is accepted either when a venous (non-pulsatile) spurt is seen, when there is fresh bleeding from the oesophageal–gastric junction in the presence of varices or when there is fresh blood in the fundus when gastric varices are present. In the absence of active bleeding (approximately in 50% of cases) either a 'white nipple sign' or the presence of varices in the absence of other lesions suggests varices as the source of haemorrhage [6]. Gastric varices are more difficult to detect by endoscopy. Erosions and portal hypertensive gastropathy are frequently found, but are an uncommon cause of acute bleeding. If the patient is exsanguinating and varices are suspected, a Sengstaken–Blakemore tube may be passed [7].

GENERAL MANAGEMENT

Resuscitation

Resuscitation follows the general rules of airway, breathing and circulation. Aspiration of blood or gastric contents place patient at risk for cardiopulmonary complications, especially in encephalopathic patients, and it is further exacerbated by endoscopic procedures. In upper gastrointestinal bleeding, cardiopulmonary complications constitute 23% to 50% of associated complications and carry an estimated 50% to 60% of mortality rate [8]. Endotracheal intubation is mandatory if there is any concern about the safety of the airway. Pulse oxymetry and oxygen are essential and adequate suction and extreme care of the airway must be maintained.

Variceal bleeding in cirrhosis is often massive; it is therefore essential to introduce at least one large-bore, 14- to 18-gauge, intravenous catheter to administer fluids and blood products if required. A central venous line may be helpful to estimate intravascular volume [9]. An internal jugular line is safer than a subclavian approach. The presence of coagulopathy and thrombocytopenia is not a contraindication to central venous access.

We recommend initial volume replacement should be with human albumin fraction or gelatine-based colloid as this has no effect on clotting or bleeding times compared to dextran [5]. Following this, specific treatment can be started with a vasopressor agent. In this respect, there is evidence from a trial using terlipressin that drug therapy should be instituted as early as possible [10].

Correcting hypovolaemia

Renal failure occurs more frequently in hospitalised cirrhotic patients with gastrointestinal haemorrhage than in non-cirrhotic patients with gastrointestinal haemorrhage. In a large series of cirrhotic patients with gastrointestinal bleeding (82% variceal), hypovolaemia and a poor liver function were the only factors independently predictive of renal failure. Moreover, this study showed that the only two independent predictors of in-hospital mortality were the presence of hypovolaemic shock and renal failure (67% mortality versus 3% in patients without either of these factors) [11]. Therefore, avoidance of hypovolaemia and maintenance of haemodynamic stability are particularly important in these patients.

Optimal volume replacement remains controversial. Over-transfusion should be avoided because it can lead to rebound portal hypertension and early rebleeding, acute pulmonary oedema and respiratory failure [12,13]. Therefore, transfusions with packed red cells should be aimed at maintaining the haematocrit between 21% and 27%, or the haemoglobin between 7 g/dL and 9 g/dL, depending on other factors such as patient's comorbidities and age, haemodynamic status and presence of ongoing bleeding clinically. However, it is important to correct anaemia progressively on the following days. All patients receiving large volumes of blood should be monitored for hypocalcaemia (citrate binding ionised calcium) and hypothermia (cold blood products). Large volume transfusion may lead to impaired haemostasis and thrombocytopenia, so that fresh frozen plasma and platelets need to be replaced [14]. Platelet transfusions are necessary to improve primary haemostasis and should be used occasionally. Transfusion decisions should be individualised according to many factors, including bleeding severity, presence of other coagulopathies, such as disseminated intravascular coagulation, and the presence of qualitative platelet defects, such as those induced by renal failure or NSAIDs.

Patients with cirrhosis often have defects in the coagulation system, the most pronounced deficiency being that of factor VII, and it is well known that coagulopathy is an important predisposing risk factor for failure to control bleeding in these patients. In this way, recombinant factor VIIa may be useful in variceal bleeding as it has been shown to normalise prothrombin time in patients with decompensated cirrhosis and variceal bleeding [15]. In fact, in a recent published randomised, double-blind trial the administration of recombinant factor VIIa significantly decreased the proportion of Child–Pugh B and C cirrhotic patients who failed to control variceal bleeding [16]. Further studies are warranted to verify this finding.

Prevention of complications and deterioration in liver function

Infection control and treatment

Up to 20% of cirrhotics who are hospitalised secondary to gastrointestinal bleeding have bacterial infections, and an additional 50% develop an infection while hospitalised [17]. In a prospective study, admission for gastrointestinal bleeding and low serum albumin were identified as the only two variables independently associated with the development of bacterial infection [18]. The most common infections in cirrhotics with gastrointestinal bleeding are spontaneous bacterial peritonitis (SBP) and/or spontaneous bacteraemia, followed by urinary tract infections and pneumonia. The most frequently isolated micro-organisms are Gram-negative; infections by Gram-positive organisms predominate in patients with pneumonia.

Besides a higher mortality, bacterial infections are also associated with a higher rate of variceal rebleeding. Therefore it would appear logical to prevent the occurrence of these infections through the use of antibiotics. In fact, it has been demonstrated that antibiotic prophylaxis significantly increases survival (9.1% mean improvement rate, 95% confidence interval CI: 2.9–15.3%, $p = 0.004$) and increases the percentage of patients free from infection (32% mean improvement rate, 95% CI: 22–42%, $p = 0.001$) [19]. Norfloxacin, administered orally at a dose of 400 mg twice a day for 7 days, has been used in many studies [20]. A recent randomised controlled trial (RCT) has compared oral norfloxacin versus intravenous ceftriaxone in the prevention of bacterial infections in cirrhotic patients with gastrointestinal bleeding (variceal in 71% of cases) and severe liver failure, defined as the presence of at least two of the following: ascites, hepatic encephalopathy, jaundice and malnutrition. In this subset of cirrhotic patients the probability of developing bacterial infections was significantly lower in patients receiving ceftriaxone than in those treated with norfloxacin (11% versus 27%, $p = 0.02$) [21]. Thus, all cirrhotics with upper gastrointestinal bleeding should receive prophylactic antibiotics using oral quinolones or intravenous cephalosporins. Aminoglycosides should be avoided because of their renal toxicity in patients with cirrhosis.

Hepatic encephalopathy

Hepatic encephalopathy often can be precipitated by an episode of gastrointestinal bleeding in cirrhotic patients. Precipitant factors should be evaluated and corrected. The routine use of lactulose for the prevention of encephalopathy is controversial. However, it should be given (5–15 mL/6 h) by mouth or nasogastric tube in encephalopathic patients.

It is important to be forewarned about the possibility of alcohol withdrawal. Signs of encephalopathy may overlap it. Intravenous clormethiazole is useful to control acute withdrawal. When necessary, thiamine should be administered to prevent Wernicke's encephalopathy.

Ascites and renal function

Renal function should be supported by adequate fluid and electrolyte replacement (saline infusions should be avoided) and should be monitored with strict attention to fluid balance. The urine output should be maintained at over 40 mL/h; an output below 20 mL/h indicates poor renal perfusion and impending renal failure. In fact, renal failure may be precipitated by a variceal bleed. The intravascular volume should be maintained and nephrotoxic drugs should be avoided, particularly aminoglycosides and NSAIDs. Tense ascites should be treated by paracentesis, preferably with albumin replacement. This has been shown to decrease portal and variceal pressure [22].

Nutrition

Malnutrition is very frequent in cirrhosis [23], particularly with advanced liver failure and may contribute to an increased susceptibility to infections and to impaired renal function. The suppression of oral intake during the acute bleeding episode worsens the nutritional state. Therefore feeding should be resumed as soon as a 24-h interval free of bleeding has been achieved. Enteral nutrition is always preferable, as parenteral nutrition further complicates the fluid balance, and leads to an added risk of infection.

Prognosis

Variceal bleeding is a life-threatening complication of liver cirrhosis. A poor outcome – either failure to control bleeding, early recurrent bleeding or death – occurs in 15–30% of cases. Several factors predictive of a poor outcome have been identified in various studies, including severity of initial bleeding, renal dysfunction, bacterial infection, spurting varices, degree of liver dysfunction, HVPG, complications of endoscopic treatment, alcoholic aetiology of cirrhosis, portal vein thrombosis and the presence of hepatocellular carcinoma [24].

VASOACTIVE DRUGS FOR VARICEAL BLEEDING IN CIRRHOSIS

The aim of a specific treatment for variceal bleeding is to stop the haemorrhage, to prevent early rebleeding and to reduce mortality. The first-line specific treatment of variceal bleeding consists of vasoactive drugs and/or endoscopic therapy.

The reason to use vasoactive drugs is the assumption that a reduction in portal pressure is associated with a better control of the variceal haemorrhage [25]. Villanueva *et al.* performed HVPG measurements during active bleeding in patients with or without natural somatostatin [26]. Those who failed were those patients in which a reduction in portal pressure was not obtained. The study further confirmed that a HVPG above 20 mmHg was associated with a bad prognosis [4].

In favour of vasoactive drugs is that they are safe and do not require skilful personnel. As such specific treatment can be started on suspicion of variceal bleeding, in the absence of contraindications treatment can be started even at home or during transfer to the hospital, which is important, since about a quarter of deaths occur very early after bleeding onset [27]. Furthermore, if used before endoscopy it may make endotherapy easier, with fewer side effects [28]. In addition, infusion of vasoactive drugs prevented the increase in portal pressure caused by blood transfusion in an experimental model [29].

The therapeutic value of the different drugs available are difficult to compare: the therapeutic schedules are heterogeneous, different methods are compared in a different way (versus placebo, another vasoactive drug or a combined treatment), the duration of the administration of the drugs might differ, the time points when vasoactive drugs are administered with regards to endotherapy are different (before or after endotherapy) and the primary aims of the studies are different.

Since the previous Baveno meeting, few new trials have been published. Excellent meta-analyses by D'Amico *et al.* of emergency sclerotherapy versus vasoactive drugs [30] and Bãnares *et al.* about the value of combining vasoactive drugs with endotherapy [31] have recently been published.

The different vasoactive drugs

Two different classes of medication that are currently used are terlipressin and natural somatostatin or its analogues.

Terlipressin

Terlipressin is a long-acting derivate of vasopressin with considerably fewer cardiovascular side effects. Terlipressin reduces portal pressure and this effect is still significant 4 h after administration [32–34]. Meta-analyses have demonstrated that terlipressin is more effective than placebo for control of variceal bleeding and that it improves survival of patients [35–37]. There is indirect evidence that terlipressin might prevent bleeding-induced renal impairment and that in animals it protects the liver in case of septic shock [38]. Terlipressin can provoke ischaemic complications and the drug is contraindicated in case of a history of ischaemic heart disease, cardiac rhythm disorders, arteriopathy of the lower limbs and a history of cerebral vascular accidents [39].

Before starting terlipressin, an ECG is mandatory and cardiac monitoring is necessary for high-risk patients. Terlipressin is given every 4 h intravenously depending on the weight: 1 mg if the weight is below 50 kg; 1.5 mg if the weight is between 50 and 70 kg and 2 mg above a weight of 70 kg. The dose is halved after bleeding has been controlled for 24 h, and may be maintained for 5 days to prevent early rebleeding. Terlipressin may offer an additional benefit to emergency sclerotherapy when given before endoscopy [10].

Somatostatin

Natural somatostatin reduces portal pressure and has been proven to reduce HVPG during active bleeding [26,40–42].

Natural somatostatin is probably more effective than placebo for the control of variceal bleeding [28,42,43]. No studies demonstrate an effect on mortality. On the other hand, its efficacy on control of bleeding, prevention of early rebleeding and mortality is probably similar to terlipressin [39]. Side effects are extremely rare. Somatostatin is administered intravenously with a perfusion rate of 250 μg/h after a bolus of 250 μg/h. The infusion is maintained for 1–5 days.

Haemodynamic investigations have suggested that higher doses of somatostatin might be more effective since a dose of 500 μg/h has a more pronounced effect on portal pressure [40] and one study suggested that a doses of 500 μg/h was more effective for control of bleeding when active bleeding was identified at endoscopy [44]. Natural somatostatin has also been shown to offer an additional beneficial effect when the drug is started before endotherapy [28].

Octreotide

Octreotide is a synthetic analogue of natural somatostatin. Octreotide is used in some countries especially because of availability. Octreotide is effective in studies where it has been used together with an endoscopic treatment to prevent early rebleeding [45–47]. Octreotide was not effective in the study in which it has been compared with placebo as initial therapy [48].

There is controversy about the effect of the drug on portal pressure. It appears that its effect on HVPG is not prolonged [49,50]. This can be explained by a tachyphylaxis or a rapid desensitisation [51]. It is well established that octreotide prevents an increase in portal pressure after a meal [52,53].

Side effects with octreotide are rare and the drug is given in a continuous infusion of 25–50 μg/h intravenously with (or without) an initial bolus of 50 μg, for up to 5 days, although the optimal dose has never been intensively explored. No placebo-controlled trials have been published in the clinical setting in which the drug is frequently used: before endotherapy.

Other analogues of somatostatin

Vapreotide and lanreotide are two analogues of somatostatin with a comparable affinity for the somatostatin receptors [54]. One study showed that vapreotide used before endotherapy is more effective than placebo to control variceal bleeding [55]. Lanreotide failed to improve the results of endoscopic therapy in a very large cooperative, double-blind, placebo-controlled trial which remains unpublished.

Still unsolved questions

Duration of pharmacological treatment

Vasoactive drugs have to be given at least until variceal haemorrhage has been controlled, which means 24 h after the last signs of active bleeding. Since vasoactive drugs are useful to prevent early rebleeding and this event occurs most frequently within the first days after the start of the bleeding, it is rational to continue vasoactive drugs for 5 days, and many studies documenting benefit have administered the drugs for 5 days. However, the optimal duration of therapy has not been investigated adequately, especially considering that most patients are treated with both vasoactive drugs and endoscopic therapy.

Adapting doses

It has been suggested that increased doses of natural somatostatin are more effective than standard doses when active bleeding is seen at endoscopy. So the question arises whether doses of vasoactive drugs should be varied in relation to early predictors of failure to control bleeding (e.g. active bleeding at the time of endoscopy, high baseline portal pressure).

Conclusions

Vasoactive drugs are the first line treatment of variceal bleeding. They are effective and safe. They should be used systematically and as soon as possible in patients with suspicion of variceal bleeding. The available data regarding terlipressin and somatostatin and its analogues do not permit conclusions regarding the superiority of one vasoactive drug over the other.

ENDOSCOPY IN DIAGNOSIS AND THERAPY OF VARICEAL BLEEDING

Timing of endoscopy

Early endoscopy is generally recommended in patients who present with major upper GI bleeding, as defined by haemodynamic instability (e.g. tachycardia, hypotension, orthostatic changes in pulse or blood pressure). Haemodynamic instability, comorbidities and age are the three pre-endoscopic independent predictors of rebleeding and death [56]. Although early endoscopy (variably defined as 2–24 h after presentation) has been documented to lower costs when performed in low-risk patients (by allowing early discharge or lower level of care if low-risk lesions are identified), benefit in clinical outcomes has not been documented [57]. The significant benefit of endoscopic therapy in high-risk patients suggests early endoscopy is beneficial in those with high-risk clinical features, but this is unproven in RCTs.

Some investigators also suggest that any patient with upper GI bleeding and the potential for variceal bleeding (e.g. known cirrhosis) should undergo early endoscopy. This is based on several factors. Patients with varices not uncommonly bleed from non-variceal sources and the outcome with bleeding from varices is much worse than with bleeding from non-variceal, non-malignant sources. Therefore, documentation of the source (variceal versus non-variceal) may provide important prognostic information and influence management. Also, as mentioned, comorbidities such as cirrhosis increase the risk of further bleeding and death. Endoscopic therapy is documented to significantly improve outcome in variceal bleeding, so the presumption is that earlier application of this therapy may be beneficial. However, no RCTs provide evidence regarding early endoscopy in patients with the potential for variceal bleeding.

Sclerotherapy

Endoscopic sclerotherapy controls active bleeding from varices in 62–100% of patients and appears to be more effective than sham therapy or medical therapy with vasopressin or balloon tamponade. A meta-analysis of five studies ($n = 251$) [58–62] comparing sclerotherapy with sham, balloon tamponade and/or vasopressin in patients with documented active bleeding revealed significant benefits of sclerotherapy in terms of cessation of acute bleeding (OR = 8.5, 95% CI: 3.6–20.0), rebleeding during hospitalisation or 2 weeks (OR = 0.36, 0.21–0.62) and mortality (OR = 0.57, 0.33–0.98) (Laine L, personal communication). Thus, sclerotherapy does appear to be beneficial in the acute treatment of patients with oesophageal variceal bleeding.

More recent studies which compare sclerotherapy with somatostatin or octreotide in acute variceal bleeding do not demonstrate significant differences in favour of sclerotherapy in the initial control of oesophageal variceal bleeding [30]. A recent meta-analysis included eight studies comparing sclerotherapy to octreotide infusion given for 12 h to 5 days (except one study that used subcutaneous octreotide) and five studies comparing sclerotherapy to somatostatin infusion given for 2 days to 5 days [30]. The absolute risk differences for sclerotherapy versus octreotide (failure to control bleeding: −3%, 95% CI, −8% to 2%, mortality: 0, −5% to 5%) and versus somatostatin (failure to control bleeding, −1%, −7% to 5%, mortality: −3%, −10% to 5%) were not significant. In three somatostatin studies the difference in serious adverse events favoured somatostatin (7%, 1% to 13%). Other studies have documented however, that the addition of octreotide [45–47,63] or somatostatin [28] improves the efficacy of sclerotherapy [28,45,47,63] and ligation [46], and that the addition of sclerotherapy improves the efficacy of somatostatin [64] in the treatment of acute oesophageal variceal bleeding.

Ligation versus sclerotherapy

Ligation is now considered to be more effective than sclerotherapy for treatment of oesophageal varices. However, relatively little information is available addressing this comparison in patients with active bleeding. A meta-analysis looking at haemostasis in patients with actively bleeding oesophageal varices revealed no significant difference (RR: 1.1, 95% CI: 0.4–2.9) [65]. However, the actively bleeding patients represented small subsets from within larger studies and thus were not truly from RCTs in this population. A single published randomised trial directly compares ligation with sclerotherapy specifically in the population of patients presenting with actively bleeding oesophageal varices [66]. Continued active bleeding (during the 1st 72 h) was significantly more frequent in the sclerotherapy group (24% versus 3%; RRR = 88%, ARR = 21% (95% CI: 6–36%), NNT = 5).

Ligation can sometimes be difficult to accomplish in patients with large amounts of blood in the oesophagus. The outer cylinder placed on the tip of the endoscope for ligation therapy may decrease the field of view, and blood may fill the cylinder, further obscuring the endoscopist's view. Therefore, the initial treatment of patients with actively bleeding varices may sometimes be more easily accomplished with sclerotherapy than with ligation. Ligation therapy can then be instituted at subsequent treatment sessions. In a randomised study comparing ligation to sclerotherapy after initial control of haemorrhage with sclerotherapy, ligation was found to have significantly less rebleeding, fewer complications, and achieved eradication with fewer sessions [67].

Tissue adhesives

Since the prior Baveno workshop, RCTs have been published that suggest that tissue adhesives such as N-butyl-cyanoacrylate should be used for the treatment of acute gastric variceal bleeding. Lo *et al.* randomly assigned 60 patients with bleeding gastric varices to N-butyl-2-cyanoacrylate therapy or ligation [68]. Haemostasis was significantly better with cyanoacrylate among the 26 patients presenting with acute variceal bleeding, and other longer-term end points (rebleeding, transfusions, mortality) were also improved in the overall group with tissue adhesive. Another randomised trial comparing N-butyl-2-cyanoacrylate with sclerotherapy in 37 patients had a subset of 17 patients with actively bleeding gastric varices [69]. Non-significant trends in favour of tissue adhesive also were seen in this small group, and variceal obliteration was significantly more common in the overall group (100% versus 44%).

Conclusions

Early endoscopy is appropriate in patients with haemodynamically significant upper GI bleeding and also perhaps in those with the potential for variceal bleeding (e.g. known cirrhosis). Ligation should be the initial endoscopic therapy employed in patients with acute or active oesophageal variceal bleeding. If technical difficulty is encountered, sclerotherapy can then be attempted; ligation should be used at subsequent treatment sessions. Cotherapy with somatostatin or octreotide for 2–5 days appears to be beneficial as compared to endoscopic therapy alone. Cyanoacrylate therapy appears to be the treatment of choice for acute gastric variceal bleeding, if technical expertise for this modality is available.

COMBINED PHARMACOLOGICAL AND ENDOSCOPIC THERAPY

Endoscopic therapy, involving either injection sclerosis or band ligation, is considered as one of the first choice interventions for acute variceal bleeding [70]. On the other hand, vasoactive drugs, such as somatostatin and terlipressin, are as effective as endoscopic sclerotherapy for the arrest of the acute episode of bleeding, prevention of early rebleeding, need for blood transfusions and mortality [30]. Therefore, the combination of both modalities of treatment is a theoretically attractive therapeutic alternative. Combination therapy adds the portal pressure lowering effect of drugs to the local haemostatic effects of injection sclerosis or ligation. In the last few years several trials have been developed aimed to answer the question as to whether drugs may improve the outcomes of endoscopic therapy (Table 42). In addition, two systematic reviews and meta-analyses have recently been published [30,31].

Comparison of endoscopic therapy versus combined pharmacological and endoscopic therapy

Effect of combined therapy on initial haemostasis

Initial haemostasis is not uniformly defined across all randomised studies. Only one study defined this variable – as recommended at the Baveno consensus meetings – as a 24 h bleeding-free period within the first 48 h after randomisation. In a recent meta-analysis, due to the lack of a homogeneous definition in the RCTs [31], initial haemostasis was defined as the clinical absence of continued bleeding within 6–48 h of treatment and was assessed in four trials involving 559 patients [45–47,55].

Table 42 Randomised controlled trials comparing endoscopic treatments with combined endoscopic and pharmacological treatments.

Study, year	Drug	Endoscopic procedure	Initial haemostasis: Drug* (P)† (CI)	Initial haemostasis: Control* (P)† (CI)	Initial haemostasis: RR (CI)	5-day haemostasis: Drug (P) (CI)	5-day haemostasis: Control (P) (CI)	5-day haemostasis: RR (CI)	5-day mortality: Drug (P) (CI)	5-day mortality: Control (P) (CI)	5-day mortality: RR (CI)
Besson, 1995	**OCT 25 µg/h IV × 5 days**	**Injection sclerosis**	**95/98 (0.97)** (0.91–0.99)	**86/101 (0.85)** (0.77–0.91)	**1.14** (1.04–1.24)	**87/98 (0.89)** (0.81–0.94)	**76/101 (0.75)** (0.66–0.83)	**1.18** (1.03–1.35)	**7/98 (0.07)** (0.03–0.14)	**10/101 (0.10)** (0.05–0.17)	**0.72** (0.29–1.82)
Sung, 1995	OCT 50 µg bolus then 50 µg/h × 5 days	Band ligation	45/47 (0.96) (0.35–0.99)	44/47 (0.94) (0.82–0.99)	1.02 (0.93–1.13)	41/47 (0.87) (0.74–0.95)	26/47 (0.55) (0.40–0.70)	1.58 (1.19–2.08)	–	–	–
Signorelli, 1996	OCT 100 µg/8 h SC × 5 days SMS 3.5 µg/kg.h IV × 5 days	Injection sclerosis	–	–	–	50/64 (0.78) (0.66–0.87)	19/30 (0.63) (0.44–0.80)	1.23 (0.91–1.67)	9/64 (0.14) (0.07–0.25)	5/30 (0.17) (0.06–0.35)	0.84 (0.31–2.30)
Ceriani, 1997	OCT 12.5 µg/h IV × 2 days	Injection sclerosis	–	–	–	22/28 (0.79) (0.59–0.92)	16/27 (0.59) (0.39–0.78)	1.33 (0.92–1.92)	4/28 (0.14) (0.04–0.33)	4/27 (0.15) (0.04–0.34)	0.96 (0.27–3.47)
Signorelli, 1997	OCT 50 µg bolus then 25 µg/h IV × 5 days	Injection sclerosis	–	–	–	37/44 (0.84) (0.70–0.93)	30/42 (0.71) (0.55–0.84)	1.18 (0.93–1.48)	–	–	–
Avgerinos, 1997	SMS 500 µg bolus then 250 µg/h IV × 5 days	Injection sclerosis	–	–	–	42/73 (0.58) (0.45–0.69)	24/72 (0.33) (0.23–0.45)	1.73 (1.18–2.53)	3/73 (0.04) (0.01–0.12)	7/72 (0.10) (0.04–0.19)	0.42 (0.11–1.57)
Zuberi, 2000	OCT 50 µg/h IV × 5 days	Injection sclerosis	33/35 (0.94) (0.31–0.99)	30/35 (0.86) (0.70–0.95)	1.10 (0.94–1.29)	31/35 (0.89) (0.73–0.97)	22/35 (0.63) (0.45–0.79)	1.41 (1.06–1.87)	1/35 (0.03) (0.00–0.15)	1/35 (0.03) (0.00–0.15)	1.00 (0.07–15.36)
Cales, 2001	VP 50 µg bolus then 50 µg/h IV × 5 days	Injection sclerosis or band ligation	72/98 (0.73) (0.54–0.82)	53/98 (0.54) (0.44–0.64)	1.36 (1.09–1.69)	65/98 (0.66) (0.56–0.76)	49/98 (0.50) (0.40–0.60)	1.33 (1.04–1.69)	5/98 (0.05) (0.02–0.11)	7/98 (0.07) (0.03–0.14)	0.71 (0.23–2.17)
Pooled data			245/278 (0.88) (0.34–0.92)	213/281 (0.76) (0.70–0.81)	1.10 (1.04–1.17)††	375/487 (0.77) (0.73–0.81)	262/452 (0.58) (0.53–0.63)	1.28 (1.18–1.39)	29/396 (0.07) (0.05–0.10)	34/363 (0.09) (0.07–0.13)	0.73 (0.45–1.18)

RR, Relative risk; CI, 95 % confidence interval; OCT, octreotide; SMS, somatostatin; VP, vapreotide

* Values are expressed as rate of events/number of patients

†Proportion with the outcome

††Fixed effect model

Initial control of bleeding was more frequently achieved after combined treatment than after isolated endoscopic therapy (88% versus 76%, RR: 1.12, 95% CI: 1.02–1.23), although significant heterogeneity among studies was found.

Effect of combined therapy on 5-day haemostasis

Five-day haemostasis was evaluated in eight different randomised trials [45–47,28,55,71,72] including 939 patients. The proportion of patients who achieved control of bleeding at 5 days was greater in the combined therapy group (77 versus 58%, RR: 1.28, 95% CI: 1.18–1.39). The beneficial impact of combined therapy can be quantified by the number needed to treat, which in this case was 5 (95% CI: 4–8). These data strongly suggest that combination therapy improves the control of variceal bleeding. Sensitivity analyses have shown that the beneficial effect persisted after exclusion of trials with a substantial proportion of alcoholics or low-risk cirrhotic patients, confirming the robustness of the overall estimation. The beneficial effect of combined treatment on 5-day haemostasis seems to be greater than that observed on initial haemostasis, suggesting that the principal contribution of the additional drug therapy is related to the prevention of early rebleeding.

Although the estimated overall effect includes different drugs and different dosage regimes, which makes the interpretation of the beneficial effect of a particular drug difficult, the lack of modification of the pooled effect after sensitivity analysis makes the estimation robust.

Effect of combined therapy on blood transfusion requirements

According to the recommendations of the Reston consensus meeting [70], the estimation of differences of blood transfusion requirements between therapeutic arms is an important outcome when assessing the efficacy of a therapeutic approach. However, the results of the randomised trials do not allow to obtain an overall estimation of differences in transfusion requirements.

Effect of combined therapy on mortality

The effect of combined endoscopic and drug therapy on mortality has been assessed in two meta-analyses [31,73], assessing 5-day and 42-day mortality.

When assessing 5-day mortality, after pooling six RCTs (total number of patients = 759), no significant reduction in mortality was observed when comparing endoscopic versus combined therapy (RR: 0.65,

95% CI: 0.35–1.20) [31]. Similarly, no differences were observed when evaluating 42-day mortality (RR: 0.86, 95% CI: 0.68–1.07) [73].

Table 42 summarises the overall estimation of effects of combined therapy on haemostasis and survival.

Influence of combined therapy on adverse events

Adverse events were only adequately reported in three RCTs. The overall number of severe adverse effects was similar in the combined and in the endoscopic arm. In no case were severe adverse events associated to either drug administration or required discontinuation of the drug. Inferences to be drawn from available data on adverse effects were limited by a lack of detailed information in the majority of trials. Further limiting factors were a lack of uniform defining criteria and reporting side effects as total numbers instead of on a per-patient basis. However it seems clear that the addition of somatostatin and its derivatives is safe in the context of acute variceal bleeding.

Interestingly, endoscopic sclerotherapy increases the risk of adverse events when compared with somatostatin administration (absolute risk difference: 0.14, CI: 95% 0.07–0.22, number needed to be treated for harm: 7, CI: 95% 4–14). Taking into account this important issue, the comparison of the combination of endoscopic and pharmacological therapy with pharmacological therapy alone may be clinically relevant.

Comparison of pharmacological therapy versus combined pharmacological and endoscopic therapy

Only two RCTs have compared these treatments [64,74]. The pooled results showed that combined therapy improved control of bleeding (RR: 3.1, 95% CI: 1.2–8.3) with no influence on mortality (RR: 0.80, 95% CI: 0.37–1.74). However, more adverse events were found in the combined therapy group. These results should be confirmed in large-scale clinical trials.

Influence of endoscopic procedures on the outcomes of combined therapy

Variceal band ligation represents the current clinical practice [75,76] for the endoscopic therapy of acute variceal bleeding and therefore the influence of combined therapy in patients treated with band ligation should be specifically assessed. Such combined therapy with band ligation and vasoactive drugs has been compared only in two RCTs, preventing any firm conclusion in this issue.

Other aspects

Other important issues related to variceal bleeding such as cost of interventions, duration of hospital stay, intensive care requirements and additional intervention have not been uniformly assessed among the different RCTs. Clearly, these aspects should be specifically assessed in the design of new trials.

Conclusions and prospects for the future

Individual RCTs and systematic reviews have shown that the efficacy of endoscopic therapy in achieving initial control of bleeding and 5-day haemostasis is significantly improved when pharmacological treatment is added to the therapeutic regime. However, this beneficial effect is not associated to a decrease in mortality. Therefore, more trials are needed to determine further the advantages of combined therapy. The design of these future trials should be aimed at comparing immediate combined therapy versus combined therapy only when medical treatment fails. Another possible approach is to examine if the addition of vasoactive drugs to band ligation improves the efficacy of band ligation alone. These trials should take into account not only control of bleeding, but also mortality, need of blood transfusions, cost, intensive care unit requirements, and rescue therapy for rebleeding.

TRANSJUGULAR INTRAHEPATIC PORTOSYSTEMIC SHUNTS (TIPS) IN ACUTE VARICEAL BLEEDING

The first clear indication for TIPS was for 'salvage' therapy for patients with uncontrolled variceal bleeding, and this still remains the indication for which there seems little dispute. TIPS has controlled bleeding in 90–95% of patients when used in this way, and 4-week survival has been approximately 50–60% [7].

However, until now there has been little evidence to guide the clinician as to where in the management pathway TIPS should be placed: after one episode of therapeutic endoscopy? or two?, and should it be used earlier in patients with advanced liver disease who are more likely to rebleed, but are also more likely to decompensate as a consequence of the shunt. The large number of trials using TIPS for secondary prophylaxis against variceal bleeding identified no survival benefit, and most randomised patients will rebleed early, between 5 days and 7 days following the index bleed, so one is talking about a situation even earlier in the bleeding episode.

These questions have been thrown into sharp focus by the groundbreaking study of Monescillo *et al.* [78]. This group measured HVPG in

116 patients admitted with cirrhosis between 1997 and 2000 within 24 h of admission with a variceal bleed. Those patients with an HVPG > 20 mmHg (a value previously identified as the best predictor of treatment failure and 1-year survival) [4] were then randomised into standard therapy (β-blockade as secondary prophylaxis, and further sclerotherapy if there was an episode of rebleeding) or TIPS procedure. In the non-TIPS high-risk group, TIPS was allowed as rescue therapy.

The two high-risk groups were well matched with respect to age, sex, Child–Pugh score, HVPG, volume of blood transfused prior to study and so on. Early (uncovered) TIPS placement resulted in 3 (12%) versus 13 (50%) treatment failures ($p = 0.003$). Early TIPS placement also significantly reduced in-hospital and 1-year mortality: 11% versus 38% and 31% versus 65%, $p = 0.02$ and $p = 0.01$ respectively. The authors state that the incidence of *de novo* encephalopathy was not different between the two groups. Of note, mortality at 6 weeks and 1 year in the low-risk group was 3% and 6%.

The significance of this trial can be highlighted at three different levels. First, it prospectively confirms the utility of early HVPG measurement, as well as the validity of a HVPG threshold predicting patients at high risk. Second, this is the only study that has measured HVPG, and then instituted a change in management in patients at high risk. Finally, it confirms the role of early portal decompression in the management of variceal bleeding, as originally proposed by Orloff [79].

This study clearly needs repeating, because if confirmed, it will signal a real shift in the management of patients with variceal bleeding, and a significant increase in the number of TIPS being placed. The question remains whether it is 'applicable' to routine clinical practice – this was a very intensive study and most hospitals would be unable to measure HVPG within 24 h, in which case the patient will need to be transferred.

Alternatively, new trials using early TIPS can focus on a high-risk groups selected according to clinical criteria, rather than on the less applicable measurement of admission HVPG. Other areas of concern with the study were the complete absence of banding, and perhaps the non-use of nitrates in combination with β-blockers for secondary prevention. A minor, but for those doing this procedure an important practical point, was that three patients developed acute respiratory failure due to sedation for TIPS insertion. It is the authors' opinion that TIPS is better placed under general anaesthetic, and that sedation alone does not provide a safe or comfortable environment for operator or patient.

Stent technology has also evolved and PTFE covered stents (WL Gore, Flagstaff, AZ) have been shown to have a significantly improved 1-year

Table 43 Baveno IV – What are the most important areas of uncertainty in acute variceal bleeding.

Five more voted:
1 Early TIPS and covered stents;
2 Best treatment for gastric varices (specially glue versus TIPS);
3 Potential of rFVIIa;
4 Treatment of patients with no active bleeding at time of endoscopy/under drug therapy;
5 Prognostic factors/models for acute bleeding.

primary patency in an RCT compared with uncovered stents [80]. After a median follow-up of 300 days, the clinical/haemodynamic event rates were 8/13% in the covered group and 29/44% in the uncovered group. Perhaps surprisingly, encephalopathy rates were trending towards lower rates in the patients with covered stents. These stents are more expensive, and the economics of using covered stents in the emergency setting (where there remains a high 40-day mortality) can be debated. Nonetheless, all reports confirm a significantly reduced stenosis rate [81], and this new technology would seem to add to the move towards early (?routine) TIPS placement in patients with variceal bleeding who are deemed to be at high risk of rebleeding.

Finally, in the context of acute variceal bleeding, a retrospective study on the management of ectopic varices has recommended the use of TIPS plus variceal embolisation for these often difficult cases, even when the portal pressure gradient has been reduced to < 12 mmHg [82].

AREAS OF UNCERTAINTY

Despite the advances made over the 5-years elapsed since Baveno III, there remain important areas of uncertainty. Table 43 reports the five more important, as voted by the participants at Baveno IV. It is clear that the answer to these important questions will require the joint effort of many of the groups present at this meeting, preferentially through cooperative RCTs. Some of these (early TIPS, rVIIa, etc.) are already being conducted and results will be available in the next couple of years. Hopefully, international meetings such as Baveno IV will foster the required cooperation to provide evidence for the remaining questions.

REFERENCES

1 D'Amico G, de Franchis R. Upper digestive bleeding in cirrhosis. Post-therapeutic outcome and prognostic indicators. *Hepatology* 2003;**38**(3): 599–612.

2 Chalasani N, Kahi C, Francois F *et al.* Improved patient survival after acute variceal bleeding: a multicenter, cohort study. *Am J Gastroenterol* 2003;**98**(3): 653–659.

3 Graham DY, Smith JL. The course of patients after variceal haemorrhage. *Gastroenterology* 1981;**80**(4): 800–809.

4 Moitinho E, Escorsell A, Bandi JC *et al.* Prognostic value of early measurements of portal pressure in acute variceal bleeding. *Gastroenterology* 1999;**117**(3): 626–631.

5 Burroughs AK. General management of the cirrhotic patient with acute variceal bleeding. In: de Franchis R (ed). *Portal hypertension III. Proceedings of the third Baveno international consensus workshop of definitions, methodology and therapeutic strategies.* Oxford; Blackwell Science, 2001; 135–142.

6 Hou MC, Lin HC, Kuo BI, Lee FY, Schmidt CM, Lee SD. Clinical implications of the white nipple sign and its role in the diagnosis of esophageal variceal haemorrhage. *Am J Gastroenterol* 1996;**91**(10): 2103–2109.

7 Teres J, Planas R, Panes J *et al.* Vasopressin/nitroglycerin infusion vs. esophageal tamponade in the treatment of acute variceal bleeding: a randomised controlled trial. *Hepatology* 1990;**11**(6): 964–968.

8 Lipper B, Simon D, Cerrone F. Pulmonary aspiration during emergency endoscopy in patients with upper gastrointestinal haemorrhage. *Crit Care Med* 1991;**19**(3): 330–333.

9 Kupfer Y, Cappell MS, Tessler S. Acute gastrointestinal bleeding in the intensive care unit. The intensivist's perspective. *Gastroenterol Clin North Am* 2000;**29**(2): 275–307, v.

10 Levacher S, Letoumelin P, Pateron D, Blaise M, Lapandry C, Pourriat JL. Early administration of terlipressin plus glyceryl trinitrate to control active upper gastrointestinal bleeding in cirrhotic patients. *Lancet* 1995;**346**(8979): 865–868.

11 Cardenas A, Gines P, Uriz J *et al.* Renal failure after upper gastrointestinal bleeding in cirrhosis: incidence, clinical course, predictive factors, and short-term prognosis. *Hepatology* 2001;**34**(4 Pt 1): 671–676.

12 Kravetz D, Sikuler E, Groszmann RJ. Splanchnic and systemic haemodynamics in portal hypertensive rats during haemorrhage and blood volume restitution. *Gastroenterology* 1986;**90**(5 Pt 1): 1232–1240.

13 Castaneda B, Morales J, Lionetti R *et al.* Effects of blood volume restitution following a portal hypertensive-related bleeding in anesthetized cirrhotic rats. *Hepatology* 2001;**33**(4): 821–825.

14 Contreras M. Final statement from the consensus conference on platelet transfusion. *Transfusion* 1998;**38**(8): 796–797.

15 Ejlersen E, Melsen T, Ingerslev J, Andreasen RB, Vilstrup H. Recombinant activated factor VII (rFVIIa) acutely normalizes prothrombin time in patients with cirrhosis during bleeding from oesophageal varices. *Scand J Gastroenterol* 2001;**36**(10): 1081–1085.

16 Bosch J, Thabut D, Bendtsen F *et al.* Recombinant factor VIIa for upper gastrointestinal bleeding in patients with cirrhosis: a randomised, double-blind trial. *Gastroenterology* 2004;**127**(4): 1123–1130.

17 Soares-Weiser K, Brezis M, Tur-Kaspa R, Leibovici L. Antibiotic prophylaxis for cirrhotic patients with gastrointestinal bleeding. *Cochrane Database Syst Rev* 2002;**2**: CD002907.

18 Deschenes M, Villeneuve JP. Risk factors for the development of bacterial infections in hospitalised patients with cirrhosis. *Am J Gastroenterol* 1999;**94**(8): 2193–2197.

19 Bernard B, Grange JD, Khac EN, Amiot X, Opolon P, Poynard T. Antibiotic prophylaxis for the prevention of bacterial infections in cirrhotic patients with gastrointestinal bleeding: a meta-analysis. *Hepatology* 1999;**29**(6): 1655–1661.

20 Rimola A, Garcia-Tsao G, Navasa M *et al.* Diagnosis, treatment and prophylaxis of spontaneous bacterial peritonitis: a consensus document. International Ascites Club. *J Hepatol* 2000;**32**(1): 142–153.

21 Fernandez J, Ruiz-del-Arbol L, Serradilla R *et al.* Randomised, multicenter, controlled trial comparing oral norfloxacin vs intravenous ceftriaxone in the prevention of bacterial infections in cirrhotics with severe liver failure and gastrointestinal bleeding. *J Hepatol* 2005;**42**(suppl. 1): 4.

22 Kravetz D, Romero G, Argonz J *et al.* Total volume paracentesis decreases variceal pressure, size, and variceal wall tension in cirrhotic patients. *Hepatology* 1997;**25**(1): 59–62.

23 Loguercio C, Sava E, Marmo R, del Vecchio BC, Coltorti M. Malnutrition in cirrhotic patients: anthropometric measurements as a method of assessing nutritional status. *Br J Clin Pract* 1990;**44**(3): 98–101.

24 Mihas AA, Sanyal AJ. Recurrent variceal bleeding despite endoscopic and medical therapy. *Gastroenterology* 2004;**127**(2): 621–629.

25 Garcia-Pagan JC, Escorsell A, Moitinho E, Bosch J. Influence of pharmacological agents on portal haemodynamics: basis for its use in the treatment of portal hypertension. *Semin Liver Dis* 1999;**19**: 427–438.

26 Villanueva C, Ortiz J, Minana J *et al.* Somatostatin treatment and risk stratification by continuous portal pressure monitoring during acute variceal bleeding. *Gastroenterology* 2001;**121**(1): 110–117.

27 Nidegger D, Ragot S, Berthelemy P *et al.* Cirrhosis and bleeding: the need for very early management. *J Hepatol* 2003;**39**(4): 509–514.

28 Avgerinos A, Nevens F, Raptis S, Fevery J. Early administration of somatostatin and efficacy of sclerotherapy in acute oesophageal variceal bleeds: the European Acute Bleeding Oesophageal Variceal Episodes (ABOVE) randomised trial. *Lancet* 1997;**350**(9090): 1495–1499.

29 Morales J, Moitinho E, Abraldes JG, Fernandez M, Bosch J. Effects of the V1a vasopressin agonist F-180 on portal hypertension-related bleeding in portal hypertensive rats. *Hepatology* 2003;**38**(6): 1378–1383.

30 D'Amico G, Pietrosi G, Tarantino I, Pagliaro L. Emergency sclerotherapy versus vasoactive drugs for variceal bleeding in cirrhosis: a Cochrane meta-analysis. *Gastroenterology* 2003;**124**(5): 1277–1291.

31 Banares R, Albillos A, Rincon D *et al.* Endoscopic treatment versus endoscopic plus pharmacologic treatment for acute variceal bleeding: a meta-analysis. *Hepatology* 2002;**35**(3): 609–615.

32 Nevens F, Van Steenbergen W, Yap SH, Fevery J. Assessment of variceal pressure by continuous non-invasive endoscopic registration: a placebo controlled evaluation of the effect of terlipressin and octreotide. *Gut* 1996;**38**(1): 129–134.

33 Moreau R, Soubrane O, Hadengue A *et al.* Haemodynamic effects of the administration of terlipressin alone or combined with nitroglycerin in patients with cirrhosis. *Gastroenterol Clin Biol* 1992;**16**(8–9): 680–686.

34 Escorsell A, Bandi JC, Moitinho E *et al.* Time profile of the haemodynamic effects of terlipressin in portal hypertension. *J Hepatol* 1997;**26**(3): 621–627.

35 Walker S, Stiehl A, Raedsch R, Kommerell B. Terlipressin in bleeding esophageal varices: a placebo-controlled, double-blind study. *Hepatology* 1986;**6**(1): 112–115.

36 Freeman JG, Cobden I, Record CO. Placebo-controlled trial of terlipressin (glypressin) in the management of acute variceal bleeding. *J Clin Gastroenterol* 1989;**11**(1): 58–60.

37 Soderlund C, Magnusson I, Torngren S, Lundell L. Terlipressin (triglycyl-lysine vasopressin) controls acute bleeding oesophageal varices. A double-blind, randomised, placebo-controlled trial. *Scand J Gastroenterol* 1990;**25**(6): 622–630.

38 Moreau R, Durand F, Poynard T *et al.* Terlipressin in patients with cirrhosis and type 1 hepatorenal syndrome: a retrospective multicenter study. *Gastroenterology* 2002;**122**(4): 923–930.

39 Feu F, Ruiz DA, Banares R, Planas R, Bosch J. Double-blind randomised controlled trial comparing terlipressin and somatostatin for acute variceal haemorrhage. Variceal Bleeding Study Group. *Gastroenterology* 1996;**111**(5): 1291–1299.

40 Cirera I, Feu F, Luca A *et al.* Effects of bolus injections and continuous infusions of somatostatin and placebo in patients with cirrhosis: a double-blind haemodynamic investigation. *Hepatology* 1995;**22**(1): 106–111.

41 Nevens F, Sprengers D, Fevery J. The effect of different doses of a bolus injection of somatostatin combined with a slow infusion on transmural oesophageal variceal pressure in patients with cirrhosis. *J Hepatol* 1994;**20**(1): 27–31.

42 Burroughs AK, McCormick PA, Hughes MD, Sprengers D, D'Heygere F, McIntyre N. Randomised, double-blind, placebo-controlled trial of somatostatin for variceal bleeding. Emergency control and prevention of early variceal rebleeding. *Gastroenterology* 1990;**99**(5): 1388–1395.

43 Gotzsche PC, Gjorup I, Bonnen H, Brahe NEB, Becker U, Burcharth F. Somatostatin v placebo in bleeding oesophageal varices: randomised trial and meta-analysis. *BMJ* 1995;**310**(6993): 1495–1498.

44 Moitinho E, Planas R, Bañares R *et al.* Multicenter randomised controlled trial comparing different schedules of somatostatin in the treatment of acute variceal bleeding. *J Hepatol* 2001;**35**(6): 712–718.

45 Besson I, Ingrand P, Person B *et al.* Sclerotherapy with or without octreotide for acute variceal bleeding. *N Engl J Med* 1995;**333**(9): 555–560.

46 Sung JJ, Chung SC, Yung MY *et al.* Prospective randomised study of effect of octreotide on rebleeding from oesophageal varices after endoscopic ligation. *Lancet* 1995;**346**(8991–8992): 1666–1669.

47 Zuberi BF, Baloch Q. Comparison of endoscopic variceal sclerotherapy alone and in combination with octreotide in controlling acute variceal haemorrhage and early rebleeding in patients with low-risk cirrhosis. *Am J Gastroenterol* 2000;**95**(3): 768–771.

48 Burroughs AK. Double blind RCT of 5 day octreotide versus placebo, associated with sclerotherapy for trial/failures. *Hepatology* 1996;**24**: 352A.

49 Jenkins SA, Nott DM, Baxter JN. Pharmacokinetics of octreotide in patients with cirrhosis and portal hypertension; relationship between the plasma levels of the

analogue and the magnitude and duration of the reduction in corrected wedged hepatic venous pressure. *HPB Surg* 1998;**11**(1): 13–21.
50 Moller S, Brinch K, Henriksen JH, Becker U. Effect of octreotide on systemic, central, and splanchnic haemodynamics in cirrhosis. *J Hepatol* 1997;**26**(5): 1026–1033.
51 Escorsell A, Bandi JC, Andreu V *et al.* Desensitization to the effects of intravenous octreotide in cirrhotic patients with portal hypertension. *Gastroenterology* 2001;**120**(1): 161–169.
52 McCormick PA, Dick R, Graffeo M *et al.* The effect of non-protein liquid meals on the hepatic venous pressure gradient in patients with cirrhosis. *J Hepatol* 1990;**11**(2): 221–225.
53 Albillos A, Rossi I, Iborra J *et al.* Octreotide prevents postprandial splanchnic hyperemia in patients with portal hypertension. *J Hepatol* 1994;**21**(1): 88–94.
54 Abraldes JG, Bosch J. Somatostatin and analogues in portal hypertension. *Hepatology* 2002;**35**(6): 1305–1312.
55 Cales P, Masliah C, Bernard B *et al.* Early administration of vapreotide for variceal bleeding in patients with cirrhosis. French Club for the Study of Portal Hypertension. *N Engl J Med* 2001;**344**(1): 23–28.
56 Rockall TA, Logan RF, Devlin HB, Northfield TC. Risk assessment after acute upper gastrointestinal haemorrhage. *Gut* 1996;**38**(3): 316–321.
57 Spiegel BM, Vakil NB, Ofman JJ. Endoscopy for acute nonvariceal upper gastrointestinal tract haemorrhage: is sooner better? A systematic review. *Arch Intern Med* 2001;**161**(11): 1393–1404.
58 Paquet KJ, Feussner H. Endoscopic sclerosis and esophageal balloon tamponade in acute haemorrhage from esophagogastric varices: a prospective controlled randomised trial. *Hepatology* 1985;**5**(4): 580–583.
59 Larson AW, Cohen H, Zweiban B *et al.* Acute esophageal variceal sclerotherapy. Results of a prospective randomised controlled trial. *JAMA* 1986;**255**(4): 497–500.
60 Moreto M, Zaballa M, Bernal A, Ibanez S, Ojembarrena E, Rodriguez A. A randomised trial of tamponade or sclerotherapy as immediate treatment for bleeding esophageal varices. *Surg Gynecol Obstet* 1988;**167**(4): 331–334.
61 Westaby D, Hayes PC, Gimson AE, Polson RJ, Williams R. Controlled clinical trial of injection sclerotherapy for active variceal bleeding. *Hepatology* 1989;**9**(2): 274–277.
62 Hartigan PM, Gebhard RL, Gregory PB. Sclerotherapy for actively bleeding esophageal varices in male alcoholics with cirrhosis. Veterans Affairs Cooperative Variceal Sclerotherapy Group. *Gastrointest Endosc* 1997;**46**(1): 1–7.
63 Freitas DS, Sofia C, Pontes JM *et al.* Octreotide in acute bleeding esophageal varices: a prospective randomised study. *Hepatogastroenterology* 2000;**47**(35): 1310–1314.
64 Villanueva C, Ortiz J, Sabat M *et al.* Somatostatin alone or combined with emergency sclerotherapy in the treatment of acute esophageal variceal bleeding: a prospective randomised trial. *Hepatology* 1999;**30**(2): 384–389.
65 Laine L, Cook D. Endoscopic ligation compared with sclerotherapy for treatment of esophageal variceal bleeding. A meta-analysis. *Ann Intern Med* 1995;**123**(4): 280–287.

66 Lo GH, Lai KH, Cheng JS *et al.* Emergency banding ligation versus sclerotherapy for the control of active bleeding from esophageal varices. *Hepatology* 1997;**25**(5): 1101–1104.
67 Avgerinos A, Armonis A, Manolakopoulos S *et al.* Endoscopic sclerotherapy versus variceal ligation in the long-term management of patients with cirrhosis after variceal bleeding. A prospective randomised study. *J Hepatol* 1997;**26**(5): 1034–1041.
68 Lo GH, Lai KH, Cheng JS, Chen MH, Chiang HT. A prospective, randomised trial of butyl cyanoacrylate injection versus band ligation in the management of bleeding gastric varices. *Hepatology* 2001;**33**(5): 1060–1064.
69 Sarin SK, Jain AK, Jain M, Gupta R. A randomised controlled trial of cyanoacrylate versus alcohol injection in patients with isolated fundic varices. *Am J Gastroenterol* 2002;**97**(4): 1010–1015.
70 Grace ND, Groszmann RJ, Garcia-Tsao G *et al.* Portal hypertension and variceal bleeding: an AASLD single topic symposium. *Hepatology* 1998;**28**(3): 868–880.
71 Ceriani R, Curioni R MLRGBS. Sclerotherapy alone (ES) vs. sclerotherapy plus terlipressin (EST) vs. sclerotherapy plus octreotide (ESO) in the treatment of acute variceal bleeding. *Gastroenterology* 1997;**112**:[1238A], 1238A.
72 Signorelli S, Paris B, Negrin F, Bonelli M, Auriemma M. Esophageal varices bleeding: comparison between treatment with sclerotherapy alone vs sclerotherapy plus octreotide. *Hepatology* 1997;**26**(suppl.): 137A.
73 D'Amico G, Criscuoli V, Fili D, Mocciaro F, Pagliaro L. Meta-analysis of trials for variceal bleeding. *Hepatology* 2002;**36**(4 Pt 1): 1023–1024.
74 Novella MT, Villanueva C, Ortiz J *et al.* Octreotide vs. sclerotherapy and octreotide for acute variceal bleeding. A pilot study. *Hepatology* 1996;**24**(suppl.): [207 A], 207 A.
75 Sharara AI, Rockey DC. Gastroesophageal variceal haemorrhage. *N Engl J Med* 2001;**345**(9): 669–681.
76 Mookerjee RP, Jalan R. All that glitters is not gold. *Gut* 2002,**51**(5). 623–624.
77 Vangeli M, Patch D, Burroughs AK. Salvage tips for uncontrolled variceal bleeding. *J Hepatol* 2002;**37**(5): 703–704.
78 Monescillo A, Martinez-Lagares F, Ruiz-del-Arbol L *et al.* Influence of portal hypertension and its early decompression by TIPS placement on the outcome of variceal bleeding. *Hepatology* 2004;**40**(4): 793–801.
79 Orloff MJ, Bell RH Jr, Orloff MS, Hardison WG, Greenburg AG. Prospective randomised trial of emergency portcaval shunt and emergency medical therapy in unselected cirrhotic patients with bleeding varices. *Hepatology* 1994;**20**(4 Pt 1): 863–872.
80 Bureau C, Garcia-Pagan JC, Otal P *et al.* Improved clinical outcome using polytetrafluoroethylene-coated stents for tips: results of a randomised study. *Gastroenterology* 2004;**126**(2): 469–475.
81 Angermayr B, Cejna M, Koenig F *et al.* Survival in patients undergoing transjugular intrahepatic portosystemic shunt: ePTFE-covered stentgrafts versus bare stents. *Hepatology* 2003;**38**(4): 1043–1050.
82 Vangeli M, Patch D, Terreni N *et al.* Bleeding ectopic varices – treatment with transjugular intrahepatic porto-systemic shunt (TIPS) and embolisation. *J Hepatol* 2004;**41**(4): 560–566.

Baveno IV Consensus Statements: Treatment of the Acute Bleeding Episode

Jaime Bosch, Loren Laine (Chairpersons), Rafael Bañares, Norman Marcon, Frederik Nevens, Christine Silvain, David Patch and Ramón Planas

Blood volume restitution

• Blood volume restitution should be done cautiously and conservatively using plasma expanders to maintain haemodynamic stability and PRBC to maintain the haemoglobin at approximately 8 g/dL, depending on other factors such as patients' co-morbidities, age, haemodynamic status and presence of ongoing bleeding clinically. (1b;A)

• Recommendations regarding management of coagulopathy and thrombocytopenia cannot be made on the basis of currently available data. (5;D)

Use of antibiotics for preventing bacterial infections/spontaneous bacterial peritonitis

• Antibiotic prophylaxis is an integral part of therapy for patients presenting with variceal bleeding and should be instituted from admission. (1a;A)

Prevention of hepatic encephalopathy

• In patients who present or develop encephalopathy, this should be treated with lactulose/lactitol or other drugs. (5;D)

• There are no studies evaluating the usefulness of lactulose/lactitol for the prevention of hepatic encephalopathy. (5;D)

Assessment of prognosis

• No adequate prognostic model has been developed to predict outcomes. (2b;B)

• No individual characteristic sufficiently predicts prognosis. (2b;B)

• Child–Pugh class, active bleeding at endoscopy, hepatic venous pressure gradient (HVPG), infection, renal failure, severity of initial bleeding, presence of portal vein thrombosis or of hepatocellular carcinoma (HCC) and ALT have been identified as indicators of poor prognosis. (2b;B)

Timing of endoscopy

- Endoscopy should be performed as soon as possible after admission (within 12 h), especially in patients with clinically significant bleeding or in patients with features suggesting cirrhosis. (5;D)

Use of balloon tamponade

- Balloon tamponade should only be used in massive bleeding as a temporary 'bridge' until definitive treatment can be instituted (for a maximum of 24 h, preferably in an intensive care facility). (5;D)

Pharmacological treatment

- In suspected variceal bleeding, vasoactive drugs should be started as soon as possible – before diagnostic endoscopy. (1b;A)
- Vasoactive drug therapy (terlipressin, somatostatin, vapreotide, octreotide) should be maintained in patients with oesophageal variceal bleeding for 2 to 5 days. (1a;A)

Endoscopic treatment

- Endoscopic therapy is recommended in any patient who presents with documented upper GI bleeding and in whom oesophageal varices are the cause of bleeding. (1a;A)
- Ligation is the recommended form of endoscopic therapy for acute oesophageal variceal bleeding although sclerotherapy may be used in the acute setting if ligation is technically difficult. (1b;A)
- Endoscopic therapy with tissue adhesive (e.g. N-butyl-cyanoacrylate) is recommended for acute gastric variceal bleeding. (1b;A)
- Endoscopic treatments are best used in association with pharmacological therapy, which preferably should be started before endoscopy. (1a;A)

Management of treatment failures

- Failures of initial therapy with combined pharmacological and endoscopic therapy are best managed by a second attempt at endoscopic therapy or TIPS. (preferably with PTFE covered stents) (2b;B)

Areas requiring further study (5;D)

- Optimal duration of vasoactive drug therapy.
- Effectiveness of early TIPS placement and of covered stents.
- Best treatment for gastric varices (especially glue versus TIPS).
- The potential of rFVIIa.
- The best treatment of patients with no active bleeding at time of endoscopy on drug therapy.
- Prognostic factors/models for acute bleeding (MELD score, variceal size, age, aetiology of portal hypertension and other co-morbidities).

LECTURE

Spontaneous Bacterial Peritonitis/Infections in Cirrhosis

Miguel Navasa and Juan Rodés

SPONTANEOUS BACTERIAL PERITONITIS

Spontaneous bacterial peritonitis (SBP) is defined as the infection of a previously sterile ascitic fluid, without any apparent intraabdominal source of infection. The prevalence of SBP in unselected cirrhotic patients with ascites admitted to a hospital ranges between 10% and 30% [1]. Diagnosis of SBP is established by a polymorphonuclear (PMN) cell count in ascitic fluid higher than 250 cells/mm^3. In approximately 50% to 60% of the cases the organism responsible is isolated in ascitic fluid culture or in blood cultures. The remaining cases are considered as a variant of SBP and are treated in the same way as those with a positive culture [2]. The outcome of cirrhotic patients with SBP has dramatically improved during the last 20 years. At present, the SBP resolution rate ranges between 70% and 90% and hospital survival ranges between 50% and 70% [1]. An early diagnosis of SBP and, specially, the use of a more adequate antibiotic therapy, are the most likely reasons for the improvement in SBP prognosis. However, despite the resolution of the infection, the mortality rate of SBP is still high (30%), mainly due to the development of some complications such as renal impairment, gastrointestinal bleeding and progressive liver failure. Cirrhotic patients recovering from an episode of SBP should be considered as potential candidates for liver transplantation since the survival expectancy after this bacterial infection is very short.

Pathogenesis

Colonisation of the ascitic fluid from an episode of bacteriaemia is nowadays the most accepted hypothesis on the pathogenesis of SBP [1,3]. Although the passage of micro-organisms from the bloodstream to ascites has never been documented, it can be assumed that bacteria present in the circulation may easily pass to the ascites because of the constant fluid exchange between these two compartments. Once bacteria have reached the ascites, the development of SBP depends on the antimicrobial capacity of the ascitic fluid. Patients with a decreased defensive capacity of ascitic fluid develop SBP.

Since most organisms causing SBP are Gram-negative bacteria of enteric origin [1,2], several pathogenic mechanisms have been proposed to explain the passage of enteric organisms from the intestinal lumen to the systemic circulation: (1) Bacterial translocation, or the process by which enteric bacteria normally present in the gastrointestinal lumen can cross the mucosa and colonise the mesenteric lymph nodes (MLN) and reach the bloodstream through the intestinal lymphatic circulation. Bacterial translocation could be the consequence of the intestinal bacterial overgrowth (IBO) that leads to an increase in aerobic Gram-negative bacilli in the jejunal flora in cirrhosis and of the possible alteration in gut permeability due to portal hypertension or to circumstances decreasing mucosal blood flow (e.g. acute hypovolaemia or splanchnic vasoconstrictor drugs); (2) The depression of the hepatic reticuloendothelial system which allows the free passage of micro-organisms from the bowel lumen to the systemic circulation via the portal vein and prolongs bacteriaemia. The skin, the urinary tract and the upper respiratory tract may be the sites by which non-enteric bacteria enter the circulation and cause SBP. This pathogenic mechanism is enhanced in many cases by diagnostic or therapeutic procedures which break the natural mucocutaneous barriers. Whatever the source of the bacteria reaching the bloodstream, a bacteraemic event is more prolonged and, therefore, may more readily become clinically significant in cirrhotic than in non-cirrhotic patients, because of the marked depression of the reticuloendothelial system in the former. As indicated above, once micro-organisms have colonised the ascites, the development of SBP depends on the defensive capacity of the ascitic fluid.

Bacterial translocation

It has been shown that in CCl_4-induced cirrhotic rats with ascites there is an increased passage of bacteria from the intestinal lumen to extraintestinal sites, including regional lymph nodes and the systemic circulation [3–8]. Causes for bacterial translocation are a disruption of the intestinal permeability barrier, IBO and/or a decrease in host immune defences. The simultaneous presence of IBO and a severe disturbance in the intestinal barrier seem to be required for bacterial translocation to MLN [4,5]. The alteration in gut permeability could be partially due to portal hypertension that causes marked oedema and inflammation in the submucosa of the caecum in cirrhotic rats with ascites, thus facilitating bacterial translocation [8]. Changed permeability of the intestinal mucosa has also been seen in haemorrhagic shock, sepsis, injury or administration of endotoxin. In portal hypertensive rats [8,9] it has been shown that haemorrhagic shock is followed by increased bacterial translocation to MLN suggesting that haemorrhagic shock, a not infrequent event in cirrhotic patients, could alter the intestinal barrier in these animals. Gram-negative bacilli overgrowth has been demonstrated in the jejunal flora of cirrhotic patients [5]. The intestinal hypomotility caused by the sympathetic overactivity of cirrhotic patients could, at least partly, explain this fact [5]. The change in the intestinal flora may increase the chance of aerobic Gram-negative bacteria invading the bloodstream and cause infections of enteric origin in patients with cirrhosis. In these patients, bacterial translocation to MLN seems to be related to the presence of ascites and to the degree of hepatic insufficiency, since it is significantly increased in Child C patients [10].

Depression of activity of the reticuloendothelial system

Although the reticuloendothelial system is widely distributed throughout the body, approximately 90% of this defensive system is in the liver, where Kupffer cells and endothelial sinusoidal cells are the major components [11]. Cirrhotic patients may have marked depression of the reticuloendothelial system function. In addition, it has been shown that survival and the risk of acquiring bacteraemia and SBP in cirrhosis are directly related to the degree of dysfunction of the reticuloendothelial system in these patients [12,13].

Several mechanisms have been proposed to explain the impairment of the phagocytic activity of the reticuloendothelial system in cirrhosis, including intrahepatic shunting, a reduction in the phagocytic capacity of monocytes, which are considered as the Kupffer cell precursors, and an impaired function of macrophage Fc gamma receptors in alcoholic cirrhosis [11,14,15]. Serum opsonic activity has been found to be markedly reduced in most cirrhotic patients, probably as a consequence of a decreased serum concentration of complement and fibronectin, substances that normally stimulate the phagocytosis of micro-organisms by enhancing their adhesiveness to the reticuloendothelial cell surface.

Decreased opsonic activity of the ascitic fluid

The non-specific antimicrobial capacity of ascitic fluid in cirrhosis varies greatly from patient to patient and this variability may be involved in the pathogenesis of SBP. There is a highly significant inverse correlation between the opsonic activity of ascitic fluid and the risk of developing SBP in patients admitted to the hospital with ascites [16].

The opsonic activity of ascitic fluid in cirrhosis is directly correlated with the total protein level in ascites and with the concentration of defensive substances, such as immunoglobulins, complement and fibronectin [16–21]. Interestingly, several investigators have found that the concentration of total protein in ascitic fluid, a very easy measurement in clinical practice, correlates inversely with the risk of SBP in cirrhosis with ascites. Patients with protein concentration in ascitic fluid below 10 g/L develop peritonitis during hospital stay with a significantly higher frequency than those with a higher protein content (15% versus 2%, respectively) [17] and the cumulative 1-year probability of developing peritonitis during long-term follow-up is significantly greater in this subgroup of cirrhotic patients than in those with an ascitic protein concentration over 10 g/L (20% versus 2%, respectively) [20]. Finally, the probability of the first episode of SBP in cirrhotic patients with ascites is significantly influenced by the antimicrobial capacity of ascitic fluid and by hepatic function, being ascitic fluid protein levels, platelet count and serum bilirubin levels the most useful indicators of high-risk of spontaneous peritonitis [21,22].

The variation in the antimicrobial properties of ascites could be related (1) to the serum levels of the defensive proteins involved in antibacterial mechanisms of ascitic fluid; (2) to the degree of portal hypertension and hepatic insufficiency and (3) to the volume of water diluting ascitic fluid solutes. This last possibility is supported by the finding that diuretic-induced reduction of water in ascitic fluid increases the total protein concentration and the antibacterial capacity of ascites, and by the common observation in clinical practice that SBP occurs predominantly in cirrhotic patients with large-volume ascites.

Neutrophil leukocyte dysfunction

A high proportion of cirrhotic patients show altered neutrophil leukocyte function at different levels. The most frequent disturbance is a marked reduction of chemotaxis, probably caused by the presence of chemotactic inhibitory substances in the serum. The nature of these substances has not yet been determined. Furthermore, the phagocytic and bacterial killing capacity of neutrophils has been found to be reduced in cirrhosis [23]. However, since infections which frequently develop in patients with congenital or acquired neutrophil-function abnormalities (mainly chronic granulomatous diseases and recurrent staphylococcal and fungal infections) are very different from those developed by cirrhotic patients, it seems very unlikely that leukocyte dysfunction plays a major role in the susceptibility of cirrhosis to bacterial infections.

Iatrogenic factors

In addition to procedures well known to predispose to infection such as intravenous or urethral catheters, cirrhotic patients are frequently subjected to other diagnostic or therapeutic manoeuvres which may alter the natural defence barriers and, therefore, increase the risk of bacterial infection. Endoscopic sclerotherapy for bleeding oesophageal varices, particularly emergency sclerotherapy, is associated with bacteraemia, with an incidence ranging from 5% to 30% [22,23]. Although, in some cases, sclerotherapy has been implicated in the development of serious infectious complications such as purulent meningitis and bacterial peritonitis, bacteraemia is usually a transient phenomenon and the use of prophylactic antibiotics is not recommended. The placement of a transjugular intrahepatic portosystemic stent for the treatment of bleeding oesophageal varices is not associated with the development of significant bacterial infections. However, cirrhotic patients with a peritoneovenous shunt (LeVeen shunt) frequently develop infectious complications, particularly spontaneous bacteraemia and peritonitis. In several series, the incidence of bacterial infections after the insertion of a LeVeen shunt for the treatment of ascites was approximately 20% [1]. Finally, there is a very low risk of clinically relevant infection with other invasive techniques often performed in these patients, such as diagnostic or therapeutic paracentesis and endoscopy.

Diagnosis

Clinical characteristics

The clinical presentation of SBP probably depends on the stage at which the infection is diagnosed. Most patients present signs or symptoms clearly suggestive of peritoneal infection, although SBP may be asymptomatic, especially in the initial stages. Abdominal pain and fever are the most characteristic symptoms. Other signs and symptoms such as alterations in gastrointestinal motility (vomiting, ileus and diarrhoea), hepatic encephalopathy, gastrointestinal bleeding, renal impairment, septic shock and hypothermia may be present in a high number of patients [1,24]. Diagnostic paracentesis should be performed on hospital admission in all cirrhotic patients with ascites to investigate the presence of SBP, and in hospitalised patients with ascites whenever they present any of the following: (1) abdominal pain, vomiting, diarrhoea, ileus or rebound tenderness; (2) systemic signs of infection such as fever, leukocytosis or septic shock and (3) hepatic encephalopathy or impairment in renal function [24].

Laboratory and microbiological data

The diagnosis of SBP is based on clinical suspicion and on ascitic fluid analysis. An ascitic fluid PMN count $\geq$ 250 cells/mm^3 is nowadays considered diagnostic of SBP and constitutes an indication to empirically initiate antibiotic treatment. In patients with haemorrhagic ascites a subtraction of one PMN per 250 red blood cells should be made to adjust for the presence of blood in ascites [24].

The measurement of lactic dehydrogenase concentration, glucose levels and total protein concentration in ascitic fluid is important to establish a differential diagnosis between spontaneous and secondary peritonitis. A secondary peritonitis should be suspected when at least two of the following features are present in ascitic fluid: glucose levels $<$ 50 mg/dL, protein concentration $>$ 10 g/L, lactic dehydrogenase concentration $>$ normal serum levels.

Gram's stain of a smear of sediment obtained after centrifugation of ascitic fluid is frequently negative in SBP, as the concentration of bacteria is usually low (1 organism/mL or less). Nevertheless, it may be helpful in identifying patients with gut perforation in whom multiple types of bacteria can be seen [24].

Culture of ascitic fluid directly into blood culture bottles (aerobic and anaerobic media) at the bedside is positive in between 50% and 80% of the cases. Moreover, blood cultures are positive in a significant proportion of patients with SBP. Table 44 shows the most common organisms isolated in patients with SBP. Other alterations in systemic laboratory parameters such as, leukocytosis, azotaemia and acidosis can be seen in cirrhotic patients with SBP.

Treatment

Antibiotic therapy must be started once the diagnosis of SBP is established. Empirical treatment should cover all potential organisms responsible for SBP without causing adverse effects. At present, third generation cephalosporins are considered the gold standard in the treatment of SBP in cirrhosis. However, other antibiotics are also effective in the treatment of this infective complication (Table 45), [25–34].

Table 44 Microorganisms responsible for spontaneous bacterial peritonitis.

Culture-positive SBP	67%
Gram-negative bacilli	50%
E.coli	37%
Klebsiella sp.	6%
Others	7%
Gram-positive cocci	17%
S. pneumoniae	10%
Other streptococci	6%
S. aureus	1%
Culture negative SBP	33%

Table 45 Spontaneous bacterial peritonitis outcome depending on the different antibiotic therapy employed [25–34].

Antibiotic	SBP resolution rate (%)	Superinfection (%)	Hospital survival (%)
Cefotaxime (i.v.)			
2 g/4 h	86	0	73
2 g/6 h	77	1	69
2 g/12 h	79	1	79
2 g/8 h/5 days	93	0	67
2 g/8 h/10 days	91	0	58
Ceftriaxone (i.v.)	91	0	70
Cefonicid (i.v.)	94	0	63
Amoxicillin–clavulanic acid (i.v.)	85	7	63
Aztreonam (i.v.)	71	14	57
Ofloxacin (oral)	84	1	81

Intravenous albumin infusion in SBP

A randomised multicentre controlled trial has demonstrated that in patients with SBP, treatment with intravenous albumin in addition to an antibiotic reduces the incidence of renal impairment and improves hospital survival [35]. The study included 126 patients with SBP, who were randomly assigned to treatment with intravenous cefotaxime (63 patients) or with cefotaxime and intravenous albumin (63 patients). Albumin was given at a dose of 1.5 g per kilogram of body weight at the time of diagnosis, followed by 1 g per kilogram of body weight on day 3. Renal impairment developed in 21 patients in the cefotaxime group (33%) and in 6 in the cefotaxime-plus-albumin group (10%). The hospital mortality rate was

29% in the cefotaxime group in comparison with 10% in the cefotaxime-plus-albumin group. The results of this study suggest that cirrhotic patients with SBP should be expanded with albumin. However, further studies are needed to determine whether lower doses of albumin have the same effects on renal function and survival, and if albumin can be substituted by artificial plasma expanders. In addition, it would be important to know those patients with SBP who may benefit from albumin infusion or if this treatment should be applied to all SBP patients. In this sense it should be noted that the incidence of renal impairment among patients with a baseline bilirubin level of less than 4 mg/dL and a creatinine level of less than 1 mg/dL was very low in both treatment groups (7% and 0% in the cefotaxime and cefotaxime + albumin groups, respectively). Therefore, patients with abnormal renal function (BUN > 30 mg/dL and/or creatinine > 1.0 mg/dL) and/or high bilirubin levels (> 4mg/dL) appear to be the subgroup of patients with SBP who derive the most benefit from volume expansion with albumin. Since renal dysfunction is a result of an aggravation in vasodilatation and a decrease in effective arterial blood volume, procedures that lead to a decreased effective blood volume, such as the use of diuretics and large-volume paracentesis, should be avoided.

Prophylaxis

Current indications of selective intestinal decontamination in SBP prevention are summarised in Table 46. Cirrhotic patients with gastrointestinal haemorrhage are predisposed to develop severe bacterial infections during or immediately after the bleeding episode. Short-term intestinal decontamination is

Table 46 Indications and duration of selective intestinal decontamination for the prevention of SBP in cirrhotic patients.

Indications	Duration of prophylaxis
Cirrhotic patients recovering from a previous episode of SBP (secondary prophylaxis)	Indefinitely or until liver transplantation
Cirrhotic patients with gastrointestinal bleeding	7 days
Cirrhotic patients with ascites and low ascitic fluid protein levels (≤ 10 g/L)	During hospitalisation (no consensus)

effective in preventing SBP in cirrhotic patients with gastrointestinal haemorrhage [36,37]. The usefulness of systemic administration of prophylactic antibiotic agents in cirrhotic patients with gastrointestinal haemorrhage has also been investigated in three controlled studies. In these studies the treated groups received ofloxacin (initially intravenously and then orally) plus amoxicillin–clavulanic acid (before each endoscopy), ciprofloxacin plus amoxicillin–clavulanic acid (first intravenously and then orally once the bleeding was controlled) and oral ciprofloxacin, respectively [38–40]. The incidence of bacterial infections was significantly lower in the treated groups (10–20%) than in the corresponding control groups (45–66%). A relative limitation in these studies was the inability to assess the effect of antibiotic prophylaxis specifically on SBP since the incidence of both SBP and bacteraemia were analysed together. Nevertheless, the marked decrease in the rate of overall infections and the improvement in survival in the groups receiving antibiotic prophylaxis support such prophylaxis being strongly recommended in cirrhotic patients with gastrointestinal haemorrhage independently of their specific risk of SBP [24]. Furthermore, a meta-analysis including all the above-mentioned studies showed a significant benefit in the subgroup of cirrhotic patients with ascites and gastrointestinal haemorrhage: 95% of patients were free of SBP in the treated group versus 87% in the control group [41].

Cases with low ascitic fluid total protein concentration may be a second group of cirrhotic patients who may benefit from selective intestinal decontamination. In 63 patients admitted to hospital for the treatment of an episode of ascites with an ascitic fluid total protein concentration lower than 15 g/L, some of whom had had a previous episode of SBP, the continuous administration of norfloxacin, 400 mg/day throughout the hospitalisation period (32 patients), decreased the in-hospital incidence of SBP from 22% in the control group to 0% in the treated group [42]. In cirrhotic patients with ascitic fluid protein concentration < 15 g/L and no previous episodes of SBP, the 6-month incidence of SBP was 0% in the group of patients prophylactically treated with norfloxacin, 400 mg/day for 6 months, compared to 9% in patients treated with placebo. Nevertheless, the difference in the incidence of SBP caused by Gram-negative organisms (the only one which theoretically can be prevented by norfloxacin prophylaxis) between the two groups was not statistically significant: 0% in the norfloxacin-treated group and 5% in the placebo-treated group [43].

Other antibiotic regimes have been evaluated in the prevention of SBP in high-risk patients. A placebo-controlled study demonstrated that 6-month prophylaxis with ciprofloxacin, 750 mg weekly, was effective in reducing the incidence of SBP in cirrhotic patients with low protein concentration in ascitic fluid: 4% in the treated group and 22% in the placebo-control group [44]. In this study, patients with and without a prior history of SBP were included together and no attempt was made to evaluate the development of SBP in these two subgroups of patients separately. Trimethoprim–sulfamethoxazol (one double-strength tablet 5 days a week) is also effective in the prevention of SBP in cirrhotic patients with ascites [45]. In a randomised controlled trial with a medium follow-up of only 90 days, the incidence of SBP was 26.7% in the control group and 3.3% in the group of patients receiving trimethoprim–sulfamethoxazole prophylaxis. Again, patients with different risk for SBP were analysed together: patients with low and high ascitic fluid protein and patients who have had and patients who have not had previous SBP episodes.

Patients recovering from an episode of SBP represent a unique population to assess the effect of long-term intestinal decontamination in the prophylaxis of SBP. In a double-blind placebo-controlled trial including 80 cirrhotic patients who had recovered from an episode of SBP, the overall probability of SBP recurrence at 1 year of follow-up was 20% in the norfloxacin group and 68% in the placebo group and the probability of SBP caused by aerobic Gram-negative bacilli at 1 year of follow-up was 3% and 60%, respectively. Only one patient treated with norfloxacin experienced side effects related to treatment (oral and oesophageal candidiasis) [46]. Long-term selective intestinal decontamination, therefore, dramatically decreases the rate of SBP recurrence in patients with SBP. Three recent economic analyses have calculated that long-term antibiotic prophylaxis in cirrhotic patients is associated with a reduced cost compared with the 'diagnose and treat' strategy, suggesting that prophylaxis is cost-effective when applied to patients at high-risk of developing SBP [47–49].

Taking into account all these prophylactic studies, it can be assumed that antibiotic prophylaxis in cirrhotic patients with ascites is indicated in patients who have had a previous episode of SBP because they are at high-risk of SBP recurrence and because prophylaxis is cost-effective. In patients with low protein content in ascitic fluid who have never had SBP, the recommendation is difficult to establish due to the heterogeneity of the published studies which included patients with low and high-risk of SBP together. This is the main reason for the lack of consensus since, despite the positive results of all the studies investigating different antibiotics in the prophylaxis of SBP in patients with cirrhosis, they have been unable to identify subsets of patients who clearly benefit from this therapy. On the other hand, it should be noted that three studies have been performed assessing the incidence and predictive factors of the first episode of SBP in cirrhotic patients with ascites, and they may help in deciding whether a patient should initiate antibiotic prophylaxis. In a series of 127 patients admitted to hospital for the treatment of an episode of ascites, the probability of the appearance of the first episode of SBP was 11% at 1 year and 15% at 3 years of follow-up [20]. Five variables obtained at admission were significantly associated with a higher risk of SBP appearance during follow-up (poor nutritional status, increased serum bilirubin levels, decreased prothrombin activity, increased serum AST levels and low ascitic fluid protein concentration) but only one (low ascitic fluid protein concentration) showed an independent predictive value. The 1-year and 3-year probabilities of the first episode of SBP in patients with ascitic fluid protein content lower than 10 g/L were 20% and 24% whereas in those with ascitic fluid protein content equal to or greater than 10 g/L they were 0% and 4%, respectively. A clear conclusion from this study is that long-term prophylactic administration of antibiotics is not necessary in patients with protein content in ascitic fluid greater than 10 g/L, in whom the risk of developing SBP is negligible. In a similar study performed in 110 consecutive cirrhotic patients hospitalised for the treatment of an episode of ascites [21], six variables associated with a higher risk of first SBP appearance during follow-up were identified: serum bilirubin > 2.5 mg/do, prothrombin activity < 60%, ascitic fluid total protein concentration < 10 g/L, serum sodium concentration < 130 meq/L, platelet count < 116,000/mm^3 and serum albumin concentration < 26 g/L. However, only two (ascitic fluid protein concentration and serum bilirubin) showed an independent predictive value. In a recent study, cirrhotic patients with low ascitic fluid protein levels (< 10 g/L) and high serum bilirubin level (> 3.2 mg/dL) and/or low platelet count (< 98,000/mm^3) presented a 1-year probability of developing a first SBP of 55% in comparison with 24% of patients with only low ascitic fluid protein levels. Three studies, therefore, indicate that cirrhotic patients with ascites who are at risk of developing a first episode of SBP can be identified using routine biochemical parameters and might benefit from selective intestinal decontamination. However, the efficacy of antibiotic prophylaxis in these high-risk patients should be adequately investigated in prospective randomised trials.

A second reason for the lack of consensus in the prophylaxis of SBP, particularly in those patients who have never had a previous episode of SBP, is the problem of the development of quinolone-resistant enterobacteria. A review of the published data indicates that from an initial stage when norfloxacin prophylaxis was considered effective and not associated with the development of quinolone-resistant bacteria, we have moved to a final stage in which quinolone-resistant bacteria may cause severe infections in these patients. Initial studies suggested that the risk of developing SBP or other infections caused by quinolone-resistant strains of Gram-negative bacilli was low, since the majority of SBP recurrences in patients on norfloxacin prophylaxis were caused by Gram-positive cocci, mainly *streptococci* [46,50,51]. Thereafter, a high incidence of quinolone-resistant strains of *E. coli* in stools of cirrhotic patients undergoing long-term quinolone-prophylaxis was reported in several studies, although none of these studies reported any infection due to quinolone-resistant *E. coli*. In 1997, the first study on long-term norfloxacin prophylaxis in SBP was published, which showed a relevant emergence of infections, mainly mild urinary infections, caused by Gram-negative bacilli resistant to quinolones (90% of *E. coli* isolated were resistant to quinolones) [52]. More recently it has been shown that 39 out of 106 infections caused by *E. coli* in hospitalised cirrhotic patients were quinolone-resistant, being long-term norfloxacin prophylaxis significantly associated with the development of infections (mainly urinary tract infections (UTI)) caused by quinolone-resistant *E. coli*. However, development of SBP due to quinolone-resistant *E. coli* in decontaminated patients was scarcely reported [53].

Data from a study performed in our Liver Unit, which prospectively evaluated all bacterial infections occurring in a 2-year period, show a clear relationship between the development of SBP caused by quinolone-resistant Gram-negative bacilli and long-term treatment with norfloxacin [54]. In patients on long-term norfloxacin prophylaxis, 50% of culture-positive SBP were caused by quinolone-resistant Gram-negative bacilli, whereas only 16% of culture-positive SBP in patients not receiving this prophylaxis were caused by these resistant bacteria. Although in this study SBP caused by quinolone-resistant Gram-negative bacilli only represented 26% of the culture-positive SBP, quinolone-resistant SBP seems to emerge for the first time as a real problem in hepatology and probably, it will increase in the near future. This study also showed a high rate of culture-positive SBP caused by trimethoprim–sulfamethoxazole-resistant Gram-negative bacteria in patients on long-term treatment with norfloxacin (44%), suggesting that this antibiotic is not an alternative to norfloxacin. These results suggest that the effectiveness of norfloxacin is decreasing in the prevention of SBP in cirrhotic patients, and therefore this should be considered as an alarm signal. Actually, this situation was expected from what occurred in the general population or in neutropenic patients. An interesting point in the evolution of quinolone resistance in patients with cirrhosis receiving prophylaxis with norfloxacin has been the maintenance of its efficacy despite the evidence that norfloxacin was unable to maintain a selective intestinal decontamination. This is the main argument favouring the use of this antibiotic in the prophylaxis of infections caused by Gram-negative bacilli. Different explanations have been proposed for this phenomenon, including a reduction in the intestinal overgrowth, a diminution in the bacterial adhesion resulting in a decreased translocation capacity and a favourable effect of quinolones upon non-specific immune defences. However, it is possible that the continuous utilisation of quinolones has promoted an accumulation of factors involved in quinolone resistance. Actually, *E. coli* quinolone resistance, initially linked to mutation located in a region of *gyrA* known as the quinolone-resistance determining region, was subsequently linked to other factors responsible for quinolone resistance (double mutation in DNA gyrase A, mutations in *gyrB*, mutations in *parC* and changes in the permeation of quinolones). Therefore, it is possible that different factors involved in quinolone resistance acting together are now responsible for the decrease in its efficacy in the prophylaxis of bacterial infections in cirrhosis.

Our study also showed no significant differences in the resolution rate of infections caused by *E. coli* resistant to quinolones in comparison with the resolution rate of those due to sensitive strains. The absence of cross-resistance between quinolones and other antibiotics commonly used to treat these bacterial infections, such as third generation cephalosporins, could explain this finding (SBP resolution rate: 92% versus 91%). The fact that none of the *E. coli* isolated in patients undergoing long-term quinolone prophylaxis was resistant to third generation cephalosporins reinforces the idea that this antibiotic constitutes the elective treatment for bacterial infections not only in non-decontaminated cirrhotic patients but also in those undergoing selective intestinal decontamination with quinolones. On the other hand, the high incidence of quinolone and trimethoprim–sulfamethoxazole-resistant strains of *E. coli* isolated in decontaminated cirrhotic patients, underlines the necessity of restricting the administration of prophylactic antibiotics only to those patients at the greatest risk of SBP. The increasing emergence of infections caused by quinolone and trimethoprim–sulfamethoxazole-resistant strains of Gram-negative bacilli also suggests that the effectiveness of these antibiotics may decrease with time due to their widespread use. In this way, further studies are needed to evaluate alternative prophylactic measures such as other antibiotic regimes and non-antibiotic procedures in SBP prophylaxis. Finally, it should be kept in mind that SBP carries a poor prognosis. The 1-year and 2-year probability of survival after an episode of SBP is 30–50% and 25–30%, respectively [1]. Therefore, patients recovering from an episode of SBP should be considered as potential candidates for liver transplantation.

OTHER BACTERIAL INFECTIONS

Urinary tract infections (UTI)

Several predisposing factors have been recognised for UTI in cirrhosis: presence of urethral catheters, ascites and female sex. In most cases UTI is oligo or asymptomatic and bacteriuria alone can be present in 40% of cases. The micro-organisms usually responsible for UTI in cirrhosis are Gram-negative *bacilli* and *Enterococcus spp* in case of urinary manipulation. The empirical treatment could include third generation cephalosporins or amoxicillin–clavulanic acid. In case of treatment failure, ampicillin should be added if urinary catheterisation is in place, and ultrasonography should be performed to rule out other facilitating pathologies in the urinary tract.

Pneumonia

The distinction between community and hospital (nosocomial) acquired pneumonia is very useful. The causative organisms in case of community acquired pneumonia are the same as we can see in the general population, *Mycoplasma pneumoniae* or Legionella spp, plus *Streptococcus pneumonia*, *Haemophilus influenza*, and in addition Gram-negative bacilli, particularly *Klebsiella pneumoniae,* and anaerobic bacteria. Empirical treatment should cover these possibilities including: Clarithromycin (or a more recent derivative) + third generation cephalosporins (or amoxicillin–clavulanic acid). In case of treatment failure, the possibility of infection by *Staphylococcus aureus and Pseudomonas spp* has to be considered.

Predisposing factors for nosocomial pneumonia are tracheal intubation, hepatic encephalopathy and oesophageal tamponade, being Gram-negative bacilli (*Pseudomonas spp*) and *Staphylococcus spp* the bacteria most frequently responsible for this infection in these cases. Therefore, empirical treatment in patients with predisposing factors should include Ceftazidime or cefepime+ciprofloxacin (to cover *Pseudomonas spp*), adding vancomycin in case of tracheal intubation. In patients without predisposing factors for *Pseudomonas spp* or *Staphylococcus spp*, third generation cephalosporins are very effective and do not have significant adverse effects.

Spontaneous bacteraemia

The causative organisms are the same found in SBP, because, in theory, spontaneous bacteraemia is a preceding step in the colonisation of ascitic fluid. Therefore, the empirical treatment should cover *Gram-negative bacilli* and *non-enterococcal streptococci*, being third generation cephalosporins the most effective and safe treatment. Amoxicillin–clavulanic acid is an option. In case of treatment failure, blood cultures are very important to ascertain the susceptibility of the bacteria. A secondary origin of the bacteraemia has to be excluded.

Secondary bacteraemia

The causative bacteria can be considered according to the origin of the bacteraemia.

- Catheter sepsis: *Staphylococcus aureus and epidermidis*
- TAE: anaerobic facultative streptococci
- TIPS: Gram-positive cocci (staphylococci etc)
- Sclerotherapy: Gram-positive cocci and Gram-negative bacilli

The recommended empiric treatment for catheter-related sepsis is vancomycin and removal of the catheter. Fever after TAE is frequent and does not necessarily mean infection. In case of bacteraemia, amoxicillin–clavulanic acid is a good antibiotic choice. In different centres cefepime + vancomycin is recommended as prophylaxis during TIPS procedure.

Cellulitis and lymphangitis

Several predisposing factors have been implicated in these infections such as deficient hygienic standards, unapparent skin injuries and oedema. The empiric treatment should cover Gram-positive cocci (*Staphylococcus aureus, Streptococci)* and *Enterobacteria*. Amoxicillin–clavulanic acid or levofloxacin are good options as empirical treatments.

SUMMARY

Spontaneous bacterial peritonitis is a frequent, severe complication of cirrhotic patients with ascites. Its diagnosis is established on the basis of a PMN cell count in ascitic fluid higher than 250 cells/mm^3. The routine use of diagnostic paracentesis whenever a cirrhotic patient with ascites is admitted to hospital usually allows an early diagnosis of the infection. At present, third generation cephalosporins are considered the gold standard in the treatment of SBP. Because of the high incidence of quinolone-resistant Gram-negative bacilli isolated in cirrhotic patients on long-term norfloxacin prophylaxis, SBP in these patients should not be treated with quinolones as empirical therapy. Although SBP prognosis has improved in recent years, the mortality rate associated with this bacterial infection is still high. The development of severe complications such as renal impairment and gastrointestinal bleeding is responsible for this poor prognosis. The mechanisms involved in the pathogenesis of these complications are still unknown. Selective intestinal decontamination with quinolones has been proven to be effective in SBP prophylaxis of patients who have recovered from a previous episode of SBP and in patients with gastrointestinal bleeding. The increasing emergence of quinolone-resistant organisms clearly establishes the necessity of restricting primary prophylaxis to those subsets of patients at high-risk of developing a first episode of SBP. The identification of these patients and the evaluation of alternative prophylactic measures such as other antibiotic regimes and no antibiotic procedures are still under investigation. Because of the poor survival expectancy after this bacterial infection, cirrhotic patients recovering from an episode of SBP should be considered as potential candidates for liver transplantation. Finally, other bacterial infections in cirrhosis with the most frequent causative organisms and the empirical treatment are summarised.

REFERENCES

1 Navasa M, Rodés J. Bacterial infections in cirrhosis. *Liver Int* 2004;**24**: 277–280.

2 Runyon BA, Hoefs JC. Culture-negative neutrocytic ascites: a variant of spontaneous bacterial peritonitis. *Hepatology* 1984;**4**: 1209–1211.

3 Runyon BA, Squier S, Borzio M. Translocation of gut bacteria in rats with cirrhosis to mesenteric lymph nodes partially explains the pathogenesis of spontaneous bacterial peritonitis. *J Hepatol* 1994;**21**: 792–796.

4 Casafont Morencos F, de las Heras Castaño G, Martín Ramos L *et al.* Small bowel bacterial overgrowth in patients with alcoholic cirrhosis. *Dig Dis Sci* 1995;**40**: 1252–1256.

5 Perez-Paramo MP, Muñoz J, Albillos A *et al.* Effect of propranolol on the factors promoting bacterial translocation in cirrhotic rats with ascites. *Hepatology* 2000;**31**: 43–48.

6 Sorell WT, Quigley EMM, Jin G *et al.* Bacterial translocation in the portal-hypertensive rat: studies in basal conditions and on exposure to haemorrhagic shock. *Gastroenterology* 1993;**104**: 1722–1726.

7 Llovet JM, Bartoli R, Planas R *et al.* Bacterial translocation in cirrhotic rats. Its role in the development of spontaneous bacterial peritonitis. *Gut* 1994;**35**: 1648–1652.

8 Garcia-Tsao G, Lee FY, Barden GE *et al.* Bacterial translocation to mesenteric lymph nodes is increased in cirrhotic rats with ascites. *Gastroenterology* 1995;**108**: 1835–1841.

9 Llovet JM, Bartoli R, Planas R *et al.* Selective intestinal decontamination with norfloxacin reduces bacterial translocation in ascitic cirrhotic rats exposed to haemorrhagic shock. *Hepatology* 1996;**23**: 781–787.

10 Cirera I, Bauer TM, Navasa M *et al.* Bacterial translocation of enteric organisms in patients with cirrhosis. *J Hepatol* 2001;**34**: 32–37.

11 Jones EA, Summerfield JA. Kupffer cells. In: Arias IM, Jakoby WB, Popper H, Schacter D, Shafritz DA (eds). *The liver: biology and pathobiology.* 2nd edn New York: Raven Press, 1988; 683–704.

12 Rimola A, Soto R, Bory F *et al.* Reticuloendothelial system phagocytic activity in cirrhosis and its relation to bacterial infections and prognosis. *Hepatology* 1984;**4**: 53–58.
13 Bolognesi M, Merkel C, Bianco S *et al.* Clinical significance of the evaluation of hepatic reticuloendothelial removal capacity in patients with cirrhosis. *Hepatology* 1994;**19**: 628–634.
14 Guarner C, Runyon BA. Macrophage function in cirrhosis and the risk of bacterial infection. *Hepatology* 1995;**22**: 367–369.
15 Gomez F, Ruiz P, Schreiber AD. Impaired function of macrophage Fc gamma receptors and bacterial infection in alcoholic cirrhosis. *N Engl J Med* 1994;**331**: 1122–1128.
16 Runyon BA. Patients with deficient ascitic fluid opsonic activity are predisposed to spontaneous bacterial peritonitis. *Hepatology* 1988;**8**: 632–635.
17 Runyon BA. Low-protein-concentration ascitic fluid is predisposed to spontaneous bacterial peritonitis. *Gastroenterology* 1986;**91**: 1343–1346.
18 Tito LL, Rimola A, Gines P *et al.* Recurrence of spontaneous bacterial peritonitis in cirrhosis: frequency and predictive factors. *Hepatology* 1988;**8**: 27–31.
19 Llach J, Rimola A, Navasa M *et al.* Incidence and predictive factors of first episode of spontaneous bacterial peritonitis in cirrhosis with ascites: relevance of ascitic fluid protein concentration. *Hepatology* 1992;**16**: 724–727.
20 Andreu M, Solá R, Sitges-Serra A *et al.* Risk factors for spontaneous bacterial peritonitis. *Gastroenterology* 1993;**104**: 1133–1138.
21 Guarner C, Sola R, Soriano G *et al.* Risk of a first community-acquired spontaneous bacterial peritonitis in cirrhotics with low ascitic protein levels. *Gastroenterology* 1999;**117**: 414–419.
22 Garcia-Gonzalez M, Boixeda D, Herrero D *et al.* Effect of granulocyte-macrophage colony-stimulating factor on leukocyte function in cirrhosis. *Gastroenterology* 1993;**105**: 527–531.
23 Rolando N, Gimson A, Philpott-Howard J *et al.* Infectious sequel after endoscopic sclerotherapy of oesophageal varices: role of antibiotic prophylaxis. *J Hepatol* 1993;**18**: 290–294.
24 Rimola A, Garcia-Tsao G, Navasa M *et al.* Diagnosis, treatment and prophylaxis of spontaneous bacterial peritonitis: a consensus document. *J Hepatol* 2000;**32**: 142–153.
25 Felisart J, Rimola A, Arroyo V *et al.* Cefotaxime is more effective than is ampicillin-tobramycin in cirrhotics with severe infections. *Hepatology* 1985;**5**: 457–462.
26 Runyon BA, McHutchison JG, Antillon MR *et al.* Short-course versus long-course antibiotic treatment of spontaneous bacterial peritonitis. A randomized controlled study of 100 patients. *Gastroenterology* 1991;**100**: 1737–1742.
27 Rimola A, Salmeron JM, Clemente G *et al.* Two different dosages of cefotaxime in the treatment of spontaneous bacterial peritonitis in cirrhosis: results of a prospective, randomized, multicenter study. *Hepatology* 1995;**21**: 674–679.
28 Mercader J, Gómez J, Ruiz J *et al.* Use of ceftriaxone in the treatment of bacterial infections in cirrhotic patients. *Chemotherapy* 1989;**35**(suppl. 2): 23–26.
29 Gómez-Jimenez J, Ribera E, Gasser I *et al.* Randomized trial comparing ceftriaxone with cefonicid for treatment of spontaneous bacterial peritonitis in cirrhotic patients. *Antimicrob Ag Chemother* 1993;**37**: 1587–1592.

30 Ariza J, Xiol X, Esteve M *et al.* Aztreonam vs. cefotaxime in the treatment of gram-negative spontaneous peritonitis in cirrhotic patients. *Hepatology* 1991;**14**: 91–98.

31 Grange JD, Amiot X, Grange V *et al.* Amoxicillin-Clavulanic acid therapy of spontaneous bacterial peritonitis: a prospective study of twenty-seven cases in cirrhotic patients. *Hepatology* 1990;**11**: 360–364.

32 Ricart E, Soriano G, Novella MT *et al.* Amoxicillin-clavulanic acid versus cefotaxime in the therapy of bacterial infections in cirrhotic patients. *J Hepatol* 2000;**32**: 596–602.

33 Silvain C, Breux JP, Grollier G *et al.* Les septicémies et les infections du liquide d'ascite du cirrhotique peuvent-elles être traitées exclusivement par voie orale? *Gastroenterol Clin Biol* 1989;**13**: 335–339.

34 Navasa M, Follo A, Llovet JM *et al.* Randomized, comparative study of oral ofloxacin versus intravenous cefotaxime in spontaneous bacterial peritonitis. *Gastroenterology* 1996;**111**: 1011–1017.

35 Sort P, Navasa M, Arroyo V *et al.* Effect of intravenous albumin on renal impairment and mortality in patients with cirrhosis and spontaneous bacterial peritonitis. *N Engl J Med* 1999;**5**: 403–409.

36 Rimola A, Bory F, Terés J *et al.* Oral non-absorbable antibiotics prevent infection in cirrhosis with gastrointestinal haemorrhage. *Hepatology* 1985;5: 463–467.

37 Soriano G, Guarner C, Tomás A *et al.* Norfloxacin prevents bacterial infection in cirrhotics with gastrointestinal haemorrhage. *Gastroenterology* 1992;**103**: 1267–1272.

38 Blaise M, Pateron D, Trinchet J-C *et al.* Systemic antibiotic therapy prevents bacterial infection in cirrhotic patients with gastrointestinal haemorrhage. *Hepatology* 1994;**20**: 34–38.

39 Pauwels A, Mostefa-Kara N, Debenes B *et al.* Systemic antibiotic prophylaxis after gastrointestinal haemorrhage in cirrhotic patients with a high risk of infection. *Hepatology* 1996;**24**: 802–806.

40 Hsieh W-J, Lin H-C, Hwang S-J *et al.* The effect of ciprofloxacin in the prevention of bacterial infections in patients with cirrhosis after upper gastrointestinal bleeding. *Am J Gastroenterol* 1998;**93**: 962–966.

41 Bernard B, Grange JD, Khac EN *et al.* Antibiotic prophylaxis for the prevention of bacterial infections in cirrhotic patients with gastrointestinal bleeding: a meta-analysis. *Hepatology* 1999;**29**: 1655–1661.

42 Soriano G, Guarner C, Teixidó M *et al.* Selective intestinal decontamination prevents spontaneous bacterial peritonitis. *Gastroenterology* 1991;**100**: 477–481.

43 Grange J-D, Roulot D, Pelletier G *et al.* Norfloxacin primary prophylaxis of bacterial infections in cirrhotic patients with ascites: a double-blind randomised trial. *J Hepatol* 1998;**29**: 430–436.

44 Rolanchon A, Cordier L, Bacq Y *et al.* Ciprofloxacin and long-term prevention of spontaneous bacterial peritonitis: results of a prospective controlled trial. *Hepatology* 1995;**22**: 1171–1174.

45 Singh N, Gayowski T, Yu VL *et al.* Trimethoprim-sulfamethoxazole for the prevention of spontaneous bacterial peritonitis in cirrhosis: a randomized trial. *Ann Intern Med* 1995;**122**: 595–598.

46 Ginès P, Rimola A, Planas R *et al.* Norfloxacin prevents spontaneous bacterial peritonitis recurrence in cirrhosis: results of a double-blind, placebo-controlled trial. *Hepatology* 1990;**12**: 716–724.
47 Inadomi J, Sonnenberg A. Cost-analysis of prophylactic antibiotics in spontaneous bacterial peritonitis. *Gastroenterology* 1997; **113**: 1289–1294.
48 Younossi ZM, McHutchison JG, Ganiats TG. An economic analysis of norfloxacin prophylaxis against spontaneous bacterial peritonitis. *J Hepatol* 1997;**27**: 295–298.
49 Das A. A cost analysis of long-term antibiotic prophylaxis for spontaneous bacterial peritonitis in cirrhosis. *Am J Gastroenterol* 1998;**93**: 1895–1900.
50 Llovet JM, Rodríguez-Iglesias P, Moitinho E *et al.* Spontaneous bacterial peritonitis in patients with cirrhosis undergoing selective intestinal decontamination. *J Hepatol* 1997;**26**: 88–95.
51 Campillo B, Dupeyron C, Richardet J-P *et al.* Epidemiology of severe hospital-acquired infections in patients with liver cirrhosis: effect of long-term administration of norfloxacin. *Clin Infect Dis* 1998;**26**: 1066–1070.
52 Novella M, Solà R, Soriano G *et al.* Continuous versus inpatient prophylaxis of the first episode of spontaneous bacterial peritonitis with norfloxacin. *Hepatology* 1997;**25**: 532–536.
53 Ortiz J, Vila MC, Soriano G *et al.* Infections caused by *Escherichia coli* resistant to norfloxacin in hospitalized cirrhotic patients. *Hepatology* 1999;**29**: 1064–1069.
54 Fernández J, Navasa M, Gomez J *et al.* Bacterial infections in cirrhosis: epidemiological changes with invasive procedures and norfloxacin prophylaxis. *Hepatology* 2002;**35**: 140–148.

Prevention of Rebleeding

Brigitte Bernard-Chabert, Tilman Sauerbruch, Gin-Ho Lo, Arun J. Sanyal, J. Michael Henderson, Gamal Shiba, Han-Chieh Lin, Càndid Villanueva, Jean-Pierre Vinel and Didier Lebrec

β-Blockers versus no Treatment, β-Blockers versus Sclerotherapy and β-Blockers versus β-Blockers plus Isosorbide Mononitrate, β-Blockers plus Isosorbide-Mononitrate versus Band Ligation

The rebleeding rate is well known with the analysis of control groups in clinical trials. At 2 years, the rebleeding rate reaches 68%, with a rebleeding rate from oesophageal varices of 63%, and a mortality rate of 33% [1]. These rates are probably underestimated, because patients included in randomised trials are those with less severe disease and low risk of being lost to follow-up.

β-blockers versus no treatment

Non-cardioselective β-blockers induce a decrease in cardiac output and a splanchnic arteriolar vasoconstriction with a resultant decrease in portal venous flow and portal pressure.

In the 1980s, numerous clinical randomised trials (RCTs) have shown the efficacy of propranolol (one trial used nadolol) in the prevention of rebleeding [2–8]. Two metaanalyses have confirmed a significant reduction of rebleeding rate from 68% in non-treated patients to 48% in treated patients at 2 years [1,9]. One metaanalysis also showed a significant increase in mean survival rate of 5% (from 67 to 74% at 2 years) [1].

β-blockers versus sclerotherapy

Ten RCTs have compared the efficacy of β-blockers and sclerotherapy in the prevention of rebleeding. Most of these studies have shown identical results, which have been confirmed by 2 metaanalyses including 9 trials [9,10].

There was no difference concerning rebleeding rate from any cause (56% in patients treated with β-blockers versus 53% in patients treated with sclerotherapy) and survival rate (40% versus 37%, respectively). On the other hand, in patients treated with sclerotherapy, the variceal rebleeding rate was significantly lower (45% versus 61%, $p < 0.001$) and adverse events were significantly more frequent (44% versus 24%, $p < 0.001$).

In conclusion, β-blockers and sclerotherapy have a similar effect on rebleeding rate and mortality. Sclerotherapy is more effective in preventing rebleeding from varices, but is also responsible of more adverse events.

β-blockers versus β-blockers plus isosorbide mononitrate (ISM)

Three RCTs have compared β-blockers and combination of β-blockers and ISM [11–13], only one being published as article [11]. In this trial, which includes 95 patients, 2-years rebleeding rate was lower in patients receiving drug combination (40% versus 57%), but the difference was not significant. There was no difference concerning mortality (22% and 24%). Conversely, in the second trial which includes 104 patients, the rebleeding rate was higher in patients treated with nadolol and ISM (51% versus 39%, respectively), but the difference was not significant [12]. Moreover, the mortality rate was significantly higher in the combination group (32% versus 14%, $p = 0.02$). The only concordant result between these two trials concerned the adverse events rate, which was significantly higher in patients treated with β-blockers and ISM [11,12]. The third trial, published in the Chinese language, did not show any difference concerning rebleeding and mortality rates [13]. Although the Italian trial has not been published as an article [12], it seems that there is not enough data to recommend the association of β-blockers and ISM as first choice treatment.

β-blockers plus isosorbide mononitrate versus band ligation

Three trials have compared the efficacy of ligation and β-blockers plus nitrates [14–16]. In one trial, the rebleeding rate was significantly lower in patients receiving nadolol and nitrates: 33% versus 49% [14]. In another [15], rebleeding was significantly lower in patients treated by band ligation. In the third one [16], there was no significant difference between the two treatments concerning rebleeding. None of these studies showed a difference in survival rate. The discrepancy in the results of these trials may be explained by differences concerning the severity of liver disease, the duration of follow-up and drugs dosage. As a consequence, whether one of these treatments is superior to the other in preventing rebleeding is at present unknown.

Band ligation versus sclerotherapy and band ligation versus band ligation plus sclerotherapy

After the development of flexible endoscopy, local sclerotherapy of oesophageal varices has become the treatment of choice not only for the control of acute bleeding but also for the prevention of rebleeding.

Metaanalysis of numerous trials comparing endoscopic sclerotherapy with conservative treatment found a rebleeding rate of 43% in the sclerotherapy group and of 57% in the control group with a reduction of mortality from 54% to 46% [17].

Sclerotherapy was shown to be effective, but less than what had been assumed in early uncontrolled trials. This is mainly due to two factors: (1) Sclerotherapy requires two to eight weeks for complete obliteration of the vessels (in some patients, even up to one year). (2) During the initial phase of treatment and more often in patients with poor Child C status, many complications (e.g. ulcers, stenoses, fever, perforation, septic events) may occur [18,19]. Therefore, the introduction of elastic band ligation for the obliteration of varices by Stiegmann provided a major advantage [20,21]. It soon became evident that this method was more effective with fewer complications than injection sclerotherapy [22].

Goulis and Burroughs [23] compiled 20 studies (1,634 patients) comparing sclerotherapy to variceal ligation (11 peer-reviewed and 9 in abstract form). Variceal rebleeding and death occurred less often in patients who had received ligation.

It has repeatedly been suggested that sclerotherapy – although inferior to ligation – has one advantage in comparison to ligation, namely, more scarring and thus less recurrence of varices. Indeed, recurrence of varices was more frequent in patients treated with variceal ligation [7]. In contrast, ligation required fewer sessions for initial obliteration than sclerotherapy [18,24].

Considering the above-mentioned factors, it is obvious that ligation has replaced sclerotherapy. Nevertheless, the question arose whether ligation plus sclerotherapy is more advantageous than ligation alone. Two approaches are possible: combined therapy or sequential therapy, that is, sclerotherapy after successful ligation in order to treat small vessels not affected by sclerotherapy. This combined approach was pursued in seven trials [23,25]. There was no significant difference with respect to rebleeding, death and variceal eradication, while the combined approach caused more complications. Therefore, the combined treatment should not be adopted. The study by Lo *et al.* showed that in patients after a full term of ligation, sclerotherapy may prevent reformation of varices and lower the rebleeding rate [26].

In summary, controlled studies have distinctly demonstrated the superiority of ligation over sclerotherapy and, as a result, ligation has replaced sclerotherapy. Sclerotherapy may still play a minor role in the setting of sequential treatment with the aim to prevent the recurrence of small varices. It is important that experienced endoscopists familiar with the technique of sclerotherapy perform these therapies.

Banding ligation plus β-blockers and sucralfate versus banding ligation alone to prevent gastrooesophageal variceal rebleeding

After 1981, due to the introduction of propranolol in the prevention of variceal rebleeding, a new era is opened for the treatment of variceal rebleeding [27]. The combination of endoscopic therapy and drug therapy for portal hypertension is intriguing. Several reasons support the addition of drug therapy during endoscopic therapy. First, rebleeding rate remains high after endoscopic therapy, especially before variceal obliteration is achieved. The rebleeding rate is around 20% to 40% in patients treated with endoscopic variceal ligation (EVL). Second, portal hypertensive gastropathy may develop or worsen after endoscopic therapy [28]. An increased incidence of gastric variceal bleeding after endoscopic therapy was also noted. Third, portal pressure was noted to be elevated in approximately 70% of patients achieving variceal obliteration by either endoscopic sclerotherapy (EIS) or EVL [29]. All of these untoward effects of endoscopic therapy are expected to be alleviated by drug therapy. A number of studies have been carried out to compare the combination of propranolol and EIS with EIS alone [17]. Unfortunately, most studies did not show a benefit of combining EIS with propranolol over EIS alone. The variceal rebleeding and complication rates were similar in these studies. It is very likely that each of these studies had insufficient sample size to show a benefit of combination treatment with EIS plus propranolol. Metaanalysis suggested that the combined treatment with EIS and propranolol was significantly better than EIS alone in preventing rebleeding, but with similar survival in both treatment modalities. It was suggested that the metaanalysis results should be interpreted with caution because of qualitative heterogeneity [17].

In view of the superiority of EVL over EIS and nadolol over propranolol, an attempt was made to combine EVL with nadolol and sucralfate in comparison with EVL alone to prevent variceal rebleeding [30]. The superiority of nadolol over propranolol includes longer half-life and renal metabolism. The use of sucralfate was to reduce ulcer bleeding provoked by EVL. It would have been better to include a third arm with patients receiving EVL and nadolol only, to clarify whether sucralfate was necessary during the course of EVL. However, to achieve adequate sample size, the study was designed with two arms only. After a median follow-up of 21 months, the study showed that combination of nadolol, sucralfate and EVL was superior to EVL alone in terms of variceal rebleeding rates (12% versus 29%) and variceal recurrence (26% versus 50%). The authors presumed that the benefits of combination therapy were primarily from nadolol rather than sucralfate, since the incidence of ulcer bleeding during the course of EVL was appreciably low.

A recent study from Spain [31] also showed that EVL plus nadolol was superior to EVL alone in reducing variceal rebleeding as well as lowering the probability of variceal recurrence, similar to the results of the former trial. These data suggested that nadolol should be added in patients receiving EVL to prevent variceal rebleeding.

Endoscopic therapy versus transjugular intrahepatic portosystemic shunt for prevention of rebleeding from oesophageal varices

Transjugular intrahepatic portosystemic shunt (TIPS) has evolved as a means of achieving portal decompression and is highly effective in preventing recurrent variceal haemorrhage. However, TIPS is generally considered as a salvage treatment for those cases where bleeding recurs despite adequate EVL. Most of the literature directly comparing the utility of TIPS versus endoscopic treatment used EIS rather than EVL as the endoscopic modality. The data from studies using EVL and EIS are combined for purposes of the analysis below.

The nature and design of the clinical trials

A total of 11 randomised controlled trials [32–42] have compared the efficacy and safety of TIPS versus endoscopic treatment with or without additional β-blockers for the prevention of recurrent oesophageal variceal bleeding. Eight studies used EIS as the form of endoscopic treatment while four studies used EVL [32–39]. Of the eight studies using EIS, three also used propranolol along with endoscopic therapy [37–39]. One of the three studies using EVL [41] used isosorbide mononitrate and propranolol in addition to endoscopic treatment.

The studies are variable with respect to the types of sclerosant, frequency of endoscopic treatment, nature of stent and methods used to monitor stent patency. The patient populations in the studies also differed with respect to the time from active bleeding to randomisation, degree of liver failure, active alcohol consumption and duration of follow-up.

Efficacy-related outcomes

Rebleeding. The great majority of clinical trials demonstrate that TIPS is associated with a significantly lower rebleeding rate compared to endoscopic treatment. The range of rebleeding rates after TIPS varied from 9 to 23% while that after endoscopic treatment was 21–66%. In two studies, there were no significant differences in the rebleeding rates after TIPS and endoscopic treatment. In both studies, the risks of rebleeding in the TIPS arm were similar to those in other studies (22% and 19.4%, respectively). The principal difference between these studies and the other trials was the rebleeding rates in the endoscopic treatment arm (21% and 29.9%, respectively).

Mortality. With the exception of a single study [36], none of the published trial showed an improvement or worsening of mortality with TIPS. The data are fairly uniform despite the differences between the individual studies. It is interesting to note that the range of survival rates in these studies varied from 13 to 69% for TIPS and from 12 to 67% for endoscopic therapy. This may reflect the severity of the underlying liver disease. It is also noteworthy that the survival data from studies of endoscopic and pharmacological treatment were similar to those of endoscopic treatment alone. Based on these data, it may be concluded that TIPS does not improve or worsen survival compared to endoscopic therapy.

Safety related outcomes

Procedure-related complications. Of the known complications, the development of bleeding from EVL-ulcers was the most clinically relevant. Chest pain and dysphagia are other complications. Another recent study has noted an increased risk of bacterial peritonitis and bacteraemia after EVL [43].

Frequency of other (non-bleeding) complications of cirrhosis. Unfortunately, most studies do not provide data on the frequency with which all of the other complications of cirrhosis occurred in subjects undergoing endoscopic therapy versus TIPS. The best data are available for encephalopathy. The risk of hepatic encephalopathy after TIPS varies widely across the different trials. This is most likely due to the different methods used to classify and grade encephalopathy and the rigour with which encephalopathy was looked for across trials. Advanced age, shunt diameter and a history of encephalopathy prior to TIPS have been identified as risk factors for the development of encephalopathy after TIPS. Encephalopathy can usually be managed with lactulose and treatment of any precipitating factors. Rarely, the shunt has to be reduced or occluded for crippling encephalopathy. Recently, it has been reported that the risk of hepatocellular cancer may be increased after TIPS placement. These data need further corroboration before this can be confirmed.

Surgical shunts versus TIPS for refractory variceal bleeding

Variceal decompression with a shunt is reserved for patients who are refractory to first-line treatment with pharmacological and endoscopic therapy. The debate in 2005 is whether such decompression is best done with a surgical shunt, or a transjugular intrahepatic portosystemic shunt (TIPS). There are two prospective randomised controlled trials that have looked at the comparative role of surgical shunt versus TIPS: Rosemurgy *et al.* [44] have compared 8 mm portocaval H-graft shunt versus TIPS, and Henderson *et al.* [45] have compared the distal splenorenal shunt (DSRS) versus TIPS.

The 8 mm portocaval shunt versus TIPS trial has been published in several formats. This trial entered patients sequentially, rather than being truly randomised. For each patient receiving one randomised therapy, the next patient received the opposite treatment. Two-thirds of the patients had alcoholic liver disease. The results showed a significantly lower rebleeding rate ($p < 0.01$) for the surgical shunt compared to TIPS. The TIPS rebleeding rate was 18%. Significantly more patients required liver transplant in the TIPS group compared to the surgical shunt group. There was no difference in mortality. The composite endpoint of 'failures' comprising rebleeding, irrevocable shunt thrombosis, deaths and need for transplant was significantly higher for the TIPS patients when compared with the surgical shunt patients.

The second prospective randomised controlled trial was a multi-centre study funded by the NIH with five clinical centres. This study compared TIPS to DSRS in Child's class A and B patients. 57% of the patients were Child's class A, and 57% had alcoholic liver disease. The mean follow-up in the study was 43 ± 25 months, with only one patient lost to follow-up and the status of all others known to at least 21 months post-procedure.

The rebleeding rate in this trial was not significantly different between the two groups, with four patients (5.5%) in the DSRS group, and six patients (9%) in the TIPS group rebleeding ($p = 0.27$). The reintervention rate was significantly higher ($p = 0.001$) in the TIPS group (82%) compared to the

DSRS group (11%). 18 patients in the TIPS group had total shunt thrombosis compared to two in the DSRS group, with the other indications for reintervention defined as a pressure gradient > 15 mm Hg or a > 50% stenosis as adjudicated by a review group. The peak time for reinterventions was at the time of annual shunt recatheterization done on protocol: criteria for reintervention were fulfilled despite documented shunt adequacy on ultrasound.

The time to the first episode of encephalopathy was not significantly different between the DSRS and TIPS groups. At late follow-up, 50% of the patients in each group had had at least one episode of clinical encephalopathy. Half of these patients had multiple episodes. The total number of deaths in the DSRS group was 28, and 27 in the TIPS group. The survival curves show a 2-year survival of over 80%, and a 5-year survival over 60%. These are not significantly different at any time point. Seven patients in each group came to liver transplant. The conclusions from this trial were that DSRS and TIPS were equally efficacious in control of variceal rebleeding, survival, encephalopathy and progression of liver disease in Child's class A and B patients. TIPS did require significantly more reintervention to maintain patency and achieve the low rebleeding rate of this study.

These two prospective randomised trials provide the best evidence as to the relative efficacy of a surgical versus a radiological shunt. Variceal rebleeding is lower in the surgical shunt groups in both studies, but only significantly in the Rosemurgy trial. In good risk patients (Child's class A and B) surgical shunt or TIPS does not appear to significantly alter the rate or severity of encephalopathy and progress of liver disease. In neither study is survival significantly different at long-term follow-up. TIPS does need significantly more surveillance and intervention to maintain patency, and to achieve these good long-term results.

What recommendations can be made from these trials? TIPS is more widely available than surgical shunt in 2005, and as such is more widely used for patients with continued bleeding after primary therapy. However, to achieve the results outlined above, careful follow-up of TIPS with the need for reintervention is required. The excellent survival, with low rebleeding rates achieved after either procedure indicate an ongoing role for variceal decompression for Child's A and B patients who have refractory bleeding.

Prevention of variceal rebleeding in non-cirrhotic patients

Non-cirrhotic portal hypertension (NCPH) comprises a group of diseases with raised portal pressure due to intra or prehepatic lesions. Distinct diseases with NCPH include schistosomal hepatic fibrosis, non-cirrhotic portal fibrosis (NCPF), extrahepatic portal vein obstruction (EHPVO) and congenital hepatic fibrosis [46–48]. After control of the acute attack, several therapeutic options are available for prevention of rebleeding: pharmacotherapy, endoscopic management: EVL or EIS, combined endoscopic and pharmacological treatment, TIPS and surgery.

Prevention of rebleeding in schistosomal hepatic fibrosis patients

In endemic areas, pure schistosomal hepatic fibrosis comprises 13–18% of patients presenting with bleeding varices, and mixed schistosomal with posthepatitic cirrhosis comprises 60–65% of patients. They present with a relatively good hepatic reserve since 17–23% of these patients are Child A class, 53–54% Child B and 23–30% Child C.

Pharmacotherapy. Use of propranolol was shown to be highly beneficial in schistosomal hepatic fibrosis patients (rebleeding rate 80% versus 20% $p < 0.05$) when compared to placebo [49]. Isosorbide-5-Mono-nitrate (ISMN) was also used in prevention of rebleeding in these patients [50].

Endoscopic management. Both EVL and EIS were effective in prevention of rebleeding in patients with schistosomal hepatic fibrosis with fewer number of sessions needed and significantly lower complication rates in the EVL group [51].

Combination of pharmacological and endoscopic treatment. Combination of EIS and propranolol was shown to be effective in the prevention of rebleeding from oesophageal varices in patients with schistosomal hepatic fibrosis when compared to sclerotherapy alone [52]. ISMN with and without propranolol also reduces rebleeding rate and variceal recurrence after obliteration when combined with sclerotherapy [52]. In a recent randomised study EVL was compared with propranolol and combined ISMN plus propranolol for the prevention of variceal rebleeding and concluded that EVL is more effective than pharmacotherapy with a lower complication rate [53].

Gastric varices. N-butyl-2-cynoacrylate was used effectively in prevention of rebleeding from gastric varices [54]. Gastric variceal ligation was also used in GOV_1, GOV_2 and IGV_1 using the multiband ligator devices [55]. Surgical intervention was proved to be highly effective in prevention of rebleeding from gastric varices when endoscopic treatment fails.

Surgery. Splenectomy and devascularisation (Hassab) was widely practiced for prevention of rebleeding in patients with schistosomal hepatic fibrosis [56]. Distal-spleno-renal-shunt (DSRS) was later used effectively. Schistosomal patients have a better survival and a lower incidence of rebleeding and encephalopathy after DSRS than that reported in cirrhosis. When DSRS was compared with Hassab operation, DSRS was superior in prevention of variceal rebleeding in schistosomal portal hypertensive patients [57]. This was proved in a controlled randomised trial on selected haemodynamic portal flow patterns in schistosomal portal hypertension with variceal bleeding. In this setting, DSRS proved to be ideal for schistosomal patients with hepatopetal flow and splenic vein flow exceeding portal vein flow, because, in addition to eliminating the high splenic flow from the portal circulation, it decreased the pressure in the gastro-oesophageal region [58].

Prevention of rebleeding in non-cirrhotic portal fibrosis (NCPF)

Endoscopic sclerotherapy was the main treatment and can prevent rebleeding in 95% of NCPF patients [59]. The incidence of variceal rebleeding and recurrence after obliteration has been 3.1% and 22%, respectively. EVL has also been found to be quite effective in NCPF patients with success in control of acute bleeding and variceal obliteration in the range of 96%. There is no data on the use of combination of endoscopic and pharmacological treatment for prevention of rebleeding in NCPF. Also, there is not enough data on the use of TIPS in these patients.

Surgery. Only 5–10% of patients with NCPF require surgery. The present day indications include: (1) Failure of endoscopic therapy (2) Hypersplenism (3) Patients coming from very far off places and requiring a one time therapy. Devascularisation procedures are quite popular in Japan and are preferred over shunt surgery [47].

Prevention of variceal rebleeding in extrahepatic portal vein obstruction (EHPVO)

Sclerotherapy and variceal banding require fewer sessions in EHPVO patients than in cirrhotic patients, and are effective in preventing rebleeding [60,61]. Gastric varices are diagnosed in 40% of EHPVO patients [62] and rebleeding after cyanoacrylate glue injection occurs in 30% of patients, who then require surgical intervention [63]. TIPS is contraindicated in EHPVO. Proximal spleno-renal shunts and devascularisation procedures are useful in prevention of rebleeding and splenectomy could be curative in some patients with segmental portal hypertension. The 5 year survival rates have been reported to be 95%. Portal decompression surgery or biliary bypass may be required in patients with established biliopathy.

Prevention of variceal rebleeding in patients with congenital hepatic fibrosis (CHF)

There is not enough data on variceal rebleeding in patients with congenital hepatic fibrosis. A group of 12 CHF patients was followed up for 6 years using a combination of EVL and propranolol for prevention of rebleeding. They were eight males and four females with an age range of 2.5–17 years. All had biopsy-proven CHF; they were Child A class with negative viral markers. Gastric varices were diagnosed in three patients (25%). Rebleeding occurred in five patients (41.7%) in the first year of follow-up; three of them had gastric variceal rebleeding that required surgical intervention. Six year survival was 100%.

Prevention of gastric variceal rebleeding

The general measures for bleeding gastric varices are similar to those in oesophageal varices. It has been shown that antibiotic prophylaxis prevented rebleeding in cirrhotic patients with oesophageal or gastric variceal bleeding following endoscopic therapy using banding ligation or cyanoacrylate glue injection [64]. Accordingly, antibiotic prophylaxis should also be an integral part of therapy to prevent early gastric variceal rebleeding. There are several modalities that have been used in the management of gastric variceal bleeding.

Endoscopic band ligation

The study of ligation of gastric varices is sparse and initial reports only included few patients. Two non-controlled trials with larger number of cases have recently been reported [65,66]. In both studies, control of acute bleeding is greater than 80% with a high variceal obliteration rate (> 90%). The overall rebleeding rate is 18% and 10%, respectively. However, the overall recurrence rate for gastric varices reached 63% in the study by Lee *et al.* [66].

Gastric variceal obturation

This treatment was shown to be effective in the control of acute gastric variceal bleeding by many non-controlled trials. The initial haemostasis may reach 90%. Gastric variceal rebleeding rate ranged from 4 to 44%. Lo *et al.* [67] compared cyanoacrylate injection to banding ligation for the treatment of bleeding gastric varices. The initial haemostasis was 87% in the cyanoacrylate group and 45% in the ligation group ($p = 0.03$). The rebleeding rate was significantly lower in the cyanoacrylate group (31%) than in the ligation group (54%). Sarin *et al.* [68] compared the use of cyanoacrylate injection to sclerotherapy with pure alcohol in patients of isolated fundic varices (IGV1). Initial control of bleeding was achieved in 89% of the cyanoacrylate group and 62% of the alcohol injection group, but the difference was not statistically significant. The rebleeding rate was similar between the two groups (25% in the alcohol injection group and 22% in the cyanoacrylate group). The mortality rate did not differ between the two groups.

Bovine thrombin has previously been shown to provide beneficial effects in the management of bleeding gastric varices [69], but it is no longer available due to the potential for transmission of Creutzfeld-Jakob disease. Recently, two clinical trials with small numbers of patients have used human thrombin (i.e. human fibrin glue) for the management of gastric variceal bleeding [70,71]. Both of them found that human thrombin is effective in initial haemostasis with a rebleeding rate of less than 25%. Further studies are needed to evaluate the efficacy of this approach.

Transjugular intrahepatic portosystemic shunts (TIPS)

In non-controlled trials, TIPS was shown to be effective in the management of acutely bleeding gastric varices with an initial haemostatic rate of over 90% and a rebleeding rate of less than 30% [72–75].

Pharmacotherapy

A recent clinical trial has reported that, in patients with gastric variceal bleeding, neither propranolol nor isosorbide mononitrate decreased the risk of rebleeding and did not improve survival [76]. However, because this is a non-controlled retrospective study, and patients were given either propranolol or nitrate alone with fixed doses and the heart rate or haemodynamic parameters were not monitored, further RCTs are needed to evaluate the role of pharmacotherapy in bleeding gastric varices.

Balloon-occluded retrograde transvenous obliteration of gastric varices (B-RTO)

B-RTO is an interventional radiological technique that is only used in Japan. It is technically feasible only in patients with a gastrorenal shunt. A number of non-controlled trials have used B-RTO as a primary prophylaxis of gastric variceal bleeding. This approach has not been accepted as a treatment procedure outside Japan. A recent study which included 24 cirrhotic patients with gastric variceal bleeding has found that B-RTO is effective in the control of acute bleeding and in the prevention of rebleeding (overall rebleeding rate = 9%) [77]. RCTs are needed for further evaluation of the clinical relevance of this form of treatment.

Surgery

A non-controlled clinical trial has used distal splenorenal shunt to treat 30 patients with bleeding gastric varices, with satisfactory results [78]. In a recent prospective, 10-year follow-up RCT including more than 100 patients with oesophageal or gastric variceal bleeding, rebleeding from varices was less frequent and survival rate was better in patients with Child class A and B receiving H-graft portacaval shunt than in those receiving TIPS [44]. Shunt failure occurred less frequently in the surgery group than in the TIPS group. The occurrence of new-onset hepatic encephalopathy was similar between the two groups. The authors suggest that H-graft portacaval shunt may be better than TIPS for patients with good liver function suffering from bleeding varices. In addition to shunt surgery, recent clinical trials have suggested that modified gastric devascularisation with splenectomy may offer an alternative choice for gastric variceal haemorrhage, particularly for patients with IGV1 [79–81].

Prevention of rebleeding from portal hypertensive gastropathy

Portal hypertensive gastropathy (PHG) is a common finding in patients with portal hypertension and its natural history is variable. The prevention of rebleeding from PHG includes pharmacological and endoscopic options as well as derivative procedures. Acid inhibitory drugs such as proton pump inhibitors and cytoprotective agents such as sucralfate are ineffective [82]. Estrogens and progesterone have been reported anecdotally to decrease gastric perfusion but their clinical efficacy is unclear [83]. Nonselective β-blockers have been shown to reduce portal pressure and gastric mucosal blood flow [84–86]. In keeping with this, small uncontrolled studies have shown that propranolol can decrease recurrent bleeding from PHG [87]. This has been confirmed by the largest randomised controlled trial performed to date in this setting [88]. Accordingly, β-blockers may be considered the first line therapy to prevent recurrent bleeding from PHG.

Furthermore, the role of derivative treatments in patients bleeding from PHG is controversial. Both TIPS and shunt surgery have been shown to be effective in small studies [89–91]. It has also been reported that the gastric mucosal changes of PHG improve in a majority of patients following TIPS insertion for variceal bleeding or ascites. However, no controlled trial to date has evaluated derivative procedures for PHG. Taking this into account, together with the invasive nature of such treatments, it seems advisable to consider TIPS only when β-blockers fail.

Several small studies suggest that therapeutic endoscopy using injection therapy or thermal methods (including either contact or non-contact techniques) may effectively reduce GAVE-associated bleeding [92–96]. However, endoscopic therapy has rarely been investigated in PHG. A recent uncontrolled study proposed that endoscopic coagulation with argon-plasma could be effective to reduce recurrent bleeding in patients with PHG unresponsive to β-blockers and iron therapy [97]. Accordingly, it may be advisable to try endoscopic therapy before using derivative procedures, particularly when differentiation from GAVE is difficult. It should also be kept in mind that liver transplantation reverses portal hypertension and therefore effectively treats PHG.

Prevention of refractory variceal rebleeding

After a first bleeding episode, approximately 20% of the patients will die, 17% will rebleed within 6 weeks and 70% within 2 years (98). It is therefore mandatory to prevent rebleeding using β-blockers associated or not with nitrates and/or banding ligation. However, still up to 50% of the patients treated will experience rebleeding [9]. So far, the efficacy of treatments has never been assessed in the specific setting of failure in the prevention of rebleeding. The difference between 'first-line' and 'second-line' treatments lies on studies including 'first-line' patients. Therapeutic techniques which are more effective in preventing rebleeding than drugs and/or band ligation, but do not improve survival and have frequent or more severe side effects are usually considered 'second-line' treatments. Whenever possible, liver transplantation should be considered in these patients whose liver function is usually poor. When transplantation is contra-indicated, as well as in patients on the waiting list, a shunting procedure should be considered.

Seven trials compared surgical shunts to endoscopic treatment. Four were pooled in a metaanalysis which showed surgery to be more effective in preventing rebleeding. However, encephalopathy was more frequent after surgery and survival was not changed [9].

Fourteen studies compared TIPS to other treatments aiming to prevent rebleeding in portal hypertensive patients: sclerotherapy [32–36,99], band ligation [40,42,100], endoscopic treatment plus β-blockers [37–39,41] and β-blockers plus nitrates [101]. As a whole, metaanalyses [102–104], showed TIPS to be more effective in preventing rebleeding, reducing the risk by approximately 50%. But the incidence of encephalopathy was significantly greater in patients treated with TIPS and survival was not changed.

The main drawback of TIPS is a high rate of occlusion: up to 80% at 2 years. This can now be overcome using covered prostheses. With PTFE covered stents, a multicenter randomised trial reported a 12% obstruction rate at 1 year, without increased incidence of encephalopathy, probably because the risk inherent to blood shunting was overcome by a significantly smaller rate of clinical relapses and need for TIPS revision [105].

TIPS should now be preferred to surgery because it does not hamper the chance for transplantation, it avoids the complications of laparotomy and it can be reduced in diameter or occluded if needed.

CONCLUSION

Variceal rebleeding should not be systematically considered a treatment failure. The need for an alternative therapy will be decided according to the severity of the haemorrhage and of the underlying liver disease, the general status of the patient and the delay since the first bleeding episode. Drug therapy might be optimised by measuring haemodynamic response to tailor the dosage and/or add nitrates to β-blockers. The association of band ligation to drug therapy should also be considered.

If optimal 'first-line' therapy has failed, the patient should be treated by TIPS and considered for liver transplantation whenever possible.

REFERENCES

1 Bernard B, Lebrec D, Mathurin P *et al.* Beta-adrenergic antagonists in the prevention of gastrointestinal rebleeding in patients with cirrhosis. A meta-analysis. *Hepatology* 1997;**25**: 63–70.

2 Lebrec D, Poynard T, Hillon P *et al.* Propranolol for prevention or recurrent gastrointestinal bleeding in patients with cirrhosis. *N Engl J Med* 1981;**305**: 1371–1374.

3 Burroughs AK, Jenkins WJ, Sherlock S *et al.* Controlled trial of propranolol for the prevention of recurrent variceal hemorrhage in patients with cirrhosis. *N Engl J Med* 1983;**25**: 1539–1542.

4 Villeneuve JP, Pomier-Layrargues G, Infante-Rivard C *et al.* Propranolol for the prevention of recurrent variceal hemorrhage: a controlled trial. *Hepatology* 1986;**6**: 1239–1243.

5 Colombo M, De Franchis R, Tommasini M *et al.* ß-blockade prevents recurrent gastrointestinal bleeding in well-compensated patients with alcoholic cirrhosis: a multicenter randomised controlled trial. *Hepatology* 1989;**9**: 433–438.

6 Colman J, Jones P, Finch C *et al.* Propranolol in the prevention of variceal haemorrhage in alcoholic cirrhotic patients (abstract). *Hepatology* 1990;**12**: 851.

7 Garden OJ, Mills PR, Birnie GG *et al.* Propranolol in the prevention of recurrent variceal hemorrhage in cirrhotic patients. *Gastroenterology* 1990;**98**: 185–190.
8 Rossi V, Calès P, Burtin P *et al.* Prevention of recurrent variceal bleeding in alcoholic cirrhotic patients: prospective controlled trial of propranolol and sclerotherapy. *J Hepatol* 1991;**12**: 283–289.
9 D'Amico G, Pagliaro L, Bosch J. The treatment of portal hypertension: a meta-analytic review. *Hepatology* 1995;**22**: 332–353.
10 Bernard B, Lebrec D, Mathurin P *et al.* Propranolol and sclerotherapy in the prevention of gastrointestinal rebleeding in patients with cirrhosis. A meta-analysis. *J Hepatol* 1997;**26**: 312–324.
11 Gournay J, Masliah C, Martin T *et al.* Isosorbide mononitrate and propranolol compared with propranolol alone for the prevention of variceal rebleeding. *Hepatology* 2000;**31**: 1239–1245.
12 Patti R, D'Amico G, Pasta L *et al.* Isosorbide mononitrate with nadolol compared to nadolol alone for prevention of recurrent bleeding in cirrhosis. A double-blind placebo-controlled randomised trial (abstract). *J Hepatol* 1999;**30**(suppl1): 81.
13 Zhang Qyuan R, Wang H. The randomised controlled trial of isosorbide mononitrate plus propranolol compared with propranolol alone for the prevention of variceal rebleeding. *Zhonghua Yi Xue Za Zhi* 2002;**8217**: 1157–1159.
14 Villanueva C, Minana J, Ortiz J *et al.* Endoscopic ligation compared with combined treatment with nadolol plus isosorbide mononitrate to prevent recurrent variceal bleeding. *N Eng J Med* 2001;**345**: 647–655.
15 Lo GH, Chen WC, Hsu PI *et al.* Banding ligation versus nadolol and isosorbide mononitrate for the prevention of esophageal variceal bleeding. *Gastroenterology* 2002;**123**: 728–734.
16 Patch D, Sabin CA, Goulis J *et al.* A randomised, controlled trial of medical therapy versus endoscopic ligation for the prevention of variceal rebleeding in patients with cirrhosis. *Gastroenterology* 2002;**123**: 1013–1019.
17 De Franchis R, Primignani M. Endoscopic treatments for portal hypertension. *Semin Liver Dis* 1999;**19**: 439–455.
18 Sauerbruch T, Scheurlen C, Neubrand M. Endoscopic treatment of variceal bleeding. In: Tytgat GNJ, Classen M, Waye DJ, Nakazawa S (eds). Practice of therapeutic endoscopy. 2nd edn, London, Edinburgh, New York, WB Saunders, 2000; 13–29.
19 Sauerbruch T, Weinzierl M, Ansari H *et al.* Injection sclerotherapy of oesophageal variceal haemorrhage. A prospective long-term follow-up study. *Endoscopy* 1987;**19**: 181–184.
20 Stiegmann GV, Goff JS, Michaletz-Onody PA *et al.* Endoscopic sclerotherapy as compared with endoscopic ligation for bleeding esophageal varices. *N Engl J Med* 1992;**326**: 1527–1532.
21 Stiegmann GV, Sun JH, Hammond WS. Results of experimental endoscopic esophageal varix ligation. *Am Surg* 1988;**54**: 105–108.
22 Laine L, Cook D. Endoscopic ligation compared with sclerotherapy for treatment of esophageal variceal bleeding. *Ann Intern Med* 1995;**123**: 280–287.
23 Goulis J, Burroughs A. Portal hypertensive bleeding. In: McDonald JWD, Burroughs A, Feagan BG (eds). Evidence-based gastroenterology and hepatology. London, Blackwell, 2004.

24 Zargar SA, Javid G, Khan BA *et al.* Endoscopic ligation vs. sclerotherapy in adults with extrahepatic portal venous obstruction: a prospective randomised study. *GastroIntEIS Endosc* 2005;**61**: 58–66.
25 Karsan HA, Morton SC, Shekelle PG *et al.* Combination endoscopic band ligation and sclerotherapy compared with endoscopic band ligation alone for the secondary prophylaxis of esophageal variceal hemorrhage: a meta-analysis. *Dig Dis Sci* 2005;**50**: 399–406.
26 Lo GH, Lai KH, Cheng JS *et al.* The additive effect of sclerotherapy to patients receiving repeated endoscopic variceal ligation: a prospective, randomised trial. *Hepatology* 1998;**28**: 391–395.
27 Lebrec D, Poynard T, Bernuau J *et al.* A randomised controlled study of propranolol for prevention of recurrent gastrointestinal bleeding in patients with cirrhosis: a final report. *Hepatology* 1984; **4**: 355–358.
28 Lo GH, Lai KH, Cheng JS *et al.* The effects of endoscopic variceal ligation and propranolol on portal hypertensive gastropathy: a prospective, controlled trial. *GastrointEIS Endosc* 2001;**53**: 579–584.
29 Lo GH, Liang HL, Lai KH *et al.* The impact of endoscopic variceal ligation on the pressure of the portal venous system. *J Hepatol* 1996;**24**: 74–80.
30 Lo GH, Lai KH, Cheng JS *et al.* Endoscopic variceal ligation plus nadolol and sucralfate compared with ligation alone for the prevention of variceal rebleeding: a prospective, randomised trial. *Hepatology* 2000;**32**: 461–465.
31 de La Pena J, Sanchez-Hernandez E, Rivero M *et al.* Variceal ligation plus nadolol compared with ligation for prophylaxis of variceal rebleeding: a multicenter trial. *Hepatology* 2005;**41**: 572–578.
32 Cabrera J, Maynar M, Granados R *et al.* Transjugular intrahepatic portosystemic shunt versus sclerotherapy in the elective treatment of variceal hemorrhage. *Gastroenterology* 1996;**110**: 832–839.
33 Sanyal AJ, Freedman AM, Luketic VA *et al.* Transjugular intrahepatic portosystemic shunts compared with endoscopic sclerotherapy for the prevention of recurrent variceal hemorrhage. A randomised, controlled trial. *Ann Intern Med* 1997;**126**: 849–857.
34 Cello JP, Ring EJ, Olcott EW *et al.* Endoscopic sclerotherapy compared with percutaneous transjugular intrahepatic portosystemic shunt after initial sclerotherapy in patients with acute variceal hemorrhage. A randomised, controlled trial. *Ann Intern Med* 1997;**126**: 858–865.
35 Merli M, Salerno F, Riggio O *et al.* Transjugular intrahepatic portosystemic shunt versus endoscopic sclerotherapy for the prevention of variceal bleeding in cirrhosis: a randomised multicenter trial. *Hepatology* 1998;**27**: 48–53.
36 Garcia-Villarreal L, Martinez-Lagares F, Sierra A *et al.* Transjugular intrahepatic portosystemic shunt versus endoscopic sclerotherapy for the prevention of variceal rebleeding after recent variceal hemorrhage. *Hepatology* 1999;**29**: 27–32.
37 Rössle M, Deibert P, Haag K *et al.* Randomised trial of transjugular-intrahepatic-portosystemic shunt versus endoscopy plus propranolol for prevention of variceal rebleeding. *Lancet* 1997;**349**: 1043–1049.
38 Sauer P, Theilmann L, Stremmel W *et al.* Transjugular intrahepatic portosystemic stent shunt versus sclerotherapy plus propranolol for variceal rebleeding. *Gastroenterology* 1997;**11**: 1623–1631.

39 Groupe d'Etude des Anastomoses Intra-Hépatiques. TIPS vs. sclerotherapy + propranolol in the prevention of variceal rebleeding: preliminary results of a multicenter randomised trial. (abstract) *Hepatology* 1995;**22**: 297A.
40 Jalan R, ForrEIS EH, Stanley AJ *et al.* A randomised trial comparing transjugular intrahepatic portosystemic stent-shunt with variceal band ligation in the prevention of rebleeding from esophageal varices. *Hepatology* 1997;**26**: 1115–1122.
41 Sauer P, Hansmann J, Richter GM *et al.* Endoscopic variceal ligation plus propranolol vs. transjugular intrahepatic portosystemic stent shunt: a long-term randomised trial. *Endoscopy* 2002;**34**: 690–697.
42 Pomier-Layrargues G, Villeneuve JP, Deschenes M *et al.* Transjugular intrahepatic portosystemic shunt (TIPS) versus endoscopic variceal ligation in the prevention of variceal rebleeding in patients with cirrhosis: a randomised trial. *Gut* 2001;**48**: 390–396.
43 Lin OS, Wu SS, Chen YY *et al.* Bacterial peritonitis after elective endoscopic variceal ligation: a prospective study. *Am J Gastroenterol* 2000;**95**: 214–217.
44 Rosemurgy AS, Serafini FM, Zweibel BR *et al.* Transjugular intrahepatic portosystemeic shunt vs. small-diameter prosthetic H-graft portacaval shunt: extended follow-up of an expanded randomised prospective trial. *J Gastrointestinal Surgery* 2000;**4**: 589–597.
45 Henderson JM, Boyer TD, Kutner MH *et al.* and the DIVERT study group. DSRS vs. TIPS for refractory variceal bleeding: a prospective randomised controlled trial. *Hepatology* 2004;**40**: 725A.
46 Sama SK, Bhargawa S, Gopinath N *et al.* Non-cirrhotic portal fibrosis. *Am J Med* 1971;**51**: 160–169.
47 Okuda K, Obata H. Idiopathic portal hypertension. In: Okuda K, Benhamou J-P (eds). *Portal Hypertension*, Tokyo, Springer-Verlag, 1992; 271–287.
48 Hillaire S, Valla D, Lebrec D. Non-cirrhotic portal hypertension. *Clin Liv Dis* 1997;**1**: 223–240.
49 Kiire CR. Controlled trial of propranolol to prevent recurrent variceal bleeding in patients with non-cirrhotic portal fibrosis. *Br Med J* 1989;**298**: 1363–1365.
50 Shiha G, Hamid H, Askalany H *et al.* Mononitrates and combination of mononitrates plus propranolol as adjuvants to sclerotherapy for the prevention of rebleeding from esophageal varices (abstract). *Digestion* 1998;**59** (suppl3); 340: 2512.
51 Fakhry S, Omar M, Al Gannam M *et al.* Endoscopic sclerotherapy versus endoscopic variceal ligation in the management of bleeding esophageal varices: a prospective randomised study in schistosomal hepatic fibrosis. *Endoscopy Arab Edition* 2000;**1**: 39–44.
52 Elsayed SS, Shiha G, Hamid M *et al.* Sclerotherapy versus sclerotherapy and propranolol in the prevention of rebleeding from esophageal varcies: a randomised study. *Gut* 1996;**38**: 770–774.
53 Shiha G, Menesy A, Seef S *et al.* Endoscopic ligation compared with propranolol and combined isosorbide mononitrates (ISMN) and propranolol to prevent recurrent variceal bleeding: a prospective randomised trial (abstract). *Gut* 2005;**54**: A6 021.

54 Thakeb F, Salama Z, Salama H *et al.* The value of combined use of N-butyl1-2 cyanoacrylate and ethanolamine oleate in the management of bleeding oesophagogastric varices. *Endoscopy* 1995;**27**: 358–364.
55 Shiha G, Elsayed SS. Gastric variceal ligation: a new technique. *Gastrointest Endosc* 1999;**49**: 437–441.
56 Rikkers LF, Sorrell WT, Jin G. Which portosystemic shunt is best? *Gastroenterol Clin North Am* 1992;**21**: 179.
57 Salam AA, Ezzat FA, Aabu-Elmagd KM. Selective shunt in shistosomiasis in Egypt. *Am J Surg* 1990;**160**: 90–92.
58 Gawish Y, El-Hammadi HA, Kotb M *et al.* Devascularization procedure and DSRS: a controlled randomised trial on selected haemodynamic portal flow pattern in schistosomal portal hypertension with variceal bleeding. *Int Surg* 2000;**85**: 325–330.
59 Chwala YK, Dilawari JB, Dhimon RK *et al.* Schlerotherapy in non-cirrhotic portal fibrosis. *Dig Dis Sci* 1997;**42**: 1449–1453.
60 Kahn D, Terblanche J, Kitano S *et al.* Injection sclerotherapy in adult patients with extrahepatic portal venous obstruction. *Br J Surg* 1987;**74**: 600–602.
61 Sarin SK, Nanda R, Gaur Sk *et al.* Repeated endoscopic sclerotherapy for active varicel bleeding. *Ann Surg* 1985;**202**: 708–711.
62 Sarin SK, Lahoti D, Saxena SP *et al.* Prevalence, classification and natural history of gastric varices: long term follow-up study on 568 patients with portal hypertension. *Hepatology* 1992;**16**: 1343–1349.
63 Sarin SK. Non-cirrhotic portal fibrosis. *Gut* 1989;**30**: 406–415.
64 Hou MC, Lin HC, Liu TT *et al.* Antibiotic prophylaxis after endoscopic therapy prevents rebleeding in acute variceal hemorrhage: a randomised trial. *Hepatology* 2004;**39**: 746–753.
65 McKiernan PJ, Beath SV, Davison SM. A prospective study of endoscopic esophageal variceal ligation using a multiband ligator. *J Pediatr Gastroenterol Nutr* 2002;**34**: 207–211.
66 Lee MS, Chou JY, Cheon YK *et al.* Use of detachable snares and elastic bands for endoscopic control of bleeding from large gastric varices. *Gastrointest Endosc* 2002;**56**: 83–88.
67 Lo GH, Lai KH, Cheng JS *et al.* A prospective, randomised trial of butyl cyanoacrylate injection versus band ligation in the management of bleeding gastric varices. *Hepatology* 2001;**33**: 1060–1064.
68 Sarin SK, Jain AK, Jain M *et al.* A randomised controlled trial of cyanoacrylate versus alcohol injection in patients with isolated fundic varices. *Am J Gastroenterol* 2002;**97**: 1010–1015.
69 Williams SJG, Peters RA, Westaby D. Thrombin – an effective treatment for gastric variceal haemorrhage. *Gut* 1994;**35**: 1287–1289.
70 Heneghan MA, Byrne A, Harrison PM. An open pilot study of the effects of a human fibrin glue for endoscopic treatment of patients with acute bleeding from gastric varices. *Gastrointest Endosc* 2002;**56**: 422–426.
71 Yang WL, Tripathi D, Therapondos G *et al.* Endoscopic use of human thrombin in bleeding gastric varices. *Am J Gastroenterol* 2002;**97**: 1381–1385.
72 Chau TN, Patch D, Chan YW *et al.* 'Salvage' transjugular intrahepatic portosystemic shunts: gastric fundal compared with esophageal variceal bleeding. *Gastroenterology* 1998;**114**: 981–987.

73 Barabge K, Péron JM, Imani K *et al.* Transjugular intrahepatic portosystemic shunt in the treatment of refractory bleeding from ruptured gastric varices. *Hepatology* 1999;**30**: 1139–1143.
74 Tripathi D, Therapondos G, Jackson E *et al.* The role of the transjugular intrahepatic portosystemic stent shunt (TIPSS) in the management of bleeding gastric varices: clinical and haemodynamic correlations. *Gut* 2002;**51**: 270–274.
75 Stanley AJ, Jalan R, Ireland HM, Hayes PC *et al.* A comparison between gastric and oesophageal variceal haemorrhage treated with transjugular portosystemic stent shunt (TIPSS). *Aliment Pharmacol Ther* 1997;**11**: 171–176.
76 Wu CY, Yeh HZ, Chen GH. Pharmacologic efficacy in gastric variceal rebleeding and survival. *J Clin Gastroenterol* 2002;**35**: 127–132.
77 Kitamoto M, Imamura M, Kamada K *et al.* Balloon-occluded retrograde transvenous obliteration of gastric fundal varices with hemorrhage. *AJR* 2002;**178**: 1167–1174.
78 Thomas PG, D'Cruz AJ. Distal splenorenal shunting for bleeding gastric varices. *Br J Surg* 1994;**81**: 241–244.
79 Tomikawa M, Hashizumi M, Saku M *et al.* Effectiveness of gastric devascularization and splenectomy for patients with gastric varices. *J Am Coll Surg* 2000;**191**: 498–503.
80 Han HS, Yi NJ, Kim YW *et al.* New operative method for fundal variceal bleeding: Fundectomy with periesophagogastric devascularization. *World J Surg* 2004;**28**: 406–410.
81 Hsieh JS, Wang WM, Perng DS *et al.* Modified devascularization surgery for isolated gastric varices assessed by endoscopic ultrasonography. *Surg Endosc* 2004;**18**: 666–671.
82 Trevino HH, Brady CE III, Schenker S. Portal hypertensive gastropathy. *Dig Dis Sci* 1996;**14**: 258–270.
83 Panes J, Casadevall M, Fernandez M *et al.* Gastric microcirculatory changes of portal-hypertensive rats can be attenuated by long-term estrogen-progestagen treatment. *Hepatology* 1994;**20**: 1261–1270.
84 Panes J, Bordas JM, Pique JM *et al.* Effects of propranolol on gastric mucosal perfusion in cirrhotic patients with portal hypertensive gastropathy. *Hepatology* 1993;**17**: 213–218.
85 Payen JL, Cales P, Pienkowski P *et al.* Weakness of mucosal barrier in portal hypertensive gastropathy of alcoholic cirrhosis. Effects of propranolol and enprostil. *J Hepatol* 1995;**23**: 689–696.
86 Shigemori H, Iwao T, Ikegami M *et al.* Effects of propranolol on gastric mucosal perfusion and serum gastrin level in cirrhotic patients with portal hypertensive gastropathy. *Dig Dis Sci* 1994;**39**: 2433–2438.
87 Hosking SW, Kennedy HJ, Seddon I *et al.* The role of propranolol in congestive gastropathy of portal hypertension. *Hepatology* 1987;**7**: 437–441.
88 Perez-Ayuso RM, Pique JM, Bosch J *et al.* Propranolol in prevention of recurrent bleeding from severe portal hypertensive gastropathy in cirrhosis. *Lancet* 1991;**337**: 1431–1434.
89 Kamath PS, Lacerda M, Ahlquist DA *et al.* Gastric mucosal responses to intrahepatic portosystemic shunting in patients with cirrhosis. *Gastroenterology* 2000;**118**: 905–911.

90 Orloff MJ, Orloff MS, Orloff SL *et al.* Treatment of bleeding from portal hypertensive gastropathy by portacaval shunt. *Hepatology* 1995;**21**: 1011–1017.
91 Urata J, Yamashita Y, Tsuchigame T *et al.* The effects of transjugular intrahepatic portosystemic shunt on portal hypertensive gastropathy. *J Gastroenterol Hepatol* 1998;**13**: 1061–1067.
92 Gostout CJ, Ahlquist DA, Radford CM *et al.* Endoscopic laser therapy for watermelon stomach. *Gastroenterology* 1989;**96**: 1462–1465.
93 Tsai HH, Smith J, Danesh BJ. Successful control of bleeding from gastric antral vascular ectasia (watermelon stomach) by laser photocoagulation. *Gut* 1991;**32**: 93–94.
94 Bjorkman DJ, Buchi KN. Endoscopic laser therapy of the watermelon stomach. *Lasers Surg Med* 1992;**12**: 478–481.
95 Lingenfelser T, Mueller M, Marks IN *et al.* Endoscopic laser therapy in a case of gastric antral vascular ectasia (watermelon stomach). *Z Gastroenterol* 1993;**31**: 322–324.
96 Potamiano S, Carter CR, Anderson JR. Endoscopic laser treatment of diffuse gastric antral vascular ectasia. *Gut* 1994;**35**: 461–463.
97 González-Suárez B, Monfort D, Piqueras M *et al.* Endoscopic treatment with argon plasma coagulation for portal hypertensive gastropathy with no response to pharmacological therapy. (abstract) *J Hepatol* 2003;**38**(185A): 59.
98 D'Amico G, de Franchis R and a cooperative study group. Upper digestive bleeding in cirrhosis. Post-therapeutic outcome and prognostic indicators. *Hepatology* 2003;**38**: 599–612.
99 Narahara Y, Kanazawa H, Kawamata H *et al.* A randomised clinical trial comparing transjugular intrahepatic portosystemic shunt with endoscopic. *Hepatol Resl* 2001;**21**: 189–198.
100 Gulberg V, Schepke M, Geigenberger G *et al.* Transjugular intrahepatic portosystemic shunting is not superior to endoscopic variceal band ligation for prevention of variceal rebleeding in cirrhotic patients: a randomised controlled trial. *Scand J Gastroenterol* 2002;**37**: 338–343.
101 Escorsell A, Banares R, Garcia-Pagan JC *et al.* TIPS versus drug therapy in preventing variceal rebleeding in advanced cirrhosis : a randomised controlled trial. *Hepatology* 2002;**35**: 385–392.
102 Papatheodoris GV, Goulis J, Leandro G *et al.* Transjugular intrahepatic portoystemic shunt compared with endoscopic treatment for prevention of variceal rebleeding: a meta-analysis. *Hepatology* 1999;**30**: 612–622.
103 Luca A, D'Amico G, La Galla R *et al.* TIPS for prevention of recurrent bleeding in patients with cirrhosis: meta-analysis of randomised clinical trials. *Radiology* 1999;**212**: 411–421.
104 Burroughs AK, Vangeli M. Transjugular intrahepatic portosystemic shunt versus endoscopic therapy: randomised trials for secondary prophylaxis of variceal bleeding: an updated meta-analysis. *Scand J Gastroenterol* 2002;**37**: 249–252.
105 Bureau C, Garcia-Pagan JC, Pomier-Layrargues G *et al.* The use of polytetrafluoroethylene (PTFE) covered stents improve the patency of TIPS: results of a randomised study (abstract). *Hepatology* 2002;**36**: 1554.

Baveno IV Consensus Statements: Prevention of Rebleeding

Didier Lebrec, Tilman Sauerbruch (Chairpersons), Brigitte Bernard-Chabert, J. Michael Henderson, Gin-Ho Lo, Han-Chieh Lin, Arun J. Sanyal, Gamal Shiha, Càndid Villanueva and Jean-Pierre Vinel

Time to start secondary prophylaxis:

- Secondary prophylaxis should start as soon as possible from day 6 of the index variceal bleeding episode. (5;D)
- The start time of secondary prophylaxis should be documented.

Patients with cirrhosis who have not received primary prophylaxis:

- Beta blockers (1a;A), band ligation (1a;A) or both (1b;A) should be used for prevention of recurrent bleeding.
- Combination of beta blockers and band ligation is probably the best treatment (1b;A), but more trials are needed.
- Assessment of haemodynamic response to drug therapy provides prognostic information about rebleeding risk. (2b;B)

Patients with cirrhosis who are on beta blockers for primary prevention and bleed:

- Band ligation should be added. (5;D)

Patients who have contraindications or intolerance to beta blockers:

- Band ligation is the preferred treatment for prevention of rebleeding. (5;D)

Patients who fail endoscopic and pharmacological treatment for prevention of rebleeding:

- TIPS or surgical shunts (distal splenorenal shunt or 8 mm H-graft) are effective for those with Child class A/B cirrhosis and should be used. (2b;B)
- In non-surgical candidates, TIPS is the only option. (5;D)
- Transplantation provides good long-term outcomes in Child class B/C cirrhosis and should be considered (2b;B). TIPS may be used as a bridge to transplantation. (4;C)

Patients who have bled from isolated gastric varices, type 1 or gastro-oesophageal varices, type 2:

- N-butyl-cyanoacrylate (A;1b), TIPS (2b;B) or beta blockers (2b;B) are recommended.

Patients who have bled from gastro-oesophageal varices, type 1:

- May be treated with N-butyl-cyanoacrylate, band ligation of oesophageal varices or beta blockers. (2b;B)

Patients who have bled from portal hypertensive gastropathy:

- Beta blockers (1b;A) should be used for prevention of recurrent bleeding.

Patients in whom beta blockers are contraindicated or fail and who cannot be managed by non-shunt therapy:

- TIPS (4;C) or surgical shunts (4;C) should be considered.

Areas requiring further study (5;D):

- Combination of beta blockers plus nitrates.
- Use of HVPG monitoring for decision making and its effect on patients' outcome.

SESSION 7

Noncirrhotic Portal Hypertension

Dominique-Charles Valla, Shiv K. Sarin, G. Barosi, Y.C. Chawla, Elwyn Elias, Harry Janssen, Massimo Primignani and Ian R. Wanless

A session devoted to non-cirrhotic portal hypertension was introduced at Baveno IV, in view of the increasing recognition and growing interest of this clinical entity. Due to time constraints, the discussion was limited to the Budd-Chiari syndrome [BCS – hepatic venous outflow tract obstruction (HVOTO)] and to extrahepatic portal vein obstruction (EHPVO).

Budd-Chiari syndrome - hepatic venous outflow tract obstruction

Dominique-Charles Valla

INTRODUCTION

The purpose of this paper is to summarise the evidence available for the management of patients with hepatic venous outflow tract obstruction. Data from prospective studies and surveys of consecutive, or unselected, patients have been identified through a systematic literature search. The overall level of evidence is graded according to the Oxford Centre for Evidence-based Medicine [http://www.cebm.net/levels_of_evidence.asp]. This review is only intended to provide a basis for the discussion of consensus recommendations. Therefore, no attempt has been made to draw conclusions for clinical management.

DEFINITIONS

Several terms have been used in the past to designate obstruction of the hepatic venous outflow tract or its consequences [1,2]. The eponym Budd-Chiari syndrome has long been used. However, some ambiguity has arisen from its use either for obstruction at any level of the hepatic venous outflow tract, or solely at the level of the hepatic veins. 'Membranous obstruction of the inferior vena cava' has been used to name fibrous obstruction of the inferior vena cava whether it takes the aspect of a web or that of a thick fibrous occlusion. The term 'hepatocavapathy' has been recently introduced to designate obstruction of the inferior vena cava when there is involvement also of one or more hepatic vein ostia [3]. Thrombosis of the large hepatic veins often recanalises leaving the large veins and their ostia patent and apparently normal on imaging studies. Such cases may be difficult to diagnose clinically but biopsy may establish the diagnosis. On biopsy, these cases of small hepatic vein thrombosis may be distinguished from veno-occlusive disease when veins larger than 300 μm are involved. The term veno-occlusive disease has been used for an obstruction limited to the small hepatic veins occurring in a context of exposure to toxic substances; some authors have used this same term in a less restrictive fashion. Recently, as the pathogenesis of sinusoidal endothelial injury became better understood, the term of 'sinusoidal obstruction syndrome' was proposed to replace veno-occlusive disease in the context of a toxic exposure [4]. In some publications, right-sided heart failure and constrictive pericarditis have been considered as forms of hepatic venous outflow tract obstruction.

In this paper the term Budd-Chiari syndrome (BCS) is used as a synonym for 'hepatic venous outflow tract obstruction' (HVOTO), with involvement of hepatic veins anywhere in the tract from 300 μm diameter up to and including the suprahepatic vena cava, and caused by any mechanism [1]. Patients with venous or sinusoidal disease confined to vessels less than 300 μm in diameter are excluded, as they are patients with hepatic congestive disease caused by cardiac or pericardial disease. BCS is separated into 'secondary' BCS when related to compression or invasion by a lesion originating outside the veins (benign or malignant tumor, abscess, cyst, etc); and 'primary' BCS when related to a primarily venous disease (thrombosis or phlebitis).

EPIDEMIOLOGY

Available data consist of two hospital-based questionnaire surveys (one from Japan reported as a full paper [5], and one from France presented in abstract form [6]). Consistency with autopsy registry data has been checked in the Japanese survey. Both surveys yielded a similar estimate of the incidence of BCS due to pure IVC block or combined IVC/HV block. However, the incidence of pure HV block appears to be 10 times higher in France than in Japan.

Comparison of the proportions of both types of block in Western countries according to time suggests an increase in the proportion of pure HV block since the 70s [6]. As a rule, pure IVC or combined IVC/HV block predominates in Asia, whereas pure HV block predominates in western countries. There appear to be areas in Asia where pure IVC block is extremely common, representing the first cause of admission for liver disease [7]. In these areas, pure IVC block is strongly related with a poor standard of living *(Level of evidence 4).*

As a rule, whatever the geographic area, there is a predominance of females among patients with pure HV block whereas there is an equal number of females and males affected with pure IVC block [6] *(Level of evidence 4).*

CAUSAL FACTORS

Secondary Budd-Chiari syndrome

Caval involvement with a variety of tumours may cause BCS, including hepatocellular carcinoma, renal adenocarcinoma, adrenal carcinoma, leiomyosarcoma of uterus or cava and right atrial myxoma. Hydatid and non-parasitic cysts, and sarcoidal phlebitis may also cause BCS [8,9,10].

Large nodules of focal nodular hyperplasia in a central location have been reported to cause compression of the hepatic veins [11]. Surgical or blunt abdominal trauma may initiate BCS. In most cases of primary BCS no local precipitating factor is identified [12] *(Level of evidence 4).*

Primary Budd-Chiari syndrome

There are several studies where a systematic investigation for risk factors for thrombosis has been performed [13–16]. These studies yielded similar results in Asia and in western countries. Data are presented in Table 47. Myeloproliferative diseases represented the leading causal factor when diagnosis was based on sensitive tests, regardless of whether peripheral blood cell counts were suggestive or not *(Level of evidence 3b).* Among these sensitive tests, endogenous erythroid colony assessment has been mostly used [12,15,17,18]. Data presented in Table 48 show high sensitivity and specificity when control populations with liver or heart disease unrelated to BCS, or with well established myeloproliferative diseases are studied [19]. Clusters of dystrophic megakaryocytes in bone marrow biopsies may also indicate the presence of a myeloproliferative disease in these patients [20,21,22] *(Level of evidence 4).*

Many other known risk factors for venous thromboembolism have been implicated in patients with BCS *(Level of evidence 3b)*: factor V Leiden mutation (odds ratio about 12), G20210A prothrombin gene mutation (odds ratio about 2). In BCS patients, reduced serum levels of proteins synthesised by the liver, such as protein C, protein S and antithrombin, are not diagnostic of genetic deficiency of these proteins. However, after adjustment for liver insufficiency, a significant association (odds ratio about 5) between low levels of these inhibitors and BCS was observed in some but not all studies. In patients with BCS, antiphospholipid antibodies are found in about 10–15%; lupus anticoagulant and antibeta-2 glycoprotein 1 antibodies are found in 4–5% [23]. The relation between C677T MTHFR polymorphism and BCS appears to be weak. Once liver disease is established, it is difficult to interpret homocysteine plasma levels as a marker of thrombotic risk *(Level of evidence 3b).*

Some rare acquired diseases, namely paroxysmal nocturnal hemoglobinuria, Behcet's disease, hypereosinophilic syndrome, granulomatous venulitis, ulcerative colitis appear to be related to an increased risk of BCS although no case-control study is available to quantify this risk [12,24,25] *(Level of evidence 4).*

There is evidence from two case-control studies that oral contraceptive use increases the risk of BCS by 2.5 fold. Pregnancy also appears to be

Table 47 Thrombotic risk factors in BCS patients.

Country	Israel [15]	Netherlands [14]		India [16]		France [12]
	N positive/ N tested (%)	N positive/ N tested (%)	OR for BCS (95% CI)	N positive/ N tested (%)	OR for BCS (95% CI)	N positive/ N tested (%)
Myeloproliferative disorders	10/22 (45.4%)	NA	NA	NA	NA	31/61 (50.8%)
Occult	8/22 (36.4%)	NA	NA	NA	NA	15/61 (24.6%)
Classical	2/22 (9.0%)	12/43 (27.0%)	NA	NA	NA	16/61 (26.2%)
Antiphospholipid syndrome	5/22 (23.0%)	2/43 (4.6%)	NA	6/53 (11.3%)	NA	9/63 (14.3%)
Paroxysmal nocturnal hemoglobinuria	1/22(4.4%)	0/43	NA	NA	NA	1/63 (1.6%)
Factor V Leiden mutation	6/22 (27.2%)	11/43 (25.6%)	11.3 (4.6–26.5)	14/53 (26.4%)	14.4 (11.9–35.7)	20/63 (31.7%)
Factor II mutation	NA	2/43 (4.7%)	2.1 (0.4–9.6)	0/53	–	3/47 (6.4%)
Protein C deficiency	7/22 (31.8%)	4/43 (9.3%)	6.8 (1.9–24.4)	7/53 (13.2%)	8.3 (2.1–10.9)	4/21 (19.0%)
Protein S deficiency	4/22 (18.2%)	0/43	–	3/53 (5.7%)	4.4 (2.2–20.6)	2/30 (6.6%)
Antithrombin deficiency	5/22 (22.7%)	0/43	–	2/53 (3.8%)	4.4 (2.1–10.9)	0/47
Plasminogen deficiency	NA	NA	–	NA	NA	1/21 (4.7%)
Recent pregnancy	NA	NA	–	2/17 (11.7%)	NA	3/47 (6.4%)
Recent oral contraceptive use	NA	12/20 (60%)	2.4 (0.9–6.2)	1/17 (5.9%)	NA	23/47 (48.9%)

Table 48 Frequency of endogenous erythroid colonies in series of consecutive patients with BCS in whom cultures of erythroid progenitors were systematically investigated and in various control groups.

	India [18]	Israel [15]	West [12,13,15,81,82]
Patients with BCS			
Total group			
n positive/n tested	22/27	10/22	52/76
Overt Myeloproliferative disease			
n positive/n tested	5/5	2/2	15/15
Controls			
Normal subjects			
n positive/n tested	0/20	0/NA	0/NA
Portal hypertension (including cirrhosis)			
n positive/n tested	0/10	0/5	0/NA
Right-sided heart failure			
n positive/n tested		0/4	

NA: the exact number of controls was not provided

a risk factor for BCS, based on chronological association between the 2 conditions, although no case-control study has been performed to quantify this risk [14,26] *(Level of evidence 3b)*. A combination of several risk factors is demonstrated in about 25% of cases [12,14,15] *(Level of evidence 3b)*.

CLINICAL MANIFESTATIONS

Classical manifestations of BCS include fever, abdominal pain, ascites, leg oedema, jaundice, gastrointestinal bleeding and hepatic encephalopathy [27–32]. Serum transaminases and alkaline phosphatases can be normal or increased. Levels of serum albumin, serum bilirubin and prothrombin can be normal or abnormal, and in some patients they are markedly abnormal. Protein level in ascitic fluid varies from patient to patient; a protein content above 3.0 g/dL is suggestive of outflow obstruction from BCS, cardiac or pericardial disease *(Level of evidence 4)*.

Presentation ranges from complete absence of symptoms to fulminant hepatic failure, through acute (rapid) or chronic (progressive) development of symptoms over weeks to months before diagnosis is made. The absence of symptoms is strongly associated with large hepatic vein collaterals [33]. Portal venous obstruction is common in patients with severe disease [34–36].

However, the suggested role of portal venous obstruction as a determinant of prognosis has not been assessed prospectively *(Level of evidence 4)*.

The course of manifestations can be stable or marked by exacerbations and remissions. Various classification into fulminant, acute, subacute and chronic forms have been proposed [1]. However, definitions of these various forms have differed according to the authors and, with one exception [37], their prognostic value has not been demonstrated. A uniform finding has been the lack of correlation between the apparent age of the venous or hepatic lesions and the duration of symptoms [27,37,38] *(Level of evidence 4)*.

DIAGNOSIS

Demonstration of solid intraluminal material, stenosis or obliteration of the hepatic veins or inferior vena cava are firm evidence for BCS [1]. Intrahepatic or extrahepatic hepatic vein or inferior vena cava collaterals are also considered diagnostic features. Doppler-ultrasound examination of the hepatic veins and inferior vena cava is a powerful diagnostic tool when performed by an experienced operator who is aware of the possible diagnosis of BCS [39,40]. Computed tomography or magnetic resonance imaging with vascular contrast enhancement usually show the above-mentioned diagnostic features [40]. Non-visibility or tortuosity of the hepatic veins are not specific, occasionally being seen in cirrhosis of any origin. Normal appearing hepatic veins may be seen when there is a localised ostial stenosis or obstruction confined to small hepatic veins because of recanalisation of the larger veins.

Hepatic venography is usually not required to make a diagnosis of BCS. Enlarged caudate lobe and heterogeneous aspect at all phases of vascular contrast enhancement are other frequent, though non-specific features. Hepatic venography is indispensable for adequate delineation of venous lesions in planning therapy *(Level of evidence 4)*.

Classical biopsy features of BCS include sinusoidal congestion and liver cell atrophy or loss, predominantly in centrilobular areas [34,35,38]. Venocentric or veno-portal parenchymal extinction and cirrhosis can be found. Recent or old thrombosis of the small and medium sized hepatic veins or portal veins can be observed. A focal appearance of nodular regenerative hyperplasia is common. All lesions are heterogeneously distributed within the liver. None of these findings is completely specific, as they can also be observed in patients with right-sided heart failure, constrictive pericarditis, veno-occlusive disease (sinusoidal obstruction syndrome) or cirrhosis of other origin. However, in the absence of these clinical conditions, the above biopsy findings are suggestive of BCS, especially if severe. Histologic thrombus is the most specific finding [1]. Large regenerative nodules (which may resemble focal nodular hyperplasia) are found in about 60% of patients during follow-up [35,41] *(Level of evidence 4).*

THERAPY

This section will focus on treatment for primary BCS.

Underlying risk factors for thrombosis

Because oral contraceptives increase the risk of hepatic vein thrombosis, these agents are contraindicated in patients with BCS. It is not known whether some form of oral contraception (e.g. devoid of estrogens) can be used safely in this context. Although pregnancy is a likely factor for hepatic vein thrombosis, there are reports of successful and uncomplicated pregnancies in patients with BCS given anticoagulation during the whole pregnancy [42]. Therefore, it is not clear whether pregnancy should be considered contraindicated in patients whose underlying risk factors for thrombosis are controlled *(Level of evidence 5).*

It is logical to treat underlying myeloproliferative diseases. Many patients have only mild changes in peripheral blood. The threshold in blood cell counts where treatment should be initiated, as well as the target counts to be reached with therapy, are still unclear. Low-dose acetylsalicylic acid has been shown to be beneficial to prevent arterial disease in patients with polycytemia vera [43]. However, the efficacy of this agent to prevent venous thrombosis has not been proven. As acetylsalicylic acid is a risk factor for gastrointestinal bleeding in patients with portal hypertension [44], the role of this agent in patients with a myeloproliferative disease complicated by BCS is unclear *(Level of evidence 5).*

For most other risk factors for BCS (namely hereditary thrombophilias and antiphospholipid syndrome), the only available treatment is anticoagulation. Indeed, indefinite anticoagulation therapy is generally recommended after an episode of idiopathic deep venous thrombosis in patients in whom an uncorrectable risk factor is present [45] *(Level of evidence 5).*

Anticoagulation therapy

There has been no prospective randomised controlled trial of anticoagulation in patients with BCS. Two retrospective studies with multivariate analysis have attempted to evaluate the impact of anticoagulation on mortality for

BCS. In a multicentre French study reported in 1999, 120 patients admitted from 1970 to 1992 were enrolled [46]. Permanent anticoagulation was systematically administered to patients admitted from 1985. Survival data demonstrated a sharp improvement beginning in that year. In an international collaborative study reported in 2004, 171 of 237 enrolled patients (72%) had been treated with anticoagulants [47]. The use of anticoagulants did not yield a significant beneficial effect on survival in the total population (relative risk, 1.05; 95% CI, 0.62–1.76) as assessed through multivariate analysis. Results did not alter when the group on anticoagulation in combination with portosystemic shunting was taken as a separate category (relative risk, 0.80; 95% CI, 0.61–1.05). Subanalysis of the effect of anticoagulation on survival for three classes of prognosis suggested improved survival for patients with a good prognosis (relative risk, 0.14; 95% CI, 0.02–1.21), but not for those with an intermediate (relative risk, 0.88; 95% CI, 0.39–2.01) and poor prognosis (relative risk, 1.3; 95% CI, 0.50–3.04). These two retrospective studies did not analyse underlying risk factors. There have been no reports of bleeding-related death in BCS patients taking anticoagulation, but the risk has not been studied formally *(Level of evidence 4)*.

Some data on anticoagulation are derived from the experience in liver transplantation for BCS. In 1988, Campbell *et al.* reported immediate recurrence of hepatic vein thrombosis post-transplant in 1 of the 3 patients not given anticoagulation, contrasting with the absence of recurrence in 14 subsequent patients given early and life-long anticoagulation [48]. In 1990, Halff *et al.* reported lethal recurrence of hepatic vein thrombosis in one patient after discontinuing anticoagulation and in two other patients with suboptimal anticoagulation [49]. Among 108 reported BCS patients treated with permanent anticoagulation there were only 2 with recurrent hepatic vein thrombosis, one of which required retransplantation [48–53]. However, anticoagulation did not prevent post-transplant hepatic artery or portal vein thrombosis in 14 of these 108 patients (13%) *(Level of evidence 4)*.

Thrombolysis

Data on efficacy and tolerance of pharmacological thrombolysis consist of a limited number of case reports and small series of selected patients. These data have been recently reviewed [54,55]. There is some evidence that *in situ* infusion of thrombolytic agents can achieve sustained patency of recently thrombosed veins when thrombolysis is coupled with restoration of a high blood flow velocity by means of angioplasty or stenting *(Level of evidence 4)*.

Angioplasty and stenting

The rationale for recanalization is to decompress the liver without compromising, and even restoring, hepatic blood flow. Short-length stenosis of the cephalad portion of one or several of large hepatic veins is present in 25–30% of patients with pure hepatic vein block [56]. Likewise, a membranous obstruction of suprahepatic IVC is found in up to about 60% of the patients with IVC block [3]. Data on percutaneous angioplasty with or without stenting, which are limited to retrospective uncontrolled studies, have been recently reviewed [54]. In patients with pure hepatic vein block, angioplasty alone achieved recanalisation in 10 out of 10 patients but obstruction recurred in 8 of 10 patients, while angioplasty combined with stent insertion achieved recanalisation in 12 out of 14 patients, with reobstruction in 1 out of 3 patients described with sufficient details. For IVC block, angioplasty alone achieved recanalization in 103 out of 110 patients, and reobstruction occurred in 22 out of 103 patients; while angioplasty combined with stent insertion achieved recanalization in 48 out of 51 patients, and reobstruction occurred in 5 out of 48 patients described with sufficient details. Data on long-term permeability in sizeable patient populations are lacking. Factors associated with reobstruction have not been evaluated. Repeated angioplasty has been successful in some patients. Complications have been uncommon, consisting of immediate rethrombosis and migration of the stent into the heart [57]. Symptoms improve in a majority of patients when patency is maintained but recur when there is rethrombosis. The risk of reobstruction appears to be increased in patients given suboptimal anticoagulation [57]. The impact of therapeutic recanalisation on survival after adjustment on initial severity has not been assessed *(Level of evidence 4)*.

Percutaneous angioplasty with or without stenting has almost completely replaced surgical angioplasty or hepatocaval resection with hepatoatrial anastomosis (so-called Banski procedure).

Portosystemic shunting

The rationale for side-to-side portosystemic shunting is to decompress the liver using the portal venous system as an outflow tract. Depending on the permeability of the inferior vena cava and on technical limitation related to caudate lobe enlargement, several variants of surgical side-to-side shunting have been used: porto-caval shunt; mesocaval shunt with interposition venous or prosthetic grafts; portoatrial or mesoatrial, or mesoinnominate shunt with long prosthetic graft; and a combination of porto or mesocaval shunts with IVC bypass or IVC stenting. Overall perioperative mortality has been high, averaging 25% [58]. The rate of shunt dysfunction has reached 30% in series with long term follow-up [52,59]. The impact of surgical portosystemic shunting on survival has been assessed in 4 multicentre, retrospective, multivariate analyses on overlapping populations of patients. A study of 45 patients with liver biopsy available at the time of diagnosis found portosystemic shunting to be a significant factor for survival ($P = 0.008$), in addition to Pugh score and prothrombin time [60]. A study of 120 patients with patent portal vein, found surgical shunting to be of no independent prognostic value after adjustment for Pugh score, ascites and serum creatinine [46]. A study of 123 patients seen since 1985, with a patent portal vein disclosed no independent prognostic value of surgical shunting after adjustment for Pugh score, ascites, serum creatinine and the clinicopathological form (acute, chronic or acute on chronic) [37]. The most recent study of 237 patients diagnosed between 1984 and 2001, found surgical shunting to be of no independent prognostic value after adjustment for encephalopathy, ascites, prothrombin time and bilirubin (all independent determinants of survival) [47]. However, in the latter study, an improved survival with surgical shunting was suggested for patients in prognostic class II (with intermediate prognosis) (RR 0.63; 95% CI, 0.26–1.49). In these four studies, surgical shunting was considered on an intention-to-treat basis, that is without consideration of shunt permeability. Data presented in an abstract form suggest that shunt dysfunction severely impacts on survival [61] *(Level of evidence 4)*.

TIPS has been used increasingly for treatment of BCS in recent years. A total of 127 patients where TIPS insertion was considered have been reported in retrospective surveys of consecutive cases [62–71]. Indications were generally stated to be manifestations unresponsive to medical therapy, but precise criteria were generally not provided. Insertion was successful in 77 of 82 cases (94%) reported on an intention-to-treat basis. Median follow-up was approximately 18 months. Dysfunction occurred in 63 of 121 cases (52%). 1-month mortality rate was 11.4% in 114 patients. Overall mortality rate was 18.1% among the 127 reported patients. 17 out of 127 patients (13.4%) underwent liver transplantation. Overall, 40 patients (31.5%) died or were transplanted. In some centres, however, TIPS was used as a bridge to planned liver transplantation, whereas in other centres, patients whose condition improved were withdrawn from the transplantation waiting list. In most surviving patients who had not undergone transplantation, dramatic improvement in general condition, control of ascites and liver function was generally described. There has been no attempt at comparing the outcome following TIPS insertion to that following surgical shunting, after adjustment for prognostic factors. Experience from 3 different centres indicate that TIPS dysfunction is much lower when using PTFE covered stents (total number of patients 17) than uncovered stents (total number of patients 41) [63]. Moreover, PTFE covered stents appear to be associated with a lower incidence of clinically significant events than uncovered stents. An unusually high incidence of bleeding complications has been suggested following TIPS insertion for treatment of BCS as compared to TIPS insertion for treatment of portal hypertension related to cirrhosis of more common aetiology. The incidence of post-TIPS encephalopathy appears to be low but prospective evaluation has not been done. Among 92 patients from centres reporting 15–35 TIPS insertions for BCS, 1-month mortality rate was 7.6%. Among 35 patients from centres reporting 2–8 TIPS insertions, 1-month mortality rate was 17.1%. Although a learning-curve effect is conceivable, the impossibility to adjust for disease severity makes a comparison between these centres unfeasible *(Level of evidence 4).*

Liver transplantation

European Liver Transplant Registry data indicate that 380 liver transplants have been performed for BCS in Europe between January 1988 and December 2003 [http://www.eltr.org/publi/index_rv.php3]. 1-, 5- and 10-year survival rates were 74%, 70% and 64%, respectively. 1-year survival is lower than in patients transplanted for cirrhosis but 5- and 10-year survival is similar. These survival rates are difficult to interpret without knowledge of indications, previous therapy and prognostic factors at the time of listing for transplantation. In surveys of consecutive cases, 27 out of 142 patients (19%) had been transplanted following portosystemic shunting [48–51,53,62,72–75]. As discussed earlier, a favourable impact of early and prolonged anticoagulation on the results of liver transplantation has been suggested. Some data indicate that, for patients with myeloproliferative disease, a strategy combining hydroxyurea and aspirin for prevention of thrombotic events might be as effective as anticoagulation [76]. There is no indication that within 10 years of transplantation, there is a significant increase in the risk of malignant transformation of underlying myeloproliferative disease compared to the natural history of this condition in non-transplant patients *(Level of evidence 4).*

TREATMENT STRATEGY

Consensus statements have been elaborated by the European Group for the Study of Vascular Disorders of the Liver, based on the data available up to 2002 [1]. A strategy was proposed consisting of the following graded

Table 49 Mortality from Budd-Chiari syndrome in patients not selected on the basis of therapy.

First author	Year		N	Mortality 1-yr	3-yr	5-yr	10-yr
Tavill [31]	1975	1965–1972	19	31.6	89.5	89.5	
Mitchell [78]	1982	1970–1980	12	42	50	58	
Powell-Jackson [30]	1982	1971–1980	36	42	59	75	
Gupta [83]	1986	1965–1984	18	22	51	51	
Zeitoun* [46]	1999	1970–1985	66	38		50	53
Zeitoun* [46]	1999	1986–1992	54	12		25	37
Tang** [60]	2001	1984-1997	45	37		46	53
Langlet* [37]	2003	1985–1997	69	9		18	26
Murad*** [47]	2004	1984–2001	237	18		31	38

* Only patients with patent portal vein
** Only patients who undergone liver biopsy. Death or liver transplantation
*** Death or liver transplantation

approach (1) anticoagulation, treatment of underlying condition, and symptomatic treatment for complications of portal hypertension in all patients with primary BCS ; (2) in patients unresponsive to medical therapy, active search for venous lesions amenable to angioplasty/stenting; (3) in patients not suited for, or unresponsive to angioplasty/stenting, TIPS insertion; (4) when TIPS insertion is unfeasible and patients are suitable for surgery, surgical portosystemic shunt; (5) in patients unresponsive to TIPS or surgical shunting, liver transplantation. However, the definitions for response to therapy have not been precisely stated. Furthermore, the impact of this strategy on survival and quality of life has not been assessed. Moreover, many data on the medium term benefits and risks of percutaneous intervention (angioplasty, stenting and TIPS insertion) were not available at the time these consensus statements were elaborated *(Level of evidence 5)*.

OUTCOME AND PROGNOSIS

The natural history of BCS is poorly known as there has been no cohort study of untreated patients. At the time of early surveys on patients receiving none of the currently available therapies, non-invasive diagnostic procedures were not available so that patients lacking typical clinical features were missed. Data presented in Table 49 clearly show a dramatic improvement in the outcome over the last 4 decades, beginning with a reduction in late mortality, and followed by a decrease in early mortality [31,37,46,47,60,77–79]. Even

Table 50 Prognostic factors in Budd-Chiari Syndrome patients. Results from multivariate analyses.

		Zeitoun *et al.* [46]		Tang *et al.* [60]		Langlet *et al.* [37]		Murad *et al.* [47]	
		RR◇	*p*	RR◇	*p*	RC+	*p*	RR◇	*p*
Encephalopathy	*present vs absent*							3.58	< 0.001
Ascites	*present vs absent*							2.83	0.08
	*Score 1, 2 or 3**	2.11	0.04						
Prothrombin	*(INR $\leq$ 2.3 vs INR $<$ 2.3)*							2.05	0.02
Bilirubin	*μmol/L*							1.004	0.7
Pugh score		1.33	0.005	NA	0.009				
Creatinine	*μmol/L*	–	0.29						
Acute-on-chronic form	*present vs absent*					2.15	0.006		
ALT	*IU/L*			NA	0.008				
Prognostic index°						1.26	0.0001		
Portosystemic shunting	*Yes vs No*	–	0.344	NA	0.008				

◇ RR risk ratio

+ RC Regression coefficient

* Ascites score: 1 absent without diuretics, 2 absent on diuretics, 3 refractory

° Prognostic index (PI) is according to Zeitoun *et al.* [46]: PI = 0.75 ascites score + 0.28 Pugh score + 0.037 age + 0.0036 creatinine

Table 51 Prognostic scores for Budd-Chiari syndrome.

Zeitoun *et al.* [46]	0.75 ascites score* + 0.28 Pugh score + 0.037 age + 0.0036 creatinine
Langlet *et al.* [37]	0.95 ascites score (1,2 or 3)* + 0.35 Pugh score + 0.047 age (years) + 0.0045 creatinine (μmol/L) + 2.2 acute on chronic form (0 or 1)°−0.26
Murad *et al.* [47]	1.27 encephalopathy (0 or 1)° + 1.04 ascites (0 or 1)° + 0.72 prothrombin (INR) + 0.004 bilirubin (μmol/L)

* ascites score: 1 absent without diuretics, 2 absent on diuretics, 3 refractory
° 0 absent, 1 present

more recent data, available only in an abstract form, indicate that 5-year mortality rate could be as low as 15% [80]. Since this improvement coincided with the introduction of portosystemic shunting, anticoagulation, liver transplantation and percutaneous manoeuvres, it is tempting to ascribe this favourable trend to these new treatment modalities. However, earlier recognition of less advanced cases through modern imaging techniques as well as improvement in the efficacy of non-specific therapy likely participated in the improvement of outcome *(Level of evidence 4)*.

Several retrospective studies have attempted to identify prognostic factors by multivariate analysis (Table 50). Serum albumin, bilirubin, prothrombin, ascites and encephalopathy, or their combination as Pugh score, have generally been found to be independent prognostic factors [37,46,47,60]. Prognostic scores have been elaborated accordingly (see Table 51). Several groups have reported that extra or intrahepatic portal vein thrombosis was common in patients with the most severe forms of the disease [34–36]. However, extrahepatic portal vein thrombosis was not identified as a prognostic factor in a recent survey on a large number of patients [47] *(Level of evidence 2b)*.

ACKNOWLEDGEMENT

The author is indebted to the panellists of Baveno IV Session 7 for their fruitful discussion of this manuscript. Panellists included Giorgio Barosi, Yogesh C Chawla, Elwyn Elias, Harry L Janssen, Massimo Primignani, Shiv K Sarin and Ian Wanless.

REFERENCES

1 Janssen HL, Garcia-Pagan JC, Elias E, Mentha G, Hadengue A, Valla DC. Budd-Chiari syndrome: a review by an expert panel. *J Hepatol* 2003;38: 364–371.

2 Ludwig J, Hashimoto E, McGill D, Heerden Jv. Classification of hepatic venous outflow obstruction: ambiguous terminology of the Budd-Chiari syndrome. *Mayo Clin Proc* 1990;**65**: 51–55.

3 Okuda K. Inferior vena cava thrombosis at its hepatic portion (obliterative hepatocavopathy). *Semin Liver Dis* 2002;**22**: 15–26.

4 DeLeve LD, Shulman HM, McDonald GB. Toxic injury to hepatic sinusoids: sinusoidal obstruction syndrome (veno-occlusive disease). *Semin Liver Dis* 2002;**22**: 27–42.

5 Okuda H, Yamagata H, Obata H, Iwata H, Sasaki R, Imai F, Okudaira M, Ohbu M, Okuda K. Epidemiological and clinical features of Budd-Chiari syndrome in Japan. *J Hepatol* 1995;**22**: 1–9.

6 Valla D. Hepatic venous outflow tract obstruction etiopathogenesis: Asia versus West. *J Gastroenterol Hepatol* 2004;**19**: S204–S211.

7 Shrestha SM, Okuda K, Uchida T *et al.* Endemicity and clinical picture of liver disease due to obstruction of the hepatic portion of the inferior vena cava in Nepal. *J Gastroenterol Hepatol* 1996;**11**: 170–179.

8 Khuroo MS, Datta DV, Khoshy A, Mitra SK, Chhuttani PN. Alveolar hydatid disease of the liver with Budd-Chiari syndrome. *Postgrad Med J* 1980;**56**: 197–201.

9 Mehrotra G, Singh RP, Krishna A, Singh BK. Pyogenic liver abscess causing acute Budd-Chiari syndrome. *Ann Trop Paediatr* 1992;**12**: 451–453.

10 Uddin W, Ramage JK, Portmann B, Wilson P, Benjamin I, Tan KC, Williams R. Hepatic venous outflow obstruction in patients with polycystic liver disease: pathogenesis and treatment. *Gut* 1995;**36**: 142–145.

11 Rangheard AS, Vilgrain V, Audet P *et al.* Focal nodular hyperplasia inducing hepatic vein obstruction. *AJR Am J Roentgenol* 2002;**179**: 759–762.

12 Deltenre P, Denninger MH, Hillaire S *et al.* Factor V Leiden related Budd-Chiari syndrome. *Gut* 2001;**48**: 264–268.

13 Denninger MH, Chait Y, Casadevall N *et al.* Cause of portal or hepatic venous thrombosis in adults: the role of multiple concurrent factors. *Hepatology* 2000;**31**: 587–591.

14 Janssen HL, Meinardi JR, Vleggaar FP *et al.* Factor V leiden mutation, prothrombin gene mutation, and deficiencies in coagulation inhibitors associated with budd-chiari syndrome and portal vein thrombosis: results of a case-control study. *Blood* 2000;**96**: 2364–2368.

15 Hirshberg B, Shouval D, Fibach E, Friedman G, Ben-Yehuda D. Flow cytometric analysis of autonomous growth of erythroid precursors in liquid culture detects occult polycythemia vera in the Budd-Chiari syndrome. *J Hepatol* 2000;**32**: 574–578.

16 Mohanty D, Shetty S, Ghosh K, Pawar A, Abraham P. Hereditary thrombophilia as a cause of Budd-Chiari syndrome: a study from Western India. *Hepatology* 2001;**34**: 666–670.

17 De Stefano V, Teofili L, Leone G, Michiels JJ. Spontaneous erythroid colony formation as the clue to an underlying myeloproliferative disorder in patients with Budd-Chiari syndrome or portal vein thrombosis. *Semin Thromb Hemost* 1997;**23**: 411–418.

18 Dayal S, Pati HP, Pande GK, Sharma MP, Saraya AK. Multilineage hemopoietic stem cell defects in Budd Chiari syndrome. *J Hepatol* 1997;**26**: 293–297.

19 Berlin NI. Polycythemia vera. *Semin Hematol* 1997;**34**: 1–80.

20 Chait Y, Condat B, Cazals-hatem D *et al.* Relevance of the criteria commonly used to diagnose myeloproliferative disorder in patients with splanchnic vein thrombosis. *Br J Haematology* 2005;In press.
21 Georgii A, Buhr T, Buesche G, Kreft A, Choritz H. Classification and staging of Ph-negative myeloproliferative disorders by histopathology from bone marrow biopsies. *Leuk Lymphoma* 1996;**22**(Suppl 1): 15–29.
22 Thiele J, Kvasnicka HM, Diehl V. Bone marrow features of diagnostic impact in erythrocytosis. *Ann Hematol* 2005.
23 Espinosa G, Font J, Garcia-Pagan JC *et al.* Budd-Chiari syndrome secondary to antiphospholipid syndrome: clinical and immunologic characteristics of 43 patients. *Medicine* (Baltimore) 2001;**80**: 345–354.
24 Bayraktar Y, Balkanci F, Bayraktar M, Calguneri M. Budd-Chiari syndrome: a common complication of Behcet's disease. *Am J Gastroenterol* 1997;**92**: 858–862.
25 Bismuth E, Hadengue A, Hammel P, Benhamou JP. Hepatic vein thrombosis in Behcet's disease. *Hepatology* 1990;**11**: 969–974.
26 Valla D, Le MG, Poynard T, Zucman N, Rueff B, Benhamou JP. Risk of hepatic vein thrombosis in relation to recent use of oral contraceptives. A case-control study. *Gastroenterology* 1986;**90**: 807–811.
27 Dilawari JB, Bambery P, Chawla Y *et al.* Hepatic outflow obstruction (Budd-Chiari syndrome). Experience with 177 patients and a review of the literature. *Medicine* (Baltimore) 1994;**73**: 21–36.
28 Mahmoud AEA, Mendoza AEA, Meshokhes AN *et al.* Clinical spectrum, investigations and treatment of Budd-Chiari syndrome. *Q J Med* 1996;**89**: 37–43.
29 Maddrey WC. Hepatic vein thrombosis (Budd-Chiari syndrome). *Hepatology* 1984;**4**: 44S–46S.
30 Powell-Jackson PR, Melia W, Canalese J, Pickford RB, Portmann B, Williams R. Budd-Chiari Syndrome: clinical patterns and therapy. *Q J Med* 1982;**51**: 79–88.
31 Tavill AS, Wood EJ, Kreel L, Jones EA, Gregory M, Sherlock S. The Budd-Chiari syndrome: correlation between hepatic scintigraphy and the clinical, radiological, and pathological findings in nineteen cases of hepatic venous outflow obstruction. *Gastroenterology* 1975;**68**: 509–518.
32 Singh V, Sinha SK, Nain CK *et al.* Budd-Chiari syndrome: our experience of 71 patients. *J Gastroenterol Hepatol* 2000;**15**: 550–554.
33 Hadengue A, Poliquin M, Vilgrain V, Belghiti J, Degott C, Erlinger S, Benhamou JP. The changing scene of hepatic vein thrombosis: recognition of asymptomatic cases. *Gastroenterology* 1994;**106**: 1042–1047.
34 Tanaka M, Wanless IR. Pathology of the liver in Budd-Chiari syndrome: portal vein thrombosis and the histogenesis of veno-centric cirrhosis, veno-portal cirrhosis, and large regenerative nodules. *Hepatology* 1998;**27**: 488–496.
35 Cazals-Hatem D, Vilgrain V, Genin P, Denninger MH, Durand F, Belghiti J, Valla D, Degott C. Arterial and portal circulation and parenchymal changes in Budd-Chiari syndrome: a study in 17 explanted livers. *Hepatology* 2003;**37**: 510–519.
36 Mahmoud AEA, Helmy AS, Billingham S, Elias E. Poor prognosis and limited therapeutic options in patients with Budd-Chiari syndrome and portal venous system thrombosis. *Eur J Gastroenterol Hepatol* 1997;**9**: 485–489.

37 Langlet P, Escolano S, Valla D *et al.* Clinicopathological forms and prognostic index in Budd-Chiari syndrome. *J Hepatol* 2003;**39**: 496–501.
38 Parker RGF. Occlusion of the hepatic veins in man. *Medicine* (Baltimore) 1959;**38**: 369–402.
39 Millener P, Grant EG, Rose S *et al.* Color Doppler imaging findings in patients with Budd-Chiari syndrome: correlation with venographic findings. *AJR Am J Roentgenol* 1993;**161**: 307–312.
40 Miller WJ, Federle MP, Straub WH, Davis PL. Budd-Chiari syndrome: imaging with pathologic correlation. *Abdom Imaging* 1993;**18**: 329–335.
41 Vilgrain V, Lewin M, Vons C *et al.* Hepatic nodules in Budd-Chiari syndrome: imaging features. *Radiology* 1999;**210**: 443–450.
42 Vons C, Smadja C, Franco D, Valla D, Rueff B, Benhamou JP. Successful pregnancy after Budd-Chiari syndrome. *Lancet* 1984;**2**: 975.
43 Landolfi R, Marchioli R, Kutti J, Gisslinger H, Tognoni G, Patrono C, Barbui T. Efficacy and safety of low-dose aspirin in polycythemia vera. *N Engl J Med* 2004;**350**: 114–124.
44 De Ledinghen V, Heresbach D, Fourdan O *et al.* Anti-inflammatory drugs and variceal bleeding: a case-control study. *Gut* 1999;**44**: 270–273.
45 Bates SM, Ginsberg JS. Clinical practice. Treatment of deep-vein thrombosis. *N Engl J Med* 2004;**351**: 268–277.
46 Zeitoun G, Escolano S, Hadengue A *et al.* Outcome of Budd-Chiari syndrome: a multivariate analysis of factors related to survival including surgical portosystemic shunting. *Hepatology* 1999;**30**: 84–89.
47 Murad SD, Valla DC, de Groen PC *et al.* Determinants of survival and the effect of portosystemic shunting in patients with Budd-Chiari syndrome. *Hepatology* 2004;**39**: 500–508.
48 Campbell DA, Rolles K, Jamieson N, O'Grady J, Wight D, Williams R, Calne R. Hepatic transplantation with perioperative and long term anticoagulation as treatment for Budd-Chiari syndrome. *Surg Gynecol Obstet* 1988;**166**: 511–518.
49 Halff G, Todo S, Tzakis AG, Gordon RD, Starzl TE. Liver transplantation for the Budd-Chiari syndrome. *Ann Surg* 1990;**211**: 43–49.
50 Ringe B, Lang H, Oldhafer KJ, Gebel M, Flemming P, Georgii A, Borst HG, Pichlmayr R. Which is the best surgery for Budd-Chiari syndrome: venous decompression or liver transplantation? A single-center experience with 50 patients. *Hepatology* 1995;**21**: 1337–1344.
51 Shaked A, Goldstein RM, Klintmalm GB, Drazan K, Husberg B, Busuttil RW. Portosystemic shunt versus orthotopic liver transplantation for the Budd-Chiari syndrome. *Surg Gynecol Obstet* 1992;**174**: 453–459.
52 Hemming AW, Langer B, Greig P, Taylor BR, Adams R, Heathcote EJ. Treatment of Budd-Chiari syndrome with portosystemic shunt or liver transplantation. *Am J Surg* 1996;**171**: 176–180; discussion 180–181.
53 Srinivasan P, Rela M, Prachalias A *et al.* Liver transplantation for Budd-Chiari syndrome. *Transplantation* 2002;**73**: 973–977.
54 Barrault C, Plessier A, Valla D, Condat B. Non surgical treatment of Budd-Chiari syndrome: a review. *Gastroenterol Clin Biol* 2004;**28**: 40–49.
55 Sharma S, Texeira A, Texeira P, Elias E, Wilde J, Olliff SP. Pharmacological thrombolysis in Budd Chiari syndrome: a single centre experience and review of the literature. *J Hepatol* 2004;**40**: 172–180.

56 Valla D, Hadengue A, el Younsi M *et al.* Hepatic venous outflow block caused by short-length hepatic vein stenoses. *Hepatology* 1997;**25**: 814–819.

57 Fisher NC, McCafferty I, Dolapci M, Wali M, Buckels JA, Olliff SP, Elias E. Managing Budd-Chiari syndrome: a retrospective review of percutaneous hepatic vein angioplasty and surgical shunting. *Gut* 1999;**44**: 568–574.

58 Langlet P, Valla D. Is surgical portosystemic shunt the treatment of choice in Budd-Chiari syndrome? *Acta Gastroenterol Belg* 2002;**65**: 155–160.

59 Panis Y, Belghiti J, Valla D, Benhamou JP, Fekete F. Portosystemic shunt in Budd-Chiari syndrome: long-term survival and factors affecting shunt patency in 25 patients in Western countries. *Surgery* 1994;**115**: 276–281.

60 Tang TJ, Batts KP, de Groen PC, van Hoek B, Haagsma EB, Hop WC, Janssen HL. The prognostic value of histology in the assessment of patients with Budd-Chiari syndrome. *J Hepatol* 2001;**35**: 338–343.

61 Bachet JB, Condta B, Hagège H, Plessier A, Belghiti J, Valla D. Long term survival after portosystemic shunting for Budd-Chiari syndrome. Shunt patency is determinant. *Hepatology* 2003;**38**: 416A.

62 Ryu RK, Durham JD, Krysl J *et al.* Role of TIPS as a bridge to hepatic transplantation in Budd-Chiari syndrome. *J Vasc Interv Radiol* 1999;**10**: 799–805.

63 Hernandez-Guerra M, Turnes J, Rubinstein P, Olliff S, Elias E, Bosch J, Garcia-Pagan JC. PTFE-covered stents improve TIPS patency in Budd-Chiari syndrome. *Hepatology* 2004;**40**: 1197–1202.

64 Rossle M, Olschewski M, Siegerstetter V, Berger E, Kurz K, Grandt D. The Budd-Chiari syndrome: outcome after treatment with the transjugular intrahepatic portosystemic shunt. *Surgery* 2004;**135**: 394–403.

65 Mancuso A, Fung K, Mela M, Tibballs J, Watkinson A, Burroughs AK, Patch D. TIPS for acute and chronic Budd-Chiari syndrome: a single-centre experience. *J Hepatol* 2003;**38**: 751–754.

66 Ganger DR, Klapman JB, McDonald V *et al.* Transjugular intrahepatic portosystemic shunt (TIPS) for Budd-Chiari syndrome or portal vein thrombosis: review of indications and problems. *Am J Gastroenterol* 1999;**94**: 603–608.

67 Cejna M, Peck-Radosavljevic M, Schoder M *et al.* Repeat interventions for maintenance of transjugular intrahepatic portosystemic shunt function in patients with Budd-Chiari syndrome. *J Vasc Interv Radiol* 2002;**13**: 193–199.

68 Gasparini D, Del Forno M, Sponza M, Branca B, Toniutto P, Marzio A, Pirisi M. Transjugular intrahepatic portosystemic shunt by direct transcaval approach in patients with acute and hyperacute Budd-Chiari syndrome. *Eur J Gastroenterol Hepatol* 2002;**14**: 567–571.

69 Kavanagh PM, Roberts J, Gibney R, Malone D, Hegarty J, McCormick PA. Acute Budd-Chiari syndrome with liver failure: the experience of a policy of initial interventional radiological treatment using transjugular intrahepatic portosystemic shunt. *J Gastroenterol Hepatol* 2004;**19**: 1135–1139.

70 Nunez O, de la Cruz G, Molina J *et al.* Interventional radiology, angioplasty and TIPS in Budd-Chiari syndrome. *Gastroenterol Hepatol* 2003;**26**: 461–464.

71 Slakey DP, Klein AS, Venbrux AC, Cameron JL. Budd-Chiari syndrome: current management options. *Ann Surg* 2001;**233**: 522–527.

72 Henderson JM, Warren WD, Millikan WJ *et al.* Surgical options, hematologic evaluation, and pathologic changes in Budd-Chiari syndrome. *Am J Surg* 1990;**159**: 41–48; discussion 48–50.

73 Malkowski P, Michalowicz B, Pawlak J *et al.* Surgical and interventional radiological treatment of Budd-Chiari syndrome: report of nine cases. *Hepatogastroenterology* 2003;**50**: 2049–2051.

74 Attwell A, Ludkowski M, Nash R, Kugelmas M. Treatment of Budd-Chiari syndrome in a liver transplant unit, the role of transjugular intrahepatic portosystemic shunt and liver transplantation. *Aliment Pharmacol Ther* 2004;**20**: 867–873.

75 Jamieson NV, Williams R, Calne RY. Liver transplantation for Budd-Chiari syndrome, 1976–1990. *Ann Chir* 1991;**45**: 362–365.

76 Melear JM, Goldstein RM, Levy MF, Molmenti EP, Cooper B, Netto GJ, Klintmalm GB, Stone MJ. Hematologic aspects of liver transplantation for Budd-Chiari syndrome with special reference to myeloproliferative disorders. *Transplantation* 2002;**74**: 1090–1095.

77 Powell-Jackson PR, Ede RJ, Williams R. Budd-Chiari syndrome presenting as fulminant hepatic failure. *Gut* 1986;**27**: 1101–1105.

78 Mitchell MC, Boitnott JK, Kaufman S, Cameron JL, Maddrey WC. Budd-Chiari syndrome: etiology, diagnosis and management. *Medicine* (Baltimore) 1982;**61**: 199–218.

79 Gupta S, Barter S, Phillips GW, Gibson RN, Hodgson HJ. Comparison of ultrasonography, computed tomography and 99mTc liver scan in diagnosis of Budd-Chiari syndrome. *Gut* 1987;**28**: 242–247.

80 Plessier A, Sibert A, Consigny Y *et al.* Assessment of a therapeutic strategy in Budd-Chiari syndrome. *Liver International* 2004;**24**: 30.

81 Valla D, Casadevall N, Lacombe C *et al.* Primary myeloproliferative disorder and hepatic vein thrombosis. A prospective study of erythroid colony formation in vitro in 20 patients with Budd-Chiari syndrome. *Ann Intern Med* 1985;**103**: 329–334.

82 Pagliuca A, Mufti GJ, Janossa-Tahernia M *et al.* In vitro colony culture and chromosomal studies in hepatic and portal vein thrombosis–possible evidence of an occult myeloproliferative state. *Q J Med* 1990;**76**: 981–989.

83 Gupta S, Blumgart LH, Hodgson HJ. Budd-Chiari syndrome: long-term survival and factors affecting mortality. *Q J Med* 1986;**60**: 781–791.

Extrahepatic portal vein obstruction

Shiv K. Sarin

INTRODUCTION

Extrahepatic Portal Vein Obstruction (EHPVO) is a common cause of portal hypertension in the developing countries and is second to cirrhosis in the West. It is characterised by obstruction in the prehepatic portion of the portal vein. This could be accompanied with thrombosis of the splenic or superior mesenteric veins. However, isolated thrombosis of the splenic or superior mesenteric veins with patent portal vein is not included in this terminology. Portal vein thrombosis is a known complication of liver cirrhosis, and if the term EHPVO is used in this context, it should be specifically mentioned whether it is associated with cirrhosis or hepatocellular carcinoma or not.

EHPVO is often associated with portal hypertension. In the Western countries, such patients comprise 5–10% of all patients with portal hypertension [1,2]. In developing countries however, the proportion may be as high as 20% [3]. EHPVO is also the most common cause of major upper gastrointestinal bleeding in children [3–6]. In children, EHPVO is usually an isolated condition presenting as portal hypertension and variceal bleeding. In adults, the diagnosis is generally made when the patient is being investigated for another disease.

The commonest site of block is at the site of portal vein formation (90%) (Fig. 46) and total block of the splenoportal axis is seen in only 10% [7].

TERMINOLOGY

EHPVO could present as an acute or a chronic event. The presentation does also differ in children and adults. Some investigators recommend the use of the term portal vein thrombosis (PVT). However, this term has several drawbacks; first it does not exclude the intrahepatic portal vein thrombosis due to cirrhosis of the liver or invasion by hepatocellular carcinoma. Second, the term does not include formation of portal cavernoma and development of portal hypertension, inherent to long-standing disease. Moreover, the obstruction to the portal vein may not always be due to thrombosis. The issue of terminology was discussed at length at the recent Baveno IV conference, and the unanimous consensus was to accept the term EHPVO.

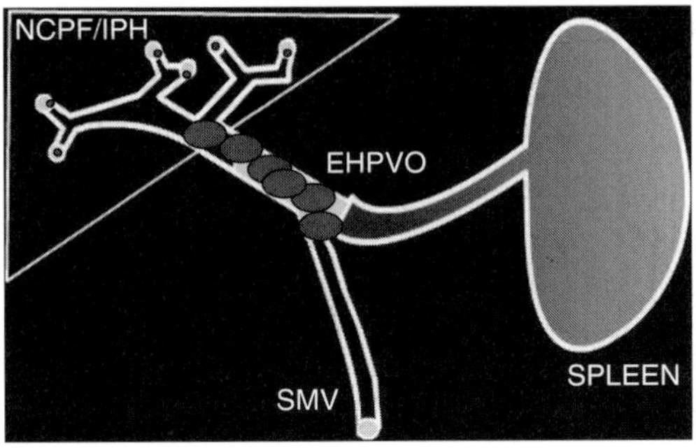

Fig. 46 Schematic diagram showing the two common causes of noncirrhotic portal hypertension; extrahepatic portal vein obstruction (EHPVO) and noncirrhotic portal fibrosis (NCPF) or idiopathic portal hypertension. The block in the former is in the main portal vein and branches while in the latter, in the small branches of the portal vein.

DEFINITION

EHPVO is defined as obstruction of the extrahepatic portal vein, with or without involvement of the intrahepatic portal veins. It mostly manifests as portal cavernoma, which is a network of porto-porto collaterals that develops as a sequel of portal vein obstruction. Isolated thrombosis of the splenic vein or superior mesenteric vein with patent portal vein is excluded. For the sake of clarity and management strategies, the definition of EHPVO should be augmented by a statement of the presence or absence of cirrhosis and hepatocellular carcinoma.

It is well known that isolated thrombosis of the superior mesenteric vein could produce collaterals in the gut and is therefore considered as a separate entity.

The overview presented at the Baveno IV consensus meeting and discussed below relates to EHPVO as a distinct disease entity and not as an association of any primary liver disease.

AETIOLOGY

EHPVO is a heterogeneous group of diseases and the aetiology varies according to the age of presentation, the population studied and the investigative approaches adopted.

EHPVO in children

The aetiology of EHPVO in children has not been well investigated. Various hypotheses postulated include congenital malformation of the portal vein, acquired thrombosis following umbilical sepsis, trauma, and prothrombotic states [3,8–10]. Thrombosis is alleged to be the most important mechanism for obstruction of the portal vein [3,9,10]. While most people believe that EHPVO in children has a primary component of phlebosclerosis with thrombosis as a secondary event, others suggest that there could be a primary thrombotic disorder.

Infection. Omphalitis and neonatal umbilical sepsis have been alleged to cause inflammation in the umbilical stump before normal obliteration of these veins. This inflammation probably proceeds proximally to involve the portal venous system. Infection may be overt or go unrecognised. Umbilical vein cannulation for exchange transfusion could add to this. Larroche found that 40% of neonates having umbilical vein catheterisation developed portal vein thrombi after 25–48 h and 100% after three days [11]. However, other workers could not confirm these observations [12]. Thompson *et al.* [2] found no cases of portal vein occlusion among 470 neonates having umbilical vein catheterisation. None of their 80 patients with umbilical sepsis developed portal vein thrombosis. Similarly, none of the 11 patients in our series with septicaemia and/or umbilical sepsis developed portal vein thrombosis [12]. In a review of 11 major studies, a positive history of umbilical vein catheterisation was available in 9% and of umbilical sepsis, in another 9% of patients with EHPVO [12]. The determinants of low positive history of umbilical sepsis could be hospitalisation and liberal antibiotic therapy.

Repeated abdominal infections, sepsis, abdominal surgery and trauma in childhood could also lead to EHPVO. Role of other factors, such as dehydration and high altitude has also been suggested.

Developmental anomaly. EHPVO can result from developmental abnormality of the portal venous system [13]. Obstruction can occur anywhere along the line of left and right vitelline veins from which the portal vein develops [14]. Other congenital defects usually of the cardiovascular system can also be associated. Odievre *et al.* [13] reported congenital defects in 12 of 30 patients with EHPVO of unknown cause.

Prothrombotic state. As the occurrence of venous thrombosis of the splenoportal axis is the predominant pathology, presence of a prothrombotic state is suggested in this condition. These disorders are often occult and are more common in adulthood [15,16]. Studies in children are limited and the frequency of these disorders is low.

While one study has shown normal coagulation function [10], other studies [18] have reported abnormal prothrombin time, partial thromboplastin time and platelet function, possibly from mild compensated disseminated intravascular coagulation secondary to portosystemic shunting [19].

Iatrogenic. Despite all efforts, the aetiology of blocked portal vein remains obscure in about 70% of children.

EHPVO in adults

The aetiology of EHPVO in adults is quite different from that in children. Prothrombotic disorders have been alleged to be the major mechanisms in adults [15].

In a recent study, prothrombin G20210A mutation and deficiency of naturally occurring anticoagulant proteins was found to be significantly more common than in patients with deep vein thrombosis [10]. The latter could be secondary to mild hepatic derangements present in EHPVO patients. Myeloproliferative disorders were found in 35% of patients. Cardin *et al.* [16] did not observe the same incidence of overt myeloproliferative disorders and believed that their presence did not alter the prognosis. Similar observations have also been reported in other recent studies [21,22]. In a recent study in Turkish patients, prothrombotic disorders were uncommon in noncirrhotic compared with cirrhotic patients [22].

Further, since venous thrombosis is a polygenic entity, it is unlikely that mere heterozygous state of one gene could be held responsible for the thrombotic event.

PATHOLOGY

The macroscopic appearance of the liver varies from smooth to finely granular. The architectural pattern of the liver is preserved. There is concentric condensation of reticulin fibers around portal tracts and in some cases, the condensation forms septa extending from portal tracts for a variable distance into the parenchyma. This could result from inflammation as a consequence of the release of hepatocellular breakdown products, bile imbibition or extension of the extrahepatic thrombophlebitic process into the intrahepatic radicals of the portal vein [23,24].

The pathology of the portal vein in patients with EHPVO has been termed 'cavernomatous malformation of the portal vein'. It is made up of a cluster of variable sized vessels arranged haphazardly within a connective tissue support and the original portal vein cannot be identified. It is usually located at the hilum of the liver and can extend for a variable length inside and outside the liver. Although hamartomatous and neoplastic theories have been proposed [4], most authors feel that these features are an end result of thrombosis of the portal vein.

EHPVO with cirrhosis and neoplasia. The primary disease in these patients is a parenchymal liver disease, EHPVO is an accompaniment and the features of the primary disease are discernible by the imaging studies.

PHYSIOLOGY OF EHPVO

The intrahepatic block in cirrhosis leads to high hepatic sinusoidal pressure and the formation of hepatofugal collaterals. The prehepatic block of EHPVO, with normal hepatic sinusoidal pressure and a high pressure in the obstructed splanchnic bed, results in the formation of multiple hepatopetal collaterals (Plate 4, *facing p.* 201). These collaterals are seen on angiography as 'cavernous transformation' and have been shown by radionuclide flow studies to provide significant component of the total hepatic blood flow in these patients. Therefore, EHPVO is not synonymous with the absence of portal perfusion.

FUNCTIONAL STATUS OF THE LIVER

Impairment of the hepatic storage capacity and transport maximum for bromosulphaleine has been reported [24]. Quantitative liver function test using lidocaine, Monoethylglycinexylidine (MEGX) was found to be abnormal in a large number of EHPVO children [25]. Depriving the liver of portal venous blood possibly leads to decreased hepatic function.

CLINICAL PRESENTATIONS

These vary with the age (childhood or adulthood) and the mode (acute or chronic) of presentation [26]. The EHPVO in childhood is most often chronic and presents with features of variceal bleeding. On the other hand, in adults the disease could present as acute or chronic.

Childhood

EHPVO can present as early as 6 weeks after birth. The typical presenting symptoms in infancy and childhood are variceal bleeding, ascites, and growth failure.

Variceal bleeding. The most usual presentation for children with EHPVO is sudden, unexpected, and often massive hematemesis. Repeated episodes of bleeding for a long period of time is the general pattern. The children withstand the haemorrhages remarkably well without significant hepatocellular failure. The splenic size, and portal pressure do not correlate with the incidence or severity of hematemesis. Webb and Sherlock [4] had reported that the frequency of variceal bleeding is reduced after puberty. This has not been confirmed in subsequent studies [27], mainly because treatment is offered to the child at the first presentation.

Ascites. Ascites develops in a proportion of children following haemorrhage or surgery and is often transient. Webb and Sherlock in their series of 97 patients observed ascites as a presenting symptom in 13 patients [4], in seven it was transient but six patients required treatment with a low sodium diet and diuretics. Other workers have also noted the occasional association of ascites with EHPVO [28]. We had recently reported the occurrence of spontaneous ascites in about 20% of older EHPVO patients; a fair proportion of them required diuretic therapy [29].

Deterioration of liver function and fall in serum albumin with increasing age in EHPVO patients has been reported [2]. Portosystemic encephalopathy also reflecting hepatocellular failure was reported in over 50% of patients with ascites by Webb and Sherlock [4]. However, this high frequency has not been reported in several large studies [3,10,30].

Development of ascites signifies hepatic dysfunction and a hyperkinetic circulatory state [31]. There are no clear explanations for this in EHPVO. Autonomic dysfunction which contributes to cirrhotic ascites by adding to decreased peripheral vascular resistance, has been reported in a significant proportion of children with EHPVO [32]. This could play a role in the genesis of spontaneous ascites. Whether prolonged portal biliopathy leads to hepatic dysfunction is speculative at present.

Growth retardation. EHPVO occurring in the pre-pubertal period could result in growth retardation in up to 50% of young EHPVO children [33]. Our work has been substantiated by other clinical studies which have shown that there is resistance to growth hormone function in these children and insulin-like growth factor is reduced [34]. It has been shown that young rats undergoing portal vein ligation or portalsystemic shunt surgery gain significantly less body weight compared with control or sham operated animals [35]. The most likely cause seems to be reduced portal blood supply to the liver due to portal vein obstruction. The hypothesis that deprivation of portal blood leads to growth retardation is further supported by observations of Kato *et al.* who have documented a spurt in growth after shunt surgery in patients with EHPVO [36].

Jaundice. Jaundice may also be a presenting feature of portal vein occlusion. It could be caused by compression by the venous collaterals running in the vicinity of the common bile duct [37–39]. Thompson *et al.* [2] had suggested that a rise in serum bilirubin follows over the years due to an acceleration in the normal ageing process of the liver as a result of impaired blood supply. Hypoxemia because of intrapulmonary vascular dilatations has also been documented in case reports in patients with EHPVO.

Adults

The presentation could be as acute or chronic EHPVO.

Acute. These patients often present with acute abdominal pain of varying severity and duration. The diagnosis is often delayed as it is made after excluding the other common causes [3]. Sometimes fever and rarely ascites could be accompanied with abdominal pain.

A small proportion of patients with acute EHPVO due to thrombosis do present with features of intestinal ischemia and sometimes with features of intestinal obstruction due to stricture formation. The estimated incidence of mesenteric vein thrombosis with transmural intestinal infarction has been reported to be around 1.8/100,000 person years [40].

Some patients may present as protein losing enteropathy or hemorrhagic ascites.

Chronic. Variceal bleeding and hypersplenism are the other common manifestations. If the oesophageal varices have been obliterated in childhood, patients may present with bleeding from gastric, duodenal [41] or anorectal varices [3].

Portal biliopathy. The term 'Portal biliopathy' was introduced in 1992 and refers to abnormalities of the extrahepatic and intrahepatic bile ducts with or without gallbladder collaterals in patients with portal hypertension [38]. Several subsequent reports have confirmed these observations [42–44].

Biliopathy changes have been reported in 80–100% of patients with EHPVO on ERCP. The changes include indentations of paracholedochal collaterals on bile duct, localised strictures, angulation of ducts, displacement of ducts and stones in the common bile duct and focal narrowing, dilatations, irregular walls and clustering of intrahepatic branches in the hepatic ducts

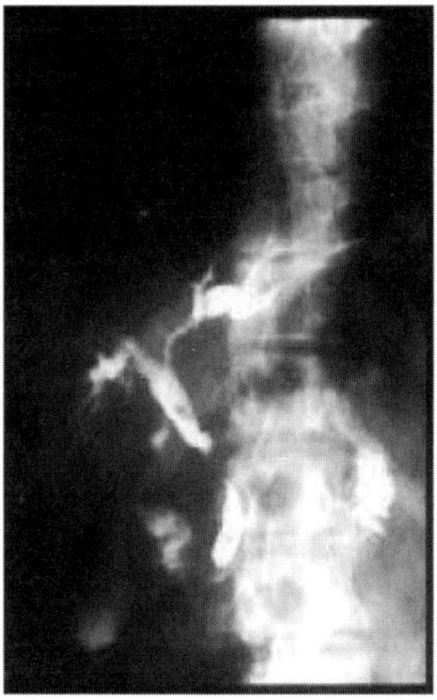

Fig. 47 Endoscopic retrograde cholangiography showing bile duct anomalies in a patient with Portal biliopathy.

(Fig. 47). The left hepatic duct is involved more commonly and severely and this may be due to formation of prominent collateral veins where the umbilical vein joins the left branch of the portal vein. The biliary abnormalities are limited to large bile ducts and spare the small bile ducts as liver histology does not demonstrate evidence of ductopenia, ductular proliferation, portal triaditis or cirrhosis.

The biliary abnormalities are common in EHPVO because paracholedochal and paracholecystic veins form the porto-portal collaterals (the predominant component of portal cavernoma) to bypass the obstructed segment of the portal vein (Fig. 47). The biliary abnormalities may be explained either by compression of bile ducts by collaterals or by ischemic injury of the bile ducts as a result of thrombosis of veins draining the bile duct [42].

Despite its common occurrence, portal biliopathy is rarely symptomatic [44], though biochemical changes may often be seen. Symptomatic patients are usually adults, indicating that portal biliopathy is a slowly progressive disease. The frequency of development of new stones and strictures has also been calculated [3].

Hepatic encephalopathy. Spontaneous hepatic encephalopathy is uncommon in EHPVO, except when large spontaneous shunts have developed. Subclinical encephalopathy has been reported in about 9% of the patients prior to surgery and in 36% of the patients after shunt surgery [3].

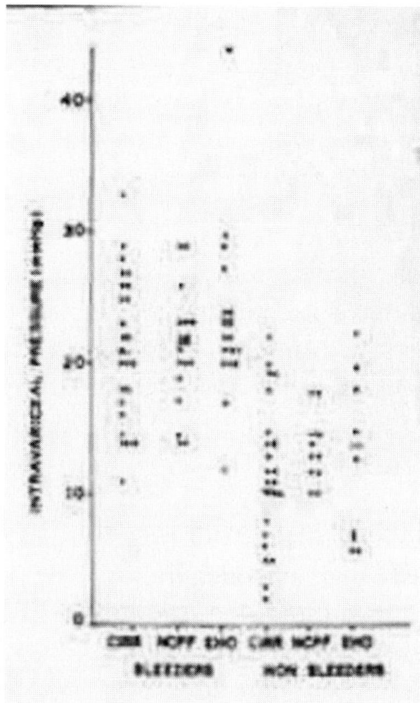

Fig. 48 Intravariceal pressure in bleeding and non-bleeding patients with extrahepatic portal vein obstruction (EHO), noncirrhotic portal fibrosis (NCPF) and cirrhosis of the liver. (Reproduced from *Gut* 1987;28: 260–266.)

Immunological anomalies. The cell-mediated immunity shows qualitatively similar defects in patients with EHPVO and chronic liver disease [45,46]. The defects in cell-mediated immunity result in part from sequestration of T-cells by the spleen and partly from the presence in serum of factors that influence the kinetics of lymphocyte response. These defects sometimes present with repeated infections and episodes of diarrhoea in children.

Hemodynamic studies in EHPVO. Wedged hepatic venous pressure (WHVP) is within normal limits and intrasplenic pressure is significantly elevated indicating the presinusoidal nature of the block [47]. Intravariceal pressure closely reflects the intrasplenic pressure (Fig. 48) and is the recommended investigation for measuring portal pressure. Due to portal vein obstruction, the hepatic blood flow is normal or decreased and is only partly compensated by increased hepatic artery flow. The functional status of the liver is likely to be determined by the extent of the increase in hepatic artery flow. Patients with EHPVO have a hyperkinetic circulatory state, with low systemic vascular resistance and increased cardiac output. It is suggested that extensive portal systemic venous collateral circulation may be responsible for this state.

Dilated cardiac chambers and hepatopulmonary syndrome [48] have been reported in a very small subset of patients.

DIAGNOSIS

Patients with EHPVO have a characteristic clinical presentation both in childhood and adulthood. An infant or child presenting with hematemesis and moderate splenomegaly in the absence of features of chronic liver disease is likely to be suffering from EHPVO. Normal liver biochemistry and absence of hepatitis viruses would further support the suspicion of EHPVO in a child.

In adults, the diagnosis of EHPVO poses several problems. First, one needs to exclude diseases such as noncirrhotic portal fibrosis and idiopathic portal hypertension, compensated cirrhosis and hepatic venous outflow tract obstruction. The presence or absence of cirrhosis and neoplasia also needs to be identified. The event is often acute and a high index of suspicion is needed. Further, EHPVO could be secondary to a disease with distinct features. The primary disease needs to be suspected and diagnosed with accompanying EHPVO.

Imaging. Imaging is the mainstay for the diagnosis of EHPVO.

Ultrasound Doppler is a reliable non-invasive technique with high degree of accuracy in the detection of portal cavernoma and is the investigation of choice [49]. Acute portal vein thrombosis could be seen as intraluminal material, sometimes even anechoic. Chronic thrombosis or obstruction would lead to cavernous transformation of the portal vein which produces a distinctive tangle of tortuous vessels in the porta hepatis.

Other radiological techniques such as CT, CT arterial portography, and MR angiography. have also been successfully used. All of them achieve high degrees of sensitivity and specificity. Splenoportography or arterial portography (selective celiac or superior mesenteric angiography) are now less employed due to their invasive nature.

Liver biopsy and biochemistry. The role of liver biopsy in the diagnosis of EHPVO is limited. Generally, the diagnosis has already been made out on the imaging study of a portal vein obstruction. Hence, liver biopsy is needed only to exclude underlying chronic liver disease or cirrhosis which could be missed by the routine imaging techniques. Its utility is also in assessing the degree of hepatic dysfunction accompanying EHPVO, especially if portal biliopathy and spontaneous ascites are present [3].

Characteristically, needle biopsy shows normal parenchyma and only venous anomalies. However, mild to moderate hepatic fibrosis has also been reported [23,24].

The tests of liver function are normal though they are likely to show derangement with the passage of time and prolonged duration of the disease [3,50].

Study of hepatitis viruses. There is no etiological association of HBV or HCV to the development of EHPVO. However, since EHPVO patients are likely to receive repeated blood transfusion, the possibility of their developing chronic hepatitis B or C exists.

Investigations for a prothrombotic state. There is evidence that a prothrombotic state does exist in a proportion of adult patients with EHPVO [15,16]. In these patients, specific investigations to detect an underlying myeloproliferative disorder need to be undertaken. Sensitive tests such as endogenous erythroid colony assessment and identification of dysmorphic megakaryocytes can distinguish polycytemia vera from secondary erythrocytosis. The test consists of demonstrating the growth of erythroid colonies, in cultures of bone marrow or peripheral blood progenitor cells, and in the absence of added erythropoietin.

There is controversial data as to whether other known risk factors for venous thromboembolism such as factor V Leiden mutation, G20210A prothrombin gene mutation and levels of natural anticoagulants, protein C, S and anti-thrombin III are altered [17,20–22]. Routine use of these tests is likely to be more rewarding in adult western patients and is not likely to be very rewarding in children.

Evaluation for varices. A careful UGI endoscopy is warranted in EHPVO patients as nearly 40% of them have gastric varices and a few have antroduodenal varices [3]. In a child presenting with lower GI bleed, proctosigmoidoscopy to detect anorectal varices should be done.

Portal biliopathy. ERCP is not recommended in the routine work-up of children with EHPVO. Only if there are features of cholangitis or obstructive jaundice, a therapeutic ERCP procedure should be planned. For assessment of biliopathy, MRCP has been shown to be comparable to ERCP [51].

MANAGEMENT

The treatment of portal venous obstruction depends very much upon the age of the patient, the site of obstruction and the clinical presentation. The management of patients with EHPVO includes treatment of variceal bleeding, hypersplenism and portal biliopathy.

Treatment of variceal bleeding

The management of variceal bleeding in patients with EHPVO has improved dramatically in the past two decades.

Treatment of acute variceal bleeding

There is limited data on the use of pharmacological agents for the control of acute bleeding in patients with EHPVO. However, based on expert opinion at the Baveno IV meeting, as in cirrhotic patients with active variceal bleeding, these vasoactive drugs could be used in EHPVO patients.

Endoscopic therapies. Acute variceal bleeding: endoscopic sclerotherapy has been found to be effective in the control of acute bleeding in several studies [52,53].

Secondary prophylaxis of variceal bleeding

There is a lack of data on the role of β-blocker therapy in the prevention of variceal rebleeding. There is an urgent need to evaluate this approach in EHPVO patients.

While both endoscopic sclerotherapy and band ligation have been found to be effective in preventing rebleeding, the latter is recommended as the treatment of choice [54].

Primary prophylaxis of variceal bleeding

The proportion of EHPVO patients with high risk oesophageal varices and no history of variceal bleeding is rather small. Although, there is no data to support the role of β-blockers in these patients, logically, these drugs should reduce the incidence of first bleed. There is however, an apprehension of further reduction in total hepatic blood flow leading to hepatic ischemia.

Surgery

Shunting procedures. Both total and selective shunts have been used [7,31,55,56]. Shunt surgery is reserved for patients who fail endoscopic therapy, have significant growth retardation in prepubertal age, symptomatic portal biliopathy and symptomatic hypersplenism. It can also be offered to patients who demand a one time treatment.

Total shunts include central splenorenal shunt with splenectomy, mesocaval, portacaval, and 'makeshift' shunts. Rebleeding rates and shunt thrombosis remain a problem. The selective shunts include distal splenorenal shunt (DSRS), distal splenocaval shunt, gastroepiploic to left renal vein shunt, and left gastric vein to left renal vein shunt [55,56].

Variceal ablative procedures. They are rarely required and should be used as rescue procedures. Splenectomy without shunt surgery should not be done unless there is only left-sided portal hypertension due to isolated splenic vein thrombosis [3].

Rex shunt or mesenterico-left portal bypass. In this shunt the mesenteric blood is redirected into the intrahepatic portal venous circulation. It not only improves the portal hypertension in EHPVO but also restores the portal blood flow to the liver [57].

Portal biliopathy

Symptomatic portal biliopathy with cholangitis and choledocholithiasis can be managed by biliary stenting, sphincterotomy and stone extraction [58]. The biliary obstruction however, often remains unrelieved and chances of recurrent stone formation remain high. For dominant biliary structures and endoscopic failures, portosystemic shunting is the initial procedure which by itself can lead to amelioration of biliary obstruction. In patients with persistent obstruction, hepaticojejunostomy may be needed to treat the biliary obstruction, access to the region being made possible by an initial portosystemic shunt [59].

Role of anticoagulant therapy

At present, the evidence on which to base recommendations for anticoagulant therapy is rather weak. However, in patients with recent EHPVO, early initiation of anticoagulation using unfractionated heparin or low molecular weight heparin could be helpful [60]. The infusion of streptokinase and/or recombinant tissue-plasminogen activator via an operatively placed multi side-hole catheter/5-Fr introducer sheath into the right portal and superior mesenteric vein clot, given within the first two weeks of thrombosis, can restore the venous patency and prevent bowel infarction [61]. It is generally believed that oral anticoagulation should be continued for at least 3 months in all such patients. However, if an underlying persistent prothrombotic state is documented, lifelong anticoagulant therapy is preferred.

In patients with chronic EHPVO, there is no consensus on the indication for anticoagulant therapy. However, in those patients with a persistent documented prothrombotic state, anticoagulant therapy can be considered.

Interventional procedures

There is some evidence that early interventional therapy such as TIPS and local thrombolysis could help in resolving thrombosis and achieve recanalisation [62–64].

Percutaneous techniques for portal recanalisation are an interesting alternative, even in non-acute thrombosis. Once flow has been restored in the portal vein, TIPS may be necessary to obtain an adequate outflow, hence facilitating and maintaining the portal flow.

In patients with EHPVO and associated cirrhosis, hepatocellular carcinoma should be excluded. There is insufficient data on which to base recommendations for giving anticoagulant therapy to these patients.

Several important areas in EHPVO require detailed investigations and long-term studies; these include aetiology and natural history of EHPVO in children as compared to adults, progression of hepatic dysfunction, portal biliopathy, thrombotic attacks and role of β-blockers and anticoagulants in the management.

In summary, EHPVO is a challenging problem due to its varied aetiology, clinical profile and management options. Early diagnosis and adequate management of variceal bleeding and judicious use of anticoagulants and thrombolytic therapy could help improve the management of these patients.

REFERENCES

1 Shaldon S, Sherlock S. Obstruction to the extraheptic portal system in childhood. *Lancet* 1962;**1**: 63–67.
2 Thompson EN, Sherlock S. The aetiology of portal vein thrombosis with particular reference to the role of infection and exchange transfusion. *QJ Med* 1964;**33**: 465–480.
3 Sarin SK, Agarwal SR. Extraheptic portal vein obstruction. *Semin Liver Dis* 2002;**22**: 43–58.

4 Webb LJ and Sherlok S. The aetiology, presentation and natural history of extrahepatic portal venous obstruction. *QJ Med* 1979;**192**: 627–639.
5 Ando H, Kaneko K, Ito F *et al.* Anatomy and aetiology of extraheptic portal vein obstruction in children leading to bleeding esophageal varices. *J Am Coll Surg* 1996;**183**: 543–547.
6 Alvarez F, Bernard O, Brunelle F *et al.* Portal obstruction in children. I. Clinical investigtions and haemorrhage risk. *J Pediatr* 1983;**103**: 696–702.
7 Mitra SK, Rao KLN, Narasimhan K *et al.* Side-to-side lienorenal shunt without splenectomy in non-cirrhotic portal hypertension in children. *J Pediatr Surg* 1993;**28**: 398–402.
8 Sarin SK, Kapoor D. Non-cirrhotic portal fibrosis: current concepts and management. *J Gastroenterol Hepatol* 2002;**17**: 526–534.
9 Ayantunde AA, Debrah SA. Portal vein thrombosis complicating appendicitis. *West Afr J Med* 2004;**23**(4): 332–334.
10 Primignani M, Martinelli I, Bucciarelli P *et al.* Risk factors for thrombophilia in extrahepatic portal vein obstruction. *Hepatology* 2005;**41**: 603–608.
11 Larroche J. Umbilical catheterization: its complications. *Biol Neonate* 1970;**16**: 101–103.
12 Yadav S, Dutta AK, Sarin SK. Do umbilical vein catheterization and sepsis lead to portal vein thrombosis? A prospective, clinical and sonographic evaluation. *J Pediatr Gastroenterol Nutr* 1993;**17**: 392–396.
13 Odievre M, Pige G, Alagille D. Congenital abnormalities associated with extraheptic portal hypertension. *Arch Dis Child* 1977;**52**: 383–385.
14 Marks C. Developmental basis of the portal venous system. *Am J Surg* 1969;**33**: 465–681.
15 Valla D, Casadevall N, Huisse MG *et al.* myeloproliferative disorders in portal vein thrombosis in adults. *Gastroenteorlogy* 1998;**94**: 1063–1069.
16 Cardin F, Graffeo M, McCormick PA, McIntyre, Burroughs A. Adult 'Idiopathic' extrahepatic venous thrombosis: Importance of putative 'Latent' myeloprolifrative disorders and comparison with cases with known aetiology. *Dig Dis* 1992;**37**: 335–339.
17 Nakase H, Kawasaki T, Itani T *et al.* Budd-Chiari syndrome and extrahepatic portal obstruction associated with congenital antithrombin III deficiency. *J Gastroenterol* 2001;**36**: 341–345.
18 Robson SC, Kruskal J, Bird AR, Kirsch RE. Abnormal hemostasis in extrahepatic portal hypertension. *Hepatology* 1993;**18**: 853–857.
19 Bajaj JS, Bhattacharjee J, Sain SK. Coagulation profile and platelet function in patients with extrahepatic portal vein obstruction and non-cirrhotic portal fibrosis. *J Gastroenterol Hepatol* 2001;**16**: 641–646.
20 Bhattacharyya M, Makharia G, Kannan M, Ahmed RP, Gupta PK, Saxena R. Inherited prothrombotic defects in Budd-Chiari syndrome and portal vein thrombosis: a study from North India. *Am J Clin Pathol* 2004;**121**: 844–847.
21 Pinto RB, Silveira TR, Bandinelli E, Rohsig L. Portal vein thrombosis in children and adolescents: the low prevalence of hereditary thrombophilic disorders. *J Pediatr Surg* 2004;**39**: 1356–1361.
22 Erkan O, Bozdayi AM, Disibeyaz S *et al.* Thrombophilic gene mutations in cirrhotic patients with portal vein thrombosis. *Eur J Gastroenterol Hepatol* 2005;**17**: 339–343.

23 Sengupta KP, Basu Mallik KC *et al.* Liver changes in extraheptic portal venous obstruction. *Ind J Med Res* 1968;**56**: 1643–1650.
24 Arora R, Mohanty M, Nundy S, Nayak NC. Phlebothrombosis as a common pathogenic denominator in noncirrhotic portal fibrosis and extrahepatic portal venous obstruciton. *Ind J Med Res* 1984;**79**: 392–403.
25 Mishra A, Guptan RC, Sarin SK. Monoethylglycinexylidine (MEGX): a sensitive non-invasive method to differentiate NCPF and Child's A chronic liver disease. *Ind J Gastroenterol* 1997;**16**(suppl. 2): 101.
26 Sobhonslidsuk A, Reddy KR. Portal vein thrombosis: a concise review. *Am J Gastroenterol* 2002;**97**: 535–541.
27 Shah SR, Mathur SK. Presentation and natural history of variceal bleeding in patients with portal hypertension due to extrahepatic portal venous obstruction. *Ind J Gastroenterol* 2003;**22**: 217–220.
28 Clatworthy HW, Boles ET. Extrahepatic portal bed block in children: pathogenesis and treatment. *Ann Surg* 1959;**150**: 371–383.
29 Rangari M, Gupta R, Jain M, Malhotra V, Sarin SK. Hepatic dysfunction in patients with extraheptic portal venous obstruction. *Liver Int* 2003;**23**: 434–439.
30 Sahni P, Pande GK, Nundy S. Extraheptic portal vein obstruction. *Br J Surg* 1990;**77**: 1201–1202.
31 Braillon A, Moreau R, Hadengus A *et al.* Hyperkinetic circulatory syndrome in patients with presinusoidal portal hypertension. Effect of propranolol. *J Hepatol* 1989;**9**: 312–318.
32 Rangari M, Sinha S, Kapoor D, Mohan JC, Sarin SK. Prevalence of Autonomic Dysfunction in Cirrhotic and Non-Cirrhotic Portal Hypertension. *Am J Gastroenterol* 2002;**97**: 707–713.
33 Sarin SK, Bansal A, Sasan S, Nigam A. Portal-vein Obstruction in Children Leads to Growth Retardation. *Hepatology* 1992;**15**: 229–233.
34 Mehrotra RN, Bhatia V, Dabadghao P, Yachha SK. Extrahepatic portal vein obstruction in children: anthropometry, growth hormone, and insulin-like growth factor I. *J Pediatr Gastroenterol Nutr* 1997;**25**: 520–523.
35 Parrel GC, Koltai A, Zaluzny L, Murry M. Effects of portal vein ligation on sex hormone metabolism in male rats: relationship to lowered hepatic cytochrome P450 levels. *Gastroenterology* 1986;**90**: 299–305.
36 Kato T, Romero R, Koutouby R, Mittal NK, Thompson JF, Schleien CL, Tzakis AG. Portosystemic shunting in children during the era of endoscopic therapy: improved postoperative growth parameters. *J Pediatr Gastroenterol Nutr* 2000;**30**: 419–425.
37 Dan SJ, Train JS, Cohen BA, Mitty MA. Common bile duct varices Cholangiographic demonstration of a hazardous portosystemic communication. *Am J Gastroenterol* 1983;**78**: 42–43.
38 Sarin SK, Bhatha V, Makwane U. 'Potal biliopathy' in extrahepatic portal vein obstruction. *Ind J Gastroenterol* 1992;**11**: A82.
39 Condat B, Vilgrain V, Asselah T *et al.* Portal cavernoma-associated cholangiopathy: a clinical and MR cholangiography coupled with MR portography imaging study. *Hepatology* 2003;**37**: 1302–1308.
40 Acosta S, Ogren M, Sternby NH, Bergqvist D, Bjorck M. Mesenteric venous thrombosis with transmural intestinal infarction: a population-based study. *J Vasc Surg* 2005;**41**: 59–63.

41 McAlister VC, Al-Saleh NA. Duodenal dearterialization and stapling for severe haemorrhage from duodenal varices with portal vein thrombosis. *Am J Surg* 2005;**189**: 49–52.

42 Dhiman RK, Puri P, Chawla Y *et al.* Biliary changes in extrahepatic portal venous obstruction: compression by collaterals or ischemic? *Gastrointest Endoscopy* 1999;**50**: 646–652.

43 Khuroo MS, Yattoo GN, Zargar SA *et al.* Biliary abnormalities associated with extrahepatic portal venous obstruction. *Hepatology* 1993;**17**: 807–813.

44 Khare R, Sikora SS, Srikanth G *et al.* Extrahepatic portal venous obstruction and obstructive jaundice: approach to management. *J Gastroenterol Hepatol* 2005;**20**: 56–61.

45 Robson SC, Kruskal J, Bird AR, Kirsch RE. Abnormal hemostasis in extrahepatic portal hypertension. *Hepatology* 1993;**18**: 853–857.

46 Webb LJ, Ross M, Markham RL *et al.* Immune function in patients with extrahepatic portal venous obstruction and the effect of splenectomy. *Gastroenterology* 1980;**79**: 99–103.

47 Sarin SK, Sethi KK, Nanda R. Measurement and correlation of wedged hepatic, intrahepatic, intrasplenic and intravariceal pressure in patients with cirrhosis & non-cirrhotic portal fibrosis. *Gut* 1987;**28**: 260–266.

48 Gupta D, Vijaya DR, Gupta R *et al.* Prevalence of hepatopulmonary syndrome incirrhosis and extrahepatic portal venous obstruction. *Am J Gastroenterol* 2001;**96**: 3395–3399.

49 Zwiebel WJ. Songraphic diagnosis of hepatic vascular disorders. Semin Ultrasound CT MRI 1995;**16**: 34–48.

50 Ogawa A, Takamori S, Kojima K, Fukasawa M, Beppu T, Futagawa S. Hemodynamics in extrahepatic portal vein obstruction and its changes during long-term follow-ups. *Hepatol Res* 2002;**24**: 141.

51 Condat B, Vilgrain V, Aselah T *et al.* Portal cavernoma-associated cholangiopathy: a clinical and MR cholangiography coupled with MR portography imaging study. *Hepatology* 2003;**37**: 1302–1308.

52 Sarin SK, Nanda R, Gaur SK, Kumar N, Vij JC, Anand BS. Repeated endoscopic sclerotherapy in active variceal bleeding. *Ann Surg* 1985;**202**: 708–711.

53 Kahn D, Terblanche J, Kitano S, Bornman P. Injection sclerotherapy in adult patients with extrahepatic portal venous obstruction. *Br J Surg* 1987;**74**: 600–602.

54 Zargar SA, Javid G, Khan BA *et al.* Endoscopic ligation compared with sclerotherapy for bleeding esophageal varices in children with extrahepatic portal venous obstruction. *Hepatology* 2002;**36**: 666–672.

55 Warren WD, Henderson JM, Millikan WJ, Galambos JT, Bryan FC. Management of variceal bleeding in patients with noncirrhotic portal vein thrombosis. *Ann Surg* 1988;**207**: 623–633.

56 Henderson JM, Millikan WJ, Galambos JT, Warren WD. Selective variceal decompression in portal vein thrombosis. *Br J Surg* 1984;**71**: 745–749.

57 Bambini DA, Superina R, Almond PS, Whitington PF, Alonso E. Experience with the Rex shunt (mesenterico-left portal bypass) in children with extrahepatic portal hypertension. *J Pediatr Surg* 2000;**35**: 13–18.

58 Chandra R, Kapoor D, Tharakan A, Chaudhary A, Sarin SK. Portal biliopathy. *J Gastroenterol Hepatol* 2001;**16**: 1086–1092.

59 Chaudhary A, Dhar P, Sarin SK *et al*. Bile duct obstruction due to portal biliopathy in extraheptic portal hypertension. Surgical management. *Br J Surg* 1988;**85**: 326–327.
60 Joh JH, KIM DI. Mesenteric and portal vein thrombosis: treated with early initiation of anticoagulation. *Eur J Vasc Endovasc Surg* 2005;**29**: 204–208.
61 Kaplan JL, Weintraub SL, Hunt JP, Gonzalez A, Lopera J, Brazzini A. Treatment of superior mesenteric and portal vein thrombosis with direct thrombolytic infusion via an operatively placed mesenteric catheter. *Am Surg* 2004;**70**: 600–604.
62 Bilbao JI, Elorz M, Vivas I, Martinez-Cuesta A, Bastarrika G, Benito A. Transjugular intrahepatic portosystemic shunt (TIPS) in the treatment of venous symptomatic chronic portal thrombosis in non-cirrhotic patients. *Cardiovasc Intervent Radiol* 2004:**27**: 474–480.
63 Stambo GW, Grauer L. Transhepatic portal venous power-pulse spray rheolytic thrombectomy for acute portal vein thrombosis after CT-guided pancreas biopsy. *Am J Roentgenol* 2005;**184**(suppl. 3): S118–S119.
64 Sze DY, O'Sullivan GJ, Johnson DL, Dake MD. Mesenteric and portal venous thrombosis treated by transjugular mechanical thrombolysis. *AJR Am J Roentgenol* 2000;**175**: 732–734.

Baveno IV Consensus Statements Noncirrhotic Portal Hypertension

Dominique-Charles Valla, Shiv K. Sarin (Chairpersons), Giovanni Barosi, Yogesh C. Chawla, Elwyn Elias, Harry Janssen, M. Primignani and I.R. Wanless

Budd-Chiari syndrome [BCS - hepatic venous outflow tract obstruction (HVOTO)]

Definition

• Budd-Chiari syndrome (BCS) is an eponym for hepatic venous outflow tract obstruction (HVOTO) which can be located from the level of the small hepatic veins to the level of the termination of inferior vena cava into the right atrium.
• BCS is an heterogeneous condition with regard to causes and pathogenesis.
• BCS is considered secondary when the mechanism for HVOTO is compression/invasion by a benign or malignant tumor, abscess or cyst.
• BCS is considered primary otherwise.
• Hepatic congestion secondary to heart failure and pericardial disease are excluded from the definition of BCS.
• Obstruction confined to small hepatic veins or sinusoids in the context of liver irradiation, chemotherapy, stem cell transplantation or exposure to toxic agents is excluded from the definition of BCS.
• The terms veno-occlusive disease and sinusoidal obstruction syndrome require further definition.

Aetiology

• Primary BCS is frequently associated with one or several risk factors for thrombosis. These underlying disorders are often occult at presentation with BCS.
• Myeloproliferative disorders should be investigated in any patient with BCS, irrespective of the peripheral blood picture.
• When liver synthetic function is impaired, low plasma levels of antithrombin, protein C and protein S are not specific for an inherited defect.

Diagnosis

• BCS is diagnosed by the demonstration of an obstruction of the venous lumen, or by the presence of hepatic vein collaterals.

• Liver biopsy is not necessary to make a diagnosis of BCS when vascular imaging has demonstrated obstruction of the hepatic venous outflow tract.
• Liver biopsy is the only means to make a diagnosis of BCS of the small intrahepatic veins.
• Clinical trials for therapy of BCS have not been performed so that current therapy is based on less rigorous information.

Treatment

On the basis of current expert opinion (5;D)
• Anticoagulation should be recommended to all patients, in the absence of major contra-indications. However, there is no consensus on the optimal duration of anticoagulation.
• Previous bleeding related to portal hypertension is not considered a major contra-indication for anticoagulation, provided appropriate prophylaxis for recurrent bleeding is initiated.
• Complications of portal hypertension may be treated as recommended for the other types of liver diseases.
• Stenoses that are amenable to percutaneous angioplasty/stenting should be actively looked for, and treated accordingly.
• TIPS insertion should be attempted when angioplasty/stenting is not feasible, and when the patient does not improve on medical therapy.
• Liver transplantation should be considered in patients with manifestations refractory to the above procedures.

Areas requiring further studies (5;D)

• Accurate diagnostic tests for myeloproliferative disorder and antiphospholipid syndrome.
• Benefit and risk of prolonged anticoagulation therapy.
• Benefit and risk of pharmacological therapy for portal hypertension.
• Optimal timing of angioplasty and TIPS with respect to severity of symptoms.
• Indications for thrombolysis.

Extra-hepatic portal vein obstruction (EHPVO)

Definition

• EHPVO is defined by obstruction of the extrahepatic portal vein with or without involvement of the intra-hepatic portal veins.

• EHPVO often manifests as portal cavernoma, which is a network of porto-porto collaterals and develops as a sequel of portal vein obstruction.
• Isolated thrombosis of the splenic vein or superior mesenteric vein with patent portal vein is excluded.
• The definition should be augmented by a statement of presence or absence of cirrhosis and neoplasia.

Aetiology

• EHPVO is a heterogeneous entity with regards to causes and pathogenesis, particularly between children and adults.
• EHPVO in adults is frequently associated with one or several risk factors for thrombosis which may be occult at presentation.
• Presence of cirrhosis, neoplasia and other intra-abdominal causes such as inflammation, trauma, etc. do not exclude the presence of systemic risk factors.

Clinical presentation

• EHPVO can be acute or chronic.
• EHPVO can be assumed to be recent when patients present with symptoms such as abdominal pain, ascites, fever or symptoms suggestive for intestinal ischaemia, in the absence of portal cavernoma and porto-systemic collaterals.
• Chronic EHPVO is associated with portal cavernoma and may present with variceal bleed, splenomegaly, abnormal blood cell counts and occasionally jaundice. A proportion of children have growth retardation.

Diagnosis

• EHPVO is diagnosed by imaging techniques like Doppler US, CT or MRI which demonstrate portal vein obstruction, presence of intraluminal material or portal vein cavernoma.

Natural history

• Most patients with EHPVO in the absence of cirrhosis and neoplasia have a relatively benign course.
• Morbidity is mainly related to variceal bleed, recurrent thrombosis, symptomatic portal biliopathy and hypersplenism.

• The natural course of EHPVO is mainly determined by the presence or absence of associated diseases such as cirrhosis or neoplasia.

Treatment (in the absence of cirrhosis and neoplasia)

• Chronic EHPVO.
• For primary prophylaxis of variceal bleeding there is insufficient data on whether β-blockers or endoscopic therapy should be preferred.
• For the control of acute variceal bleeding, endoscopic therapy is effective (1b;A). In the absence of specific data on patients with EHPVO it is presumed that the same treatments used in bleeding cirrhotic patients could be applied (5;D).
• For secondary prophylaxis, endoscopic therapy is effective (1b;A). There is insufficient evidence to recommend β-blockers.
• There is no consensus on the indication for anticoagulant therapy.
• However, in those patients with a persistent documented prothrombotic state, anticoagulant therapy can be considered.
• There is insufficient evidence in favor of interventional therapy such as TIPS and local thrombolysis.
• Decompressive surgery should only be considered for patients with failure of endoscopic therapy. (5;D)
• For portal biliopathy with obstructive jaundice, endoscopic therapy is recommended (5;D). In case of failure, shunt surgery may be considered (5;D).
• *Recent EHPVO*.
• Recent EHPVO rarely resolves spontaneously.
• The evidence on which to base recommendations for anticoagulant therapy is weak.
On the basis of current expert opinion (5;D), in patients with *recent EHPVO*:
• Anticoagulation should be given for at least 3 months in all patients.
• When an underlying persistent prothrombotic state has been documented, life-long anticoagulant therapy is recommended.
• In patients with EHPVO and *associated* cirrhosis, hepatocellular carcinoma should be excluded. There is insufficient data on which to base recommendations for giving anticoagulant therapy to these patients.

Areas requiring further studies (5;D)

• Natural history in children versus adults: hepatic dysfunction, portal biliopathy, growth retardation.
• Aetiology – role of various prothrombotic states in EHPVO (in the East), identification of susceptible population.

- Assessment of thrombosis, progression and recurrence.
- Definitions of variceal bleeding and predictors of 1st bleed and rebleed.
- Role of β-blockers and comparison with endoscopic therapy.
- Usefulness of long-term anticoagulants, TIPS, shunt surgery.
- Development of good experimental models.

LECTURE

Quality of Randomised Clinical Trials in Portal Hypertension and Other Fields of Hepatology

Christian Gluud, Sarah Louise Klingenberg and Lise Lotte Gluud

INTRODUCTION

The hierarchy of evidence regarding the benefits of preventive, diagnostic or therapeutic interventions is established [1–3]. Randomised trials are the gold standard for intervention comparisons [1–9]. Cohort studies and case-control studies are unreliable designs to estimate intervention effect unless the latter is dramatic [10,11]. Dramatic intervention effects are rare. Logistic regression analysis may increase rather than decrease the risks of over and underestimation of intervention effects [10]. Expert opinions, case reports and experimental models can be as misleading as cohort and case-control studies – or worse. Therefore, they rank lowest in the evidence hierarchy [1–3].

Accordingly, randomised clinical trials are increasingly being used to guide evidence-based clinical practice. The quality of randomised trials has therefore been discussed vigorously, especially during the last 10 years. One needs to address one central question before considering if trial results can be used for patients: are the results valid? Result validity depends on the internal validity of the trial. The internal validity of a trial depends on the risks of random errors [6,12] and the risks of systematic errors (i.e. bias) [4–9,12,13]. Conducting randomised clinical trials with many participants and outcomes decrease the risks of random errors [12]. Conducting randomised clinical trials with high methodological quality, avoiding selection, performance, assessment, attrition and other biases, decreases the risks of systematic errors [4–9,12,13]. External validity should only be considered if internal validity is adequate. If the internal validity is inadequate the discussion on external validity becomes irrelevant.

Systematic reviews with meta-analyses of several randomised trials are becoming more important in clinical decision-making (www.cochrane.org).

Table 52 Chronological overview of some international portal hypertension and generic activities with the aim of improving the quality of randomised clinical trials since 1986.

- 1986 Groningen
- 1990 Baveno I
- 1992 Milano
- 1993 The Cochrane collaboration
- 1995 Baveno II
- 1995 ICH – GCP
- 1996 The cochrane hepato-biliary group
- 1996 The CONSORT statement
- 1997 Reston - AASLD
- 1998 The Cochrane hepatobiliary group trial register
- 2000 Baveno III
- 2004 The Ottava statement

Therefore, the risks of publication bias (i.e. the tendency not to publish trials with neutral or negative intervention effects) have never been greater [14–18]. It is therefore necessary that all trials become registered before inclusion of the first patient with sufficient details so that one can avoid publication bias [14–18] and post hoc changes of primary outcome measures [19,20].

Many randomised trials on portal hypertension and other hepatobiliary diseases are too small and have methodological deficiencies [4,11,21–24]. Since the 1980s a number of activities have taken place in order to try to improve the quality of portal hypertension randomised trials (Table 52). The Baveno workshops [25–31], other portal hypertension workshops [32–34], The Cochrane Collaboration (www.cochrane.org), the CONSORT Statement (www.consort-statement.org), the International Committee on Harmonization – Good Clinical (Research) Practice (ICH – GCP) guidelines (www.ich.org) [35], The Cochrane Hepato-Biliary Group [36,37] and several other initiatives have been undertaken to improve the quality of randomised trials.

In this chapter we assess the sample size and the proportion with adequate quality components of portal hypertension randomised trials. We compare the findings with other fields of hepatology. Further, we analyse how the size and quality of portal hypertension randomised trials have developed during the last 20 years. Finally, we assess the number of trials having been registered in a publicly accessible trial register in a cohort of portal hypertension trials published as full paper articles during 2003 and 2004.

METHODS

Identification and selection of trials

We included trials described in two of our recent studies on the sample size and methodological quality of randomised clinical trials on portal hypertension and other fields of hepatology [23,24].

We also included full paper articles describing randomised clinical trials on interventions for portal hypertension published during 2003 and 2004. Trials were considered as randomised if some form of the word random was used to describe the allocation of patients. Articles referring to subgroups of patients from randomised trials were excluded.

The 2003 and 2004 trials were identified through hand searches of specialist journals and electronic searches (performed March 2005) of The Cochrane Hepato-Biliary Group (CHBG) Controlled Trials Register, The Cochrane Central Register of Controlled Trials on The Cochrane Library Issue 1, 2005 (www.cochrane.org) and MEDLINE. The following search strategies were used:

The CHBG Controlled Trials Register [37]: 'portal hypertensi*' OR 'bleeding varice*' OR gastropath* OR 'hepatic nephropath*' AND (#20 = 2003 OR #20 = 2004).

The Cochrane Library (www.cochrane.org): #1 hypertension portal explode all trees (MeSH), (#2 portal next hypertensi*), #3 bleeding, #4 varice*, #5 (#3 and #4), #6 (portal next hypertensive next gastropath*), #7 (hepatic next nephropath*), #8 (#1 or #2 or #5 or #6 or #7) (2003–2004).

MEDLINE: (portal hypertensi* OR Portal hypertension [MeSH] OR (varice* AND bleeding) OR portal hypertensive gastropath* OR hepatic nephropath*) AND random*, Limits: Publication Date from 2003 to 2004.

These searches identified a total of 45 references, of which 26 were full paper articles on portal hypertension trials published during 2003 and 2004 [38–63]. Additional searches on PubMed using the 'Related articles' link identified another three full paper articles on portal hypertension trials published during 2003 and 2004 [64–66].

Data extraction

We extracted type of interventions, quality, sample size calculations and number of included participants from the trials. Trial quality was assessed by whether the randomisation (allocation sequence generation and allocation concealment) and blinding methods were adequately performed and described [6]. The generation of the allocation sequence was defined as adequate if based on computer generated random numbers, table of random numbers or similar. The allocation concealment was defined as adequate if randomisation involved a central independent unit, serially numbered opaque sealed envelopes, identical coded drug bottles or similar. Trials in which investigators (outcome assessors or caretakers) and patients were kept unaware of treatment allocation by identical placebo, identically appearing active drugs or similar were classified as adequately double blinded. Data on blinding of outcome assessment or data analyses were also extracted. For trials published in 2003 and 2004 we also extracted information on any registration of the trial in a public trial register.

Statistical methods

Proportions were compared by the Chi-square for trend. Continuous variables were compared with the Kruskal-Wallis test. Significance was accepted at the $P \leq 0.05$ level.

RESULTS

Sample size

Compared to other disease areas of hepatology, portal hypertension randomised trials seem to be including relatively large samples of patients (Table 53). The median number of patients per intervention arm was 34 patients.

When evaluating the trend in portal hypertension randomised trials during the last 20 years, however, we could not find any significant signs of an improvement in the number of patients randomised (Fig. 49).

Sample size estimation

When evaluating the internal validity of a randomised trial it is important to know what the targeted sample size was. Otherwise, we do not know whether the data were reported before, at or after the targeted sample size was reached. Further, the sample size estimation can help readers to define the primary outcome measure of the trial.

Among the portal hypertension trials published in 2003 or in 2004, 19/29 (66%) reported a sample size estimation.

Table 53 Median number of patients per intervention arm in different disease areas of 616 hepato-biliary randomised trials published in 12 journals from 1985–1996. Based on Kjaergard and Gluud [23].

Disease area	Median number of patients per trial arm	5 to 95 percentiles
Alcoholic liver disease	36	6 to 149
Portal hypertension	34	9 to 88
Primary biliary cirrhosis	29	6 to 112
Hepatitis C	27	9 to 122
Hepatitis B	18	6 to 96
Cirrhosis	16	6 to 58
Hepatic encephalopathy	15	6 to 33
Miscellaneous	15	3 to 510
Autoimmune liver disease	12	6 to 41

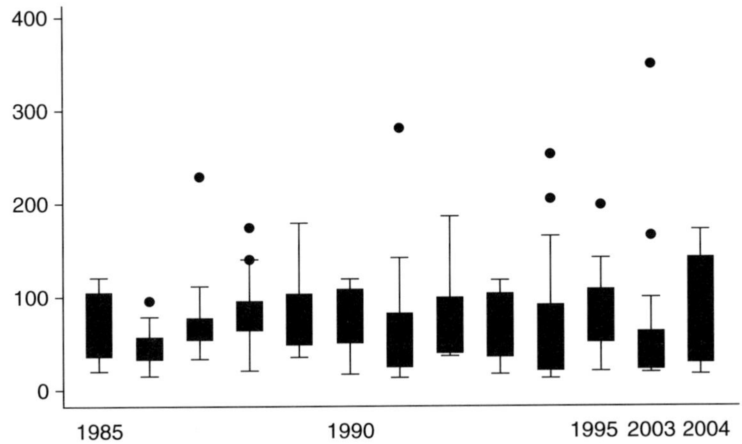

Fig. 49 Number of patients per intervention arm (bars are interquartile range, lines are 5 to 95 percentiles and dots are outliers) in 179 portal hypertension randomised trials published from 1985–2005. Data from the 150 trials published during 1985 to 1996 are from Kjaergard and Gluud [24] while data from the 29 trials published in 2003 and 2004 have been generated for this chapter.
$P = 0.25$ for trend.

Adequacy of generation of the allocation sequence

Compared to other fields of hepatology, portal hypertension randomised trials published in *Gastroenterology* seem to be the group of trials reporting

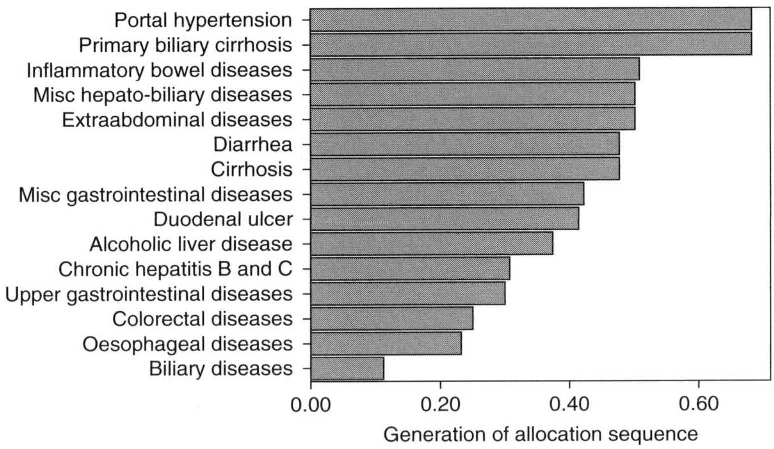

Fig. 50 Proportion of trials reporting adequate generation of allocation sequence in 383 randomised clinical trials published in gastroenterology from 1964 to 2000 stratified according to disease area. Data from Kjaergard *et al.* [23].

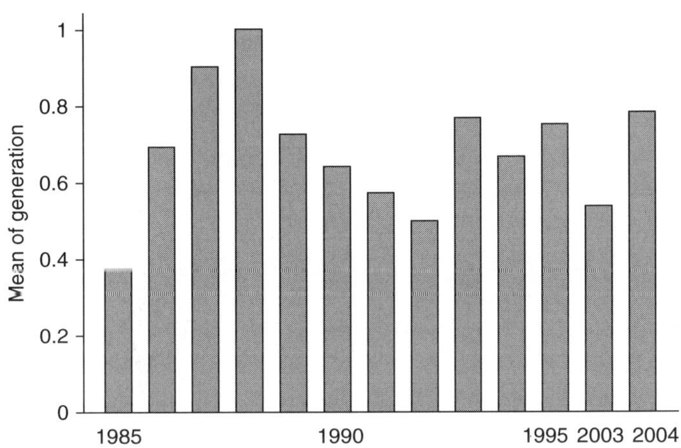

Fig. 51 Proportion of 179 portal hypertension randomised clinical trials reporting adequate generation of the allocation sequence. Data from the 150 trials published during 1985 to 1996 are from Kjaergard and Gluud [24] while data from the 29 trials published in 2003 and 2004 have been generated for this chapter. $P = 1.00$ for trend.

adequate generation of the allocation sequence most frequently, that is, 70% of the trials did so (Fig. 50).

However, the proportion of portal hypertension trials reporting adequate generation of the allocation sequence does not seem to improve significantly during the last 20 years (Fig. 51).

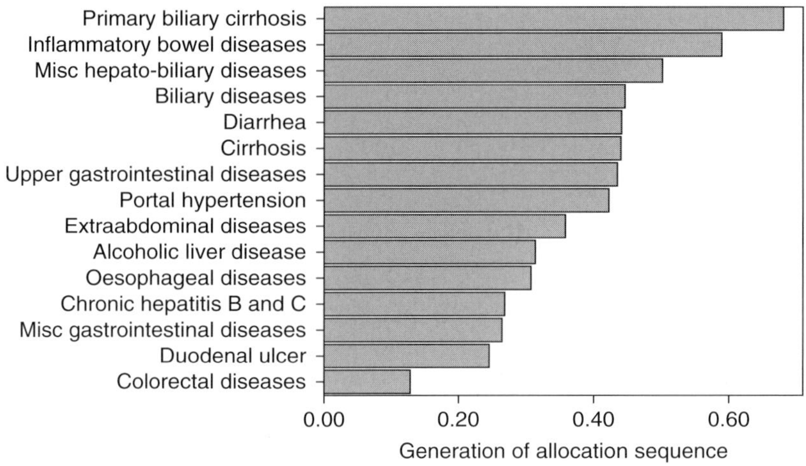

Fig. 52 Proportion of trials reporting adequate allocation concealment in 383 randomised clinical trials published in gastroenterology from 1964 to 2000 stratified according to disease area. Data from Kjaergard *et al.* [23].

Adequacy of the allocation concealment

Compared to other fields of hepatology, portal hypertension randomised trials seem to be the group of trials reporting adequate allocation concealment less frequently than a number of other disease areas, but more frequently than in other disease areas (Fig. 52).

However, the proportion of portal hypertension trials reporting adequate allocation concealment does not seem to improve significantly during the last 20 years (Fig. 53).

Balance at entry

Among the portal hypertension trials published in 2003 or in 2004, 26/29 randomised trials (90%) used significance tests for baseline comparisons.

Blinding

Compared to other fields of hepatology, portal hypertension randomised trials seem to be the group of trials reporting adequate double blinding less frequently than other disease areas, that is, only in 27% of the trials (Fig. 54).

The proportion of portal hypertension trials reporting adequate double blinding does not seem to improve significantly during the last 20 years (Fig. 55).

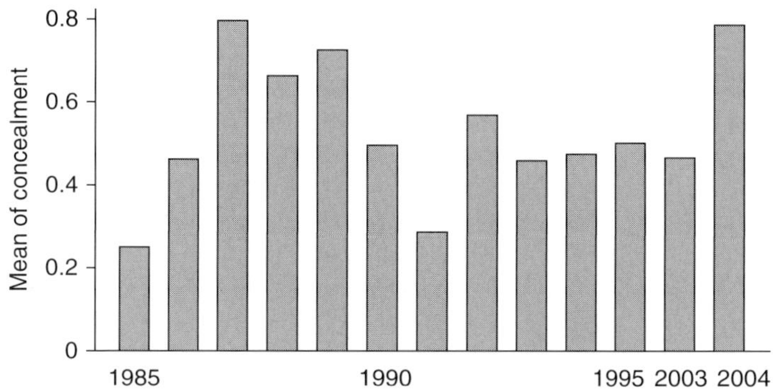

Fig. 53 Proportion of 179 portal hypertension randomised clinical trials reporting adequate allocation concealment. Data from the 150 trials published during 1985 to 1996 are from Kjaergard and Gluud [24] while data from the 29 trials published in 2003 and 2004 have been generated for this chapter. $P = 0.18$ for trend.

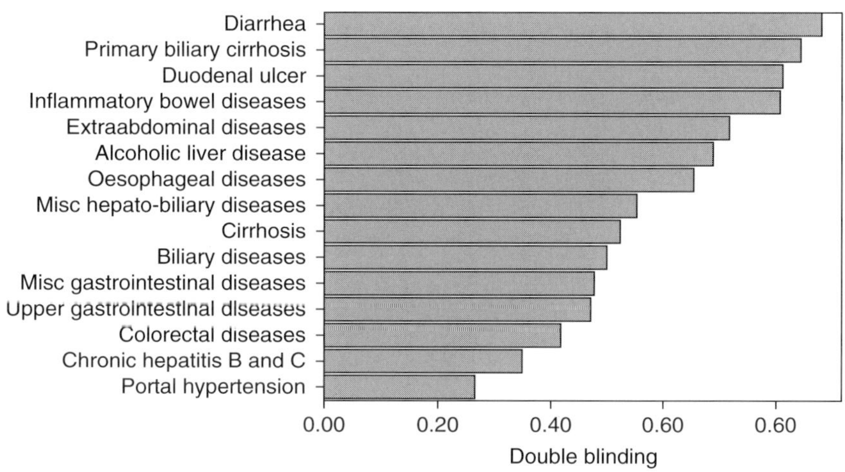

Fig. 54 Proportion of trials reporting adequate double blinding in 383 randomised clinical trials published in gastroenterology from 1964 to 2000 stratified according to disease area. Data from Kjaergard *et al.* [23].

Among the portal hypertension trials published in 2003 or in 2004, only 6/29 (21%) reported blinded outcome assessment.

ITT analysis

Among the portal hypertension trials published in 2003 or in 2004, 19/29 reported ITT analysis (66%).

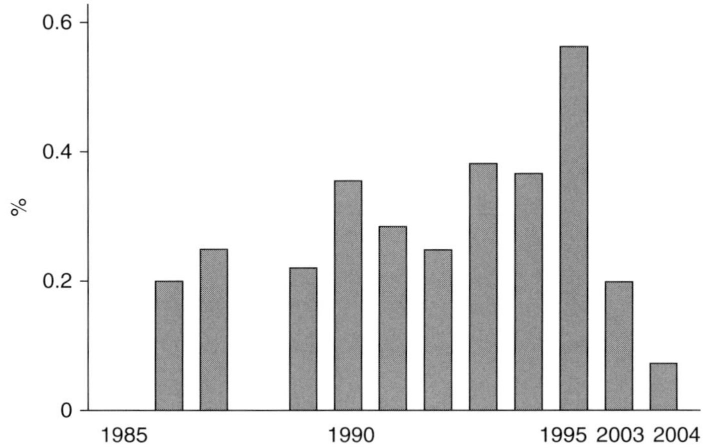

Fig. 55 Proportion of 179 portal hypertension randomised clinical trials reporting adequate double blinding. Data from the 150 trials published during 1985 to 1996 are from Kjaergard and Gluud [24] while data from the 29 trials published in 2003 and 2004 have been generated for this chapter. $P = 0.90$ for trend.

Trial registration

Among the portal hypertension trials published in 2003 or in 2004, only 1/29 reported registration at a publicly accessible trial register (3%) [59].

DISCUSSION AND CONCLUSIONS

During the last 20 years, the yearly publication rate of full paper articles on randomised clinical portal hypertension trials is about 15. This accomplishment is impressing, considering the conditions under which one conducts trials. These conditions have increased in complexity and costs during this time period. It is also very positive that about 2/3 portal hypertension randomised trials reported the sample size estimation, adequate generation of the allocation sequence and ITT analysis.

We are aware of the potential weaknesses of the present study. The number of trials assessed is relatively small, as is the span of time we have looked at. Therefore, we are not able to exclude that the reasons for us not observing a significant positive development may be due to type II errors. Our overall finding of no significant positive development over time is supported by recent findings in other studies [67,68].

The fact that 66% of portal hypertension trials reported sample size estimation is significantly better than the 7 to 26% previously reported for hepatobiliary randomised trials [30] and the 16% of 523 randomised clinical trials from a random sample of Cochrane Reviews [69]. It is also significantly better than the 27% of 519 PubMed-indexed randomised trials published in 2000 [68].

A very high proportion of portal hypertension trials – about 70% – reported adequate generation of the allocation sequence. This is significantly better than 24% of 523 randomised clinical trials from a random sample of Cochrane Reviews [69] and the 21% of 519 PubMed-indexed randomised trials published in 2000 [68].

The finding of 66% of the portal hypertension trials using ITT analyses is also better than the 27% of 523 randomised clinical trials from a random sample of Cochrane Reviews [69].

The above findings are very rewarding as they show that portal hypertension trialists conduct trials as one would hope. A number of our other findings seem, however, to leave ample room for improvements.

The median number of patients per intervention arm was only 34 patients, which showed no signs of improvement during the last 20 years. These small sample sizes are worrying. But small sample sizes are not confined to hepatobiliary trials. In 523 randomised trials from 41 randomly selected Cochrane reviews, we found a median of 52 participants per intervention arm [69]. In 519 PubMed-indexed randomised trials published in 2000, the median number was 32 participants per intervention arm [68]. With the noted median of about 34 patients, a two-group comparison has only about 40% power to detect a difference between event rates of 10% and 30% at the 0.05 significance level. The power may be further diminished by losses to follow-up. Inadequately powered trials have a high type II error rate. At the same time, small trials run the risk of type I errors due to unequal distribution of prognostically important factors in the randomised groups.

A total of 42% of the portal hypertension trials reported adequate allocation concealment. This proportion was higher in some areas of hepatology (e.g. primary biliary cirrhosis), but lower in others (e.g. hepatitis B and C). We were unable to detect any improvement in the reporting of allocation concealment in portal hypertension randomised trials during the last 20 years. In 523 randomised trials from 41 randomly selected Cochrane reviews, we found that only 28% reported adequate allocation concealment [69]. In 519 PubMed-indexed randomised trials published in 2000, only 18% reported adequate methods for allocation concealment [68]. Accordingly, it seems that portal hypertension trialists are better than a number of other fields in reporting adequately on allocation concealment, but they seem resistant to make further improvements. It has repeatedly been shown that publications of trials with unclear or inadequate allocation concealment are associated with a 20 to 30% exaggeration of the intervention effect [6–9,13]. Some studies have found that unclear reporting of allocation concealment does not necessarily mean unclear or inadequate conduct of allocation concealment, but that these studies have been on small and select groups of patients [70–72]. However, Liberati *et al.* [73] and Pildal *et al.* [74] observed that unclear reporting of allocation concealment was connected with unclear or inadequate methodology in about 80% of trials.

Only about 25% of randomised trials on portal hypertension were double blind. This is significantly less than in other disease areas of gastroenterology [23]. In 523 randomised trials from randomly selected Cochrane reviews, we found that 49% were double blind or had blinded outcome assessment [69]. In 519 PubMed-indexed randomised trials published in 2000, 60% reported any blinding [68]. Due to the nature of many interventions for portal hypertension, double blinding (i.e. blinding of both patient and caregivers) may not be feasible. Only blinding of all involved in a trial can secure that reporting bias, performance bias, assessment bias, attrition bias and other bias do not occur. All trials, which cannot blind interventions with a placebo or a sham, can use blinded outcome assessment. This may reduce assessment and attrition bias.

Balance is an important issue in the entry data of patients in a randomised clinical trial. Such balance among known and unknown prognostic indicators is sought through a sufficiently large number of patients and an adequate randomisation, that is, adequate generation of the allocation sequence and adequate allocation concealment [6–9,13]. Testing for imbalance of entry variables is not recommended [12,75]. However, 9/10 portal hypertension trials tested for entry imbalance.

We have focused on some quality measures of randomised trials. One should also know other aspects of trials, for example, who is the sponsor. Studies have shown that trial interpretation and conclusions may be influenced by the sponsor of the trial [76–79]. The whole issue of the influence of the drug and device industry on medical research has gained increasing attention in recent years [80]. Increased government funding of independent and transparent research seems urgently needed [80].

In our sample of 2003 and 2004 portal hypertension randomised trials we only observed one trial that was registered in one of the two international trial registers (www.clinicaltrials.gov and www.controlled-trials.com) that are currently supported by the WHO (http://www.who.int/ictrp/en/). Such trial registration should be considered mandatory in the future, as this is the only way we can secure that publication bias [14–18] and outcome measure bias [19,20] can be reduced in the future.

Portal hypertension trials seem to be robust to the number of conferences, workshops and publications held and written in order to improve the quality of portal hypertension trials. This has also been observed regarding randomised trials in other disease areas [67–69,81]. If international meetings, workshops, consensus conferences, guidelines and instructions for authors are not enough for changing the practice of clinical research we have to consider other measures. Ethics review boards, national and international medicines agencies, peer reviewers and medical editors could be involved more with quality assurance. There seems to be a large educational task in getting these groups to understand the importance of reducing risks of random as well as systematic errors. The CONSORT (Consolidated Standards of Reporting Trials) statement of 1996, updated in 2001, gives recommendations for reporting randomised trials and has been endorsed by the World Association of Medical Editors, the International Committee of Medical Journal Editors (ICMJE) and the Council of Science Editors [82]. In 2003, 36/167 (22%) of high impact medical journals referred to CONSORT in their advice to authors [82]. The uptake of CONSORT by leading journals is encouraging, but 11/36 referred to a superseded version of CONSORT [82]. The beneficial effects of the CONSORT statement can only be obtained if journal editors use the full and updated version of the CONSORT statement.

Competing interests: CG and LLG are editors of The Cochrane Hepato-Biliary Group. SLK is trials search coordinator of The Cochrane Hepato-Biliary Group. CG is directing the Copenhagen Trial Unit, which is a not-for-profit, public clinical trials service unit and has an interest in increasing the awareness of the scientific strengths of randomised clinical trials and meta-analyses.

REFERENCES

1 Sackett DL, Straus SE, Richardson WS, Rosenberg W, Haynes RB. *Evidence-based medicine, how to practise and teach EBM*. 2nd edn, Edingburgh, Churchill Livingstone, 2000.

2 Hayward, Robert, electronic editor. Users' guides interactive, Chicago (IL): JAMA Publishing Group; 2002 [cited 2005 05 06]. Available from: http://www.usersguides.org.

3 Gluud C, Gluud LL. Evidence based diagnostics. *BMJ* 2005;**330**: 724–726.

4 Kjaergard LL, Nikolova D, Gluud C. Randomised clinical trials in HEPATOLOGY: predictors of quality. *Hepatology* 1999;**30**: 1134–1138.

5 Schulz KF, Chalmers I, Hayes RJ, Altman DG. Empirical evidence of bias. Dimensions of methodological quality associated with estimates of treatment effects in controlled trials. *JAMA* 1995;**273**: 408–412.

6 Moher D, Pham B, Jones A, Cook DJ, Jadad AR *et al.* Does quality of reports of randomised trials affect estimates of intervention efficacy reported in meta-analyses? *Lancet* 1998;**352**: 609–613.
7 Kjaergard LL, Villumsen J, Gluud C. Reported methodological quality and discrepancies between large and small randomised trials in meta-analyses. *Ann Intern Med* 2001;**135**: 982–989.
8 Balk EM, Boris PA, Moskowitz H, Schmid CH, Ioannidis JP *et al.* Correlation of quality measures with estimates of treatment effect in meta-analyses of randomised controlled trials. *JAMA* 2002;**287**: 2973–2982.
9 Als-Nielsen B, Chen W, Gluud LL, Siersma V, Hilden J *et al.* Are trial size and quality associated with treatment effects in randomised trials? Observational study of 523 randomised trials (abstract). *12th International Cochrane Colloquium*, Ottawa 2004: 102–103.
10 Deeks JJ, Dinnes J, D'Amico R, Sowden AJ, Sakarovitch C *et al.* Evaluating non-randomised intervention studies. *Health Technol Assess* 2003;**7**(27): iii–x, 1–173.
11 Kjaergard LL, Liu J, Als-Nielsen B, Gluud C. Artificial and bioartificial support systems for acute and acute-on-chronic liver failure: a systematic review. *JAMA* 2003;**289**(2): 217–222.
12 Pocock SJ. *Clinical trials – A practical approach*. Chichester, John Wiley and Sons, 1996.
13 Als-Nielsen B, Gluud LL, Gluud C. Methodological quality and treatment effects in randomised trials – a review of six empirical studies (abstract). *12th International Cochrane Colloquium*, Ottawa 2004: 88–89.
14 Simes RJ. The case for an international registry of clinical trials. *J Clin Oncol* 1986;**4**: 1529–1541.
15 Dickersin K. Report from the panel on the case for registers of clinical trials at the Eighth Annual Meeting of the Society for Clinical Trials. *Control Clin Trials* 1988;**9**: 76–81.
16 Gluud C. 'Negative trials' are positive! *J Hepatol* 1998;**28**(4): 731–733.
17 Dickersin K, Rennie D. Registering clinical trials. *JAMA* 2003;**290**: 516–523.
18 Krleza-Jeric K, Chan AW, Dickersin K, Sim I, Grimshaw J *et al.* Principles for international registration of protocol information and results from human trials of health related interventions: Ottawa statement (part 1). *BMJ* 2005;**330**(7497): 956–958.
19 Chan AW, Hrobjartsson A, Haahr MT, Gøtzsche PC, Altman DG. Empirical evidence for selective reporting of outcomes in randomised trials: comparison of protocols to published articles. *JAMA* 2004;**291**(20): 2457–2465.
20 Chan AW, Krleza-Jeric K, Schmid I, Altman DG. Outcome reporting bias in randomised trials funded by the Canadian Institutes of Health Research. *CMAJ* 2004;**171**(7): 735–740.
21 Gluud C. Evidence based medicine in Liver. *Liver* 1999;**19**: 1–2.
22 Gluud C, Nikolova D. Quality assessment of reports on clinical trials in the Journal of Hepatology. *J Hepatol* 1998;**29**: 321–327.
23 Kjaergard LL, Frederiksen SL, Gluud C. Validity of randomised clinical trials in Gastroenterology from 1964–2000. *Gastroenterology* 2002;**122**: 1157–1160.

24 Kjaergard LL, Gluud C. Funding, disease area, and internal validity of hepatobiliary randomised clinical trials. *Am J Gastroenterol* 2002;**97**: 2708–2713.
25 De Franchis R, Pascal JP, Ancona E *et al.* Definitions, methodology and therapeutic strategies in portal hypertension. A consensus development workshop, Baveno, Lake Maggiore, Italy, April 5 and 6, 1990. *J Hepatol* 1992; **15**: 256–261.
26 De Franchis R ed. *Portal Hypertension II. Proceedings of the second Baveno international consensus workshop on definitions, methodology and therapeutic strategies.* Oxford, Blackwell Science Ltd, 1996.
27 De Franchis R ed. *Portal Hypertension III. Proceedings of the third Baveno international consensus workshop on definitions, methodology and therapeutic strategies.* Oxford, Blackwell Science Ltd, 2001.
28 Becker U, Burroughs AK, Calés P *et al.* Trials in portal hypertension: valid meta-analyses and valid randomised clinical trials. *Portal Hypertension II* (De Franchis R ed) Oxford, Blackwell Science Ltd, 1996; 180–209.
29 Gluud C, Becker U, Burroughs AK *et al.* Baveno II Consensus Statements: Trials in Portal Hypertension.*Portal Hypertension II* (de Franchis R ed) Oxford, Blackwell Science Ltd, 1996; 210.
30 Gluud C, Kjaergard LL. Quality of randomised clinical trials in portal hypertension and other fields of hepatology. *Portal Hypertension III* (de Franchis R ed) Oxford, Blackwell Science Ltd, 2001; 204–218.
31 Sørensen TIA, D'Amico G, van Buuren H *et al.* Methodology of future trials: prognostic stratification, health-related quality of life and health economics. *Portal Hypertension III* (De Franchis R ed) Oxford, Blackwell Science Ltd 2001, 219–239.
32 Burroughs AK. *Methodology and reviews of clinical trials in portal hypertension.* Amsterdam, Excerpta Medica, 1987.
33 Spina GP, Arcidiacono R, Bosch J, Pagliaro L, Burroughs AK *et al.* Gastric endoscopic features in portal hypertension: final report of a consensus conference, Milan, Italy, September 19, 1992. *J Hepatol* 1994;**21**(3): 461–467.
34 Grace ND, Groszmann RJ, Garcia-Tsao G, Burroughs AK, Pagliaro L *et al.* Portal hypertension and variceal bleeding: an AASLD single topic symposium. *Hepatology* 1998;**28**(3): 868–880.
35 International Conference on Harmonisation Steering Committee. *ICH Harmonised Tripartite Guideline. General Considerations for Clinical Trials.* http://www.ich.org/pdfICH/e8.pdf (accessed 7 May 2005).
36 Gluud C, Als-Nielsen B, D'Amico G, Gluud LL, Khan S *et al. The Cochrane Hepato-Biliary Group. About The Cochrane Collaboration (Collaborative Review Groups (CRGs)).* The Cochrane Library 2005, Issue 2.
37 Gluud C on behalf of the Cochrane Hepato-Biliary Editorial Team. The Cochrane Hepato-Biliary Group. In: Bircher J, Benhamou JP, McIntyre N *et al.* (eds). *Oxford Textbook of Clinical Hepatology 2nd edn*, Oxford, Oxford University Press, 1999; 2145–2148.
38 Abecasis R, Kravetz D, Fassio E, Ameigeiras B, Garcia D *et al.* Nadolol plus spironolactone in the prophylaxis of first variceal bleed in nonascitic cirrhotic patients: a preliminary study. *Hepatology* 2003;**37**(2): 359–365.
39 Avgerinos A, Armonis A, Stefanidis G, Mathou N, Vlachogiannakos J *et al.* Sustained rise of portal pressure after sclerotherapy, but not band ligation, in acute variceal bleeding in cirrhosis. *Hepatology* 2004;**39**(6): 1623–1630.

40 Bellis L, Berzigotti A, Abraldes JG, Moitinho E, Garcia-Pagan JC *et al.* Low doses of isosorbide mononitrate attenuate the postprandial increase in portal pressure in patients with cirrhosis. *Hepatology* 2003;**37**(2): 378–384.
41 Bosch J, Thabut D, Bendtsen F, D'Amico G, Albillos A *et al.* Recombinant factor VIIa for upper gastrointestinal bleeding in patients with cirrhosis: a randomised, double-blind trial. *Gastroenterology* 2004;**127**(4): 1123–1130.
42 Castano G, Viudez P, Riccitelli M, Sookoian S. A randomised study of losartan vs propranolol: effects on hepatic and systemic hemodynamics in cirrhotic patients. *Ann Hepatol* 2003;**2**(1): 36–40.
43 De BK, Bandyopadhyay K, Das TK, Das D, Biswas PK *et al.* Portal pressure response to losartan compared with propranolol in patients with cirrhosis. *Am J Gastroenterol* 2003;**98**(6): 1371–1376.
44 Dong YH, Lu YF, Qiu Q, Huang H, Wei H. Clinical analysis of pericardial devascularization by preserving vagus trunks in 42 patients with portal hypertension. *Asian Journal of Surgery* 2004;**27**(2): 108–113.
45 Evrard S, Dumonceau JM, Delhaye M, Golstein P, Deviere J *et al.* Endoscopic histoacryl obliteration vs. propranolol in the prevention of esophagogastric variceal rebleeding: a randomised trial. *Endoscopy* 2003;**35**(9): 729–735.
46 Garcia-Pagan JC, Morillas R, Banares R, Albillos A, Villanueva C *et al.* Propranolol plus placebo versus propranolol plus isosorbide-5-mononitrate in the prevention of a first variceal bleed: a double-blind RCT. *Hepatology* 2003;**37**(6): 1260–1266.
47 Hou MC, Lin HC, Liu TT, Kuo BI, Lee FY *et al.* Antibiotic prophylaxis after endoscopic therapy prevents rebleeding in acute variceal hemorrhage: a randomised trial. *Hepatology* 2004;**39**(3): 746–753.
48 Lee HY, Lee HJ, Lee SM, Kim JH, Kweon SW *et al.* A prospective randomised controlled clinical trial comparing the effects of somatostatin and vasopressin for control of acute variceal bleeding in the patients with liver cirrhosis. *Korean J Intern Med* 2003;**18**(3): 161–166.
49 Lin HC, Yang YY, Hou MC, Huang YT, Lee FY *et al.* Acute administration of carvedilol is more effective than propranolol plus isosorbide-5-mononitrate in the reduction of portal pressure in patients with viral cirrhosis. *Am J Gastroenterol* 2004;**99**(10): 1953–1958.
50 Lo GH, Chen WC, Chen MH, Lin CP, Lo CC *et al.* Endoscopic ligation vs. nadolol in the prevention of first variceal bleeding in patients with cirrhosis. *Gastrointest Endosc* 2004;**59**(3): 333–338.
51 Mandell MS, Durham J, Kumpe D, Trotter JF, Everson GT *et al.* The effects of desflurane and propofol on portosystemic pressure in patients with portal hypertension. *Anesth Analg* 2003;**97**(6): 1573–1577.
52 Merkel C, Marin R, Angeli P, Zanella P, Felder M *et al.* A placebo-controlled clinical trial of nadolol in the prophylaxis of growth of small esophageal varices in cirrhosis. *Gastroenterology* 2004;**127**(2): 476–484.
53 Monescillo A, Martinez-Lagares F, Ruiz-del-Arbol L, Sierra A, Guevara C *et al.* Influence of portal hypertension and its early decompression by TIPS placement on the outcome of variceal bleeding. *Hepatology* 2004;**40**(4): 793–801.
54 Rosemurgy AS, Zervos EE, Bloomston M, Durkin AJ, Clark WC *et al.* Post-shunt resource consumption favors small-diameter prosthetic H-graft portacaval

shunt over TIPS for patients with poor hepatic reserve. *Ann Surg* 2003;**237**(6): 820–827.

55 Schepke M, Kleber G, Nurnberg D, Willert J, Koch L *et al.* Ligation versus propranolol for the primary prophylaxis of variceal bleeding in cirrhosis. *Hepatology* 2004;**40**(1): 65–72.

56 Schiedermaier P, Koch L, Stoffel-Wagner B, Layer G, Sauerbruch T. Effect of propranolol and depot lanreotide SR on postprandial and circadian portal haemodynamics in cirrhosis. *Aliment Pharmacol Ther* 2003;**18**(8): 777–784.

57 Tomikawa M, Shimabukuro R, Okita K, Tsutsumi N, Akahoshi T *et al.* Propranolol alone may not be acceptable to prevent first esophageal variceal bleeding in Japanese cirrhotic patients: randomised controlled trial. *J Gastroenterol Hepatol* 2004;**19**(5): 576–581.

58 Tripathi D, Lui HF, Helmy A, Dabos K, Forrest E *et al.* Randomised controlled trial of long term portographic follow up versus variceal band ligation following transjugular intrahepatic portosystemic stent shunt for preventing oesophageal variceal rebleeding. *Gut* 2004;**53**(3): 431–437.

59 van Buuren HR, Rasch MC, Batenburg PL, Bolwerk CJ, Nicolai JJ *et al.* Endoscopic sclerotherapy compared with no specific treatment for the primary prevention of bleeding from esophageal varices. A randomised controlled multicentre trial. *BMC Gastroenterol* 2003;**3**(1): 22.

60 Venon WD, Baronio M, Leone N, Rolfo E, Fadda M *et al.* Effects of long-term Irbesartan in reducing portal pressure in cirrhotic patients: comparison with propranolol in a randomised controlled study. *J Hepatol* 2003;**38**(4): 455–460.

61 Weston BR, Chadalawada V, Chalasani N, Kwo P, Overley CA *et al.* Nurse-administered propofol versus midazolam and meperidine for upper endoscopy in cirrhotic patients. *Am J Gastroenterol* 2003;**98**(11): 2440–2447.

62 Zafra C, Abraldes JG, Turnes J, Berzigotti A, Fernandez M *et al.* Simvastatin enhances hepatic nitric oxide production and decreases the hepatic vascular tone in patients with cirrhosis. *Gastroenterology* 2004;**126**(3): 749–755.

63 Pomier-Layrargues G, Paquin SC, Hassoun Z, Lafortune M, Tran A. Octreotide in hepatorenal syndrome: a randomised, double-blind, placebo-controlled, crossover study. *Hepatology* 2003;**38**(1): 238–243.

64 Salerno F, Merli M, Riggio O, Cazzaniga M, Valeriano V *et al.* Randomised controlled study of TIPS versus paracentesis plus albumin in cirrhosis with severe ascites. *Hepatology* 2004;**40**(3): 629–635.

65 Cordoba J, Lopez-Hellin J, Planas M, Sabin P, Sanpedro F *et al.* Normal protein diet for episodic hepatic encephalopathy: results of a randomised study. *J Hepatol* 2004;**41**(1): 38–43.

66 Rosemurgy AS, Zervos EE, Clark WC, Thometz DP, Black TJ *et al.* TIPS versus peritoneovenous shunt in the treatment of medically intractable ascites: a prospective randomised trial. *Ann Surg* 2004;**239**(6): 883–891.

67 Meinert CL, Tonascia S, Higgins K. Content of reports on clinical trials: a critical review. *Control Clin Trials* 1984;**5**: 328–347.

68 Chan A-W, Altman DG. Epidemiology and reporting of randomised trials published in PubMed journals. *The Lancet* 2005;**365**: 1159–1162.

69 Als-Nielsen B, Chen W, Gluud C, Gluud LL. Characteristics of randomised clinical trials in Cochrane reviews. *Unpublished observations* 2005.

70 Hill CL, LaValley MP, Felson DT. Discrepancy between published report and actual conduct of randomised clinical trials. *J Clin Epidemiol* 2002;**55**: 783–786.
71 Devereaux PJ, Choi PT, El-Dika S, Bhandari M, Montori VM *et al.* An observational study found that authors of randomised controlled trials frequently use concealment of randomization and blinding, despite the failure to report these methods. *J Clin Epidemiol* 2004;**57**: 1232–1236.
72 Soares HP, Daniels S, Kumar A, Clarke M, Scott C *et al.* Bad reporting does not mean bad methods for randomised trials: observational study of randomised controlled trials performed by the Radiation Therapy Oncology Group. *BMJ* 2004;**328**: 22–24.
73 Liberati A, Himel HN, Chalmers TC. A quality assessment of randomised control trials of primary treatment of breast cancer. *J Clin Oncol* 1986;**4**: 942–951.
74 Pildal J, Chan A-W, Hróbjartsson A, Forfang E, Altman DG *et al.* Comparison of descriptions of allocation concealment in trial protocols and the published reports: cohort study. *BMJ* 2005;**330**: 1049.
75 Assmann SF, Pocock SJ, Enos LE, Kasten LE. Subgroup analysis and other (mis)uses of baseline data in clinical trials. *Lancet* 2000;**355**(9209): 1064–1069.
76 Kjaergard LL, Als-Nielsen B. Association between competing interests and authors' conclusions: epidemiological study of randomised clinical trials published in the BMJ. *BMJ* 2002;**325**: 249.
77 Als-Nielsen B, Chen W, Gluud C, Kjaergard LL. Association of funding and conclusions in randomised drug trials: a reflection of treatment effect or adverse events? *JAMA* 2003;**290**: 921–928.
78 Bekelman JE, Li Y, Gross CP. Scope and impact of financial conflicts of interest in biomedical research: a systematic review. *JAMA* 2003;**289**: 454–465.
79 Lexchin J, Bero LA, Djulbegovic B, Clark O. Pharmaceutical industry sponsorship and research outcome and quality: systematic review. *BMJ* 2003;**326**: 1167–1170.
80 House of Commons Health Committee. The Influence of the Pharmaceutical Industry. Fourth Report of Session 2004–05. Volume I (http://www.publications.parliament.uk/pa/cm200405/cmselect/cmhealth/42/4202.htm).
81 Gluud C. Trials and errors in clinical research. *Lancet* 1999;**354**: SIV59.
82 Altman DG. Endorsement of the CONSORT statement by high impact medical journals: survey of instructions for authors. *BMJ* 2005;**330**: 1056–1057.

LECTURE

Value and Limits of Evidence-Based Medicine (EBM)

Luigi Pagliaro

The origins and development of EBM

Concerns about medical practice

The interest around EBM has been focused by the belief that it might alleviate the concerns about health care raised in recent years [1,2]. The concerns regard the quality of medical practice, the unwarranted variation in the rates of use of medical procedures and the deterioration of the doctors' competence along their professional life, as reported in the next points.

- There is evidence that the quality of medical practice is not fully consistent with updated medical knowledge. Diagnostic and therapeutic practices of proven effectiveness are often underused, whereas others are overused in comparison with generally accepted guidelines, and misuse of both may result in avoidable complications [3,4].
- An indicator of these inconsistencies is the well demonstrated existence of wide variations in clinical practice, not explained by patients' characteristics or preferences, and related to local clinical routine, to the doctors' specialty, to the availability or lack of resources, to socio-economic differences and other factors [3–6].
- Both these problems are increased by the pace of clinical research that is faster than the translation of its products into practice, so generating a gap between research and practice [7].
- And finally, there is evidence that the doctors' competence tends to deteriorate over time [8,9], and that doctors who have been practising longer may provide lower-quality care, raising the need for better methods of continuing medical education.

EBM as a (partial) solution

- EBM, introduced in 1992 as a 'new paradigm of medicine' [10], might contribute to alleviate these problems by educating the doctors to link their

Table 54 The 5 steps of EBM (from ref. 16).

1. Asking answerable questions
2. Finding the best evidence
3. Critically appraising the evidence
4. Acting on the evidence
5. Evaluating your performance

Table 55 The 5 steps of EBM (from ref. 17).

1. Asking answerable questions
2. Finding the best evidence from prefiltered sources
3. Judging whether it applies to the health problem at hand
4. Acting on the evidence
5. Evaluating your performance

decisions to a common basis of scientific evidence, with the two-fold effect of improving the quality of medical practice and limiting its unwarranted variations. With this aim, EBM has produced a large amount of educational material, teaching how to search, appraise and use clinical studies from the medical literature [8,10–14]. Initially, the EBM Working Group assumed that 'physicians can gain the skills to make *independent* assessments of evidence, and thus evaluate the credibility of opinions being offered by experts' [10]. Thus, the initial educational target of EBM focused on the individual doctors, aiming to teach them how to link their practice with the research evidence ('the Era of Optimism' [15]), following the 5 steps of Table 54.

• The subsequent experience has shown that very few doctors have sufficient time and motivation to face the 'largely hopeless task' [17] of learning how to search and appraise *independently* the original medical literature to find out the evidence about best care [18,19]. Accordingly, the EBM advocates have changed their mind, and now propose that most doctors can practice evidence-based medicine using secondary publications, reviews and guidelines prefiltered and preassessed by experts [17–19], as shown in Table 55: 'the Era of Innocence Lost and Regained' [15].

• This change respected the principle that use of research evidence would improve the doctors' professional behaviour and the quality of practice, but neglected another principle of EBM, that is, the development of doctors' intellectual independence from an authority, a role now taken over by 'informationists' who not necessarily have clinical expertise.

• Guidelines, an increasingly published kind of prefiltered evidence, have a mixed effect on the doctors' practice. There is evidence that at least in some countries the national guidelines are followed by about 60% of general practitioners [20], and that doctors' compliance with guidelines can sometimes improve clinical practice [21]. However, there are many barriers to the physicians' guideline adherence [22]: guidelines are unlikely to be followed and are less effective when they are complex, lengthy, difficult to remember and use and lack of a local active educational input [23]. Furthermore, the attempt to standardise care by guidelines must take into account the heterogeneity of patients, and must be adapted to the local setting and the complexity of medical decisions [24].

• Finally, there is extensive evidence that isolated dissemination of information is of modest value to change the doctors' behaviour, and should be integrated in multifaceted strategies encompassing group interactive educational meetings, continuity, involvement of local opinion leaders [25–28], and perhaps a disease-specific approach, for example, not the same for diabetes and hypertension [29]. Furthermore, the doctors' behaviour is only a component of the quality of healthcare, that also depends on organization, access to care and equity of the healthcare system of a country [30].

Value and limitations of EBM in the individual patient care

Medical practice has 3 components: patient-doctor relationship, diagnosis and therapeutic decisions

• The doctors' attitude to establish a proper relationship with patients is a critical attribute of good practice [31,32], the germ of which should be conveyed to the students by the clinical teachers during the years of school, and then developed and maintained along the professional life. However, there is evidence that the natural empathy and patient-centred attitude of medical students *decline* as they progress along the clinical curriculum [33–37], and that patients frequently complain about inappropriate doctors' behaviour, stressing disrespect, poor communication and insufficient availability [36,37]. Although this area clearly requires attention, there is nothing in the EBM-related educational initiative to foster the doctors' attitude to establish a positive and humane relationship with the patients.

• The memorised knowledge of the doctors is sufficient to make diagnostic and therapeutic decisions when they are familiar with the pathology. However, in around 2 of 3 clinical encounters, mostly with patients with unfamiliar diseases or clinical presentations, the doctors need new information, and ask questions to solve the problem [38]. This is the starting point of the possible help by EBM to the individual doctor.

Table 56 Questions from primary care doctors asked in clinical encounters, and their frequency (from ref. 39).

Question	Rank	% of questions
What is the drug of choice for condition X?	1st	11
What is the cause of symptom X?	2nd	8
What test is indicated in situation X?	3rd	8
What is dose of drug X?	4th	7
How should I treat condition X (not limited to drug treatment)	5th	6
How should I manage condition X (not specifying diagnostic or therapeutic)?	6th	5
What is the cause of physical finding X?	7th	5
What is the cause of test finding X?	8th	5
Can drug X cause (adverse) finding Y?	9th	4
Could this patient have condition X?	10th	4

Doctors' needs of clinical information

• As shown in Table 56, the doctors ask a number of questions that are almost equally divided between diagnosis and therapy.

In contrast, EBM (and many guidelines) mostly provides evidence about therapy, with limited information about diagnosis, almost exclusively dealing with the choice and interpretation of diagnostic tests (Table 57).

Underrepresented in the EBM sources are issues describing the clinical presentation of diseases to be memorised and used as template to match with the findings elicited in a patient. Definitely lacking are examples of the cognitive process of diagnostic reasoning from the clinical presentation to the generation of working hypotheses, although this is a critical step to orient the search of further information [43]. The 'meat' [44] to help a clinician to reach a difficult diagnosis must be searched in other sources. A journal specialised in the publication of excellent articles describing the clinical presentation of diseases is Medicine (Baltimore) (e.g. [45,46]); useful descriptive information is more or less often reported in many journals (e.g. *New Engl J Med, Lancet, JAMA, Mayo Clin Proc* and others). Diagnostic reasoning is exemplified in the cases of the series *Clinical Problem Solving* (e.g. [47,48]) published by the *New Engl J Med*, and in those of the book on *Learning Clinical Reasoning* by Kassirer and Kopelman [43].

• The largest part of the EBM-related literature is aimed at answering questions about the choice of treatments. Prefiltered therapeutic evidence, essentially from RCTs and systematic reviews of RCTs, is summarised in Clinical

Table 57 Therapy and diagnosis in some prefiltered publications of (or recommended by) EBM.

Paper-based and/or online publication	Content
The Cochrane Database of Systematic Reviews (CDSR)	Systematic reviews (SRs, meta-analyses) of RCTs
Clinical Evidence [40]	A monthly updated compendium of treatments, based on RCTs & SRs
ACP J Club	Around 80% of summaries are about therapy; 6% are about diagnosis; the remaining are about other issues (a mean of 2003–2005 issues)
Evidence-based medicine	≅ as ACP J Club
Diagnostic strategies for common medical problems [41]	A highly valuable textbook about the diagnostic tests, produced by the American College of Physicians and 'adopted' the EBM CD-ROM Best Evidence 4 & 5
The evidence base of clinical diagnosis [42]	12 essays on the evaluation and methodology of tests (only 1 essay on the cognitive aspects of the diagnosis)

Evidence, in the commented summaries of ACP Journal Club and Evidence-Based Medicine and in other evidence-based specialty journals (e.g. E-B Mental Health, E-B Gastroenterology, E-B Obstetrics and Gynaecology, others). A source applying the principles of EBM is the Cochrane Database of Systematic Reviews (CDSR). The full text of the reviews is too long and cumbersome for clinical use; the abstracts can be of use although very brief, and are free online [49]. A disadvantage of all these sources is that the information is not systematically ordered (e.g. in chapters, as in a textbook), and its search may be lengthy and not always successful.

RCTs as an incomplete evidence

• The randomised clinical trial (RCT) is generally recognised as the most reliable instrument to determine the effect of a treatment, and is the only source of therapeutic evidence accepted by EBM. RCTs must have internal validity (i.e. must be properly designed to avoid bias), but to be clinically useful they must also have external validity (or generalisability), and their applicability to an individual patient must be contextualised [50]. The RCTs

Table 58 Some post-marketing drug withdrawals or warnings for adverse events not detected by pre-registration RCTs.

Drugs	References
Fenfluramine, Dexfenfluramine	Withdrawn, 1997; see JAMA 2000; 283: 1738–1740
Mibefradil	Circulation 1998; 98: 831–832
Cisapride	JAMA 2000; 283: 2228
Troglitazone	JAMA 2000; 283: 2228
Alosetron	Lancet 2001; 357: 1544–1545
Cerivastatin	BMJ 2001; 323: 359
Nimesulide (Finland, Spain)	BMJ 2003; 327: 18–22
Coxibs: withdrawn, or admitted with black-box warnings	N Engl J Med 2005; 352: 1283–1285

recruit selected samples of patients with a disease or a subcategory of disease, and the treatment effect in these patients may not be repeated in those encountered in real practice, for example, for differences in gender, genetic characteristics, race, severity of disease, comorbidity and clinical setting. For instance, primary prevention with aspirin lowers myocardial infarction risk in men, but not in women [51]; there is genetically determined heterogeneity in the glycaemic response to oral antidiabetic drugs [52]; the antihypertensive effect of ACE inhibitors and angiotensin-receptor blockers is blunted in blacks [53]; the benefit of endarterectomy is strongly associated with the severity of carotid stenosis [54]; chronic obstructive pulmonary disease or asthma may contraindicate β-blockers for otherwise appropriate indications; high quality of setting and operators may be crucial to obtain good patients' outcomes [50].

• RCTs are not very efficient in detecting or accurate in reporting drug adverse reactions [55,56]. Most of them emerge post marketing in the real practice, sometimes leading to the withdrawal of drugs more harmful than beneficial (Table 58). RCTs of these drugs, often enrolling cumulative sample sizes of thousands patients, had failed to detect the adverse reactions.

• EBM has published a large amount of material teaching how to appraise RCTs and systematic reviews, for example, procedure and concealment of randomisation, follow-up, analysis and others. Although indispensable, these criteria are insufficient. Most large, multicenter, multinational RCTs are sponsored by the industry, and may suffer from influences causing a systematic exaggeration of the clinical value of new treatments. This influence, that could be impossible without the participation of the academy [57,58], is manifold, for example, it may originate from the comparison of the experimental drug with an inferior comparator [59]; from composite end points, where the treatment effect on a major outcome cannot be easily discerned by the effect on others, less important [60]; from publication bias, causing the disappearance of the less favourable RCTs [61]; from outcome reporting bias, that is, the discrepancy between the protocol and the published selective results [62]; from claims in discussion unwarranted by the results [63], and other mechanisms. As a consequence, the industry-sponsored RCTs have percentages of positive results higher than those non-industry sponsored [64, 65], raising the suspect that some of them may be at least in part falsely positive.

EBM: conclusive remarks

• The two key principles of EBM are that medical decisions must be supported by valid and ready evidence from research, and that any clinical evidence presented to the doctors must report on which bases it is founded. Both these principles are fundamental, and although not new, they have been very efficiently spread and impressed on the healthcare literature by the EBM advocates.

• The EBM-sponsored dissemination of valid and ready evidence should enter into more complex educational strategies to affect the doctors' professional behaviour. Furthermore, it should be taken into account that the doctors' professional behaviour is only a component of the quality of health care, that also depends on organisational characteristics, easy access and equity. No data are available to evaluate whether EBM has modified the quality and the unwarranted variations of health care. However, there is recent evidence that both these problems are still firmly with us [4,6].

• EBM-related sources are more suitable to answer doctors' questions about therapeutic decisions. They don't deal with the doctors' attitude to establish good patient–doctor relationship, and rarely help in the generation of diagnostic hypotheses. Furthermore, the criteria of validity of RCTs taught by EBM are not sufficient to translate their results into practice: contextualisation in the setting and in the characteristics and preferences of individual patients, safety, and industry-related distortions must be taken into account.

• As clinicians and clinical researchers, the Baveno people are both *users* and *producers* of 'evidence'. As *users*, they should use the best research evidence, adapting this evidence to the peculiarities of the local setting and the heterogeneity of the patients. As *producers* of original research and prefiltered secondary sources they should maintain the transparency until now used in their relationship with the industry, and should adapt the prefiltered sources to the target segment of health operators in a plain, objective and usable style.

REFERENCES

1 Eddy DM. Evidence-based Medicine: a unified approach. *Health Affairs* 2004;**24**: 9–17.
2 Elstein AS. On the origins and development of evidence-based medicine and medical decision making. *Inflamm Res* 2004;**53**(Suppl)2: S184–S189.
3 Chassin MR, Galvin RW and the National Roundtable on Health Care Quality. The urgent need to improve Health Care Quality. Institute of Medicine Roundtable on Health Care Quality. *JAMA* 1998;**280**: 100–105.
4 McGlynn EA, Asch SM, Adams J *et al.* The quality of health care delivered to adults in the United States. *N Engl J Med* 2003;**348**: 2635–2645.
5 Chassin MR, Brook RH, Park RE *et al.* Variations in the use of medical and surgical services by the Medicare population. *N Engl J Med* 1986;**314**: 285–290.
6 Wennberg JE. Variation in the use of Medicare Services among regions and selected academic medical centers: is more better? Duncan W Clark Lecture, New York Academy of Medicine. January 24, 2005. Accessed April 6 2005, at: http://www.dartmouthatlas.org/.
7 Antman EM, Lau J, Kupelnick B *et al.* A comparison of results of meta-analyses of randomised control trials and recommendations of clinical experts. *JAMA* 1992;**268**: 240–248.
8 Sackett DL, Richardson WS, Rosenberg W, Haynes RB. Evidence-based Medicine. How to practice and teach EBM. 1st edn, London, Churchill Livingstone, 1997.
9 Choudhry NK, Fletcher RH, Soumerai SB. Systematic review: the relationship between clinical experience and quality of health care. *Ann Intern Med* 2005;**142**: 260–273.
10 Evidence-Based Medicine Working Group. Evidence-based medicine. A new approach to teaching the practice of medicine. *JAMA* 1992;**268**: 2420–2425.
11 Twenty five users' guides to the medical literature, published by JAMA, from: Oxman AD, Sackett DL, Guyatt GH for the EBM Working Group. How to get started. *JAMA* 1993;**270**: 2093–2095, to: Guyatt GH, Haynes RB, Jaeschke RZ *et al* for the EBM Working Group. XXV. Evidence based medicine: principles for applying the users' guides to patient care. *JAMA* 2000;**284**: 1290–1296.
12 Sackett DL, Straus SE, Richardson WS, Rosenberg W, Haynes RB. Evidence-based medicine. How to practice and teach EBM. 2nd edn London, Churchill Livingstone, 2000.
13 Guyatt G, Rennie D Editors. Users' Guides to the Medical Literature. A manual for Evidence-Based Clinical Practice. Chicago: *JAMA & Archives Journals*, AMA Press, 2002.
14 Oxford Centre for Evidence-based Medicine Levels of Evidence (May 2001). Accessed April 6 2005 at: http://www.cebm.net.
15 Naylor CD, Putting evidence into practice. *Am J Med* 2002; **113**: 161–163.
16 http://www.cebm.net/learning_ebm.asp.

17 Haynes RB. What kind of evidence is it that Evidence-Based Medicine advocates want health care providers and consumers to pay attention to? *BMC Health Services Research* 2002, 2:3.
18 McColl A, Smith H, White P, Field J. General practitioners' perceptions of the route to evidence-based medicine: a questionnaire survey. *BMJ* 1998;**316**: 361–365.
19 Guyatt GH, Meade OM, Jaeschke RZ, Cook DJ, Haynes RB. Practitioners of evidence based care. Not all clinicians need to appraise evidence from scratch but all need some skills. *BMJ* 2000;**320**: 954–955.
20 Grol R, Dalhuijsen J, Thomas S *et al.* Attributes of clinical guidelines that influence use of guidelines in general practice: observational study. *BMJ* 1998;**317**: 858–861.
21 Grimshaw J, Russell IT. Effect of clinical guidelines on medical practice. A systematic review of rigorous evaluation. *Lancet* 1993;**342**: 1317–1322.
22 Cabana MD, Rand CS, Powe NR *et al.* Why don't physicians follow clinical practice guidelines? A framework for improvement. *JAMA* 1999;**282**: 1458–1465.
23 Gundersen L. The effect of clinical practice guidelines on variations in care. *Ann Intern Med* 2000;**133**: 317–318.
24 Klein WW. Current and future relevance of guidelines. *Heart* 2002;**87**: 497–500.
25 Oxman AD, Thomson MA, Davis DA, Haynes RB. No magic bullets: a systematic review of 102 trials of interventions to improve professional practice. *Can Me Assoc J* 1995;**153**: 1423–1431.
26 Davis DA, Thomson MA, Oxman AD, Haynes RB. Changing physician performance: a systematic review of the effect of continuing medical education strategies. *JAMA* 1995;**274**: 700–705.
27 Davis D, O'Brien MA, Freemantle N *et al.* Impact of formal continuing medical education. Do conferences, workshops, rounds, and other traditional continuing education activities change physician behaviour or health care outcomes? *JAMA* 1999;**282**: 867–874.
28 Grol R, Grimshaw J. From best evidence to best practice: effective implementation of change in patients' care. *Lancet* 2003;**362**: 1225–1230.
29 Shojania KG, Grimshaw JM. Evidence-based quality improvement: the state of the science. *Health Affairs* 2005;**24**: 138–227.
30 De Maeseneer JM, van Driel ML, Green LA, van Weel C. The need for research in primary care. *Lancet* 2003;**362**: 1314–1319.
31 Laine C, Davidoff F. Patient-centered medicine. A professional evolution. *JAMA* 1996;**275**: 152–156.
32 Gask L, Usherwood T. ABC of psychological medicine. The consultation. *BMJ* 2002;**324**: 1567–1569.
33 Wilkes M, Milgrom E, Hoffman J. Towards more empathic medical students: a medical student hospitalization experience. *Med Educ* 2002;**36**: 528–533.
34 Hojat M, Mangione S, Nasca TJ *et al.* An empirical study of decline in empathy in medical school. *Med Educ* 2004;**38**: 934–941.
35 Woloschuk W, Harasym PH, Temple W. Attitude change during medical school: a cohort study. *Med Educ* 2004;**38**: 522–534.
36 Eisenberg L. Good technical outcome, poor service experience: a verdict on contemporary medical care? *JAMA* 2001;**285**: 2639–2641.

37 Wofford MM, Wofford JL, Bothra J *et al.* Patient complaints about physician behaviours: a qualitative study. *Acad Med* 2004;**79**: 134–138.
38 Wyatt JC. Clinical questions and information need. *J R Soc Med* 2000;**93**: 168–171.
39 Ely JW, Osheroff JA, Gorman PN *et al.* A taxonomy of generic clinical questions: classification study. *BMJ* 2000; **321**: 429–432.
40 www.clinicalevidence.com, a BMJ-related, monthly updated compendium.
41 Black ER, Bordley DR, Tape TG, Panzer RJ. Diagnostic strategies for common medical problems. 2nd edn. Philadelphia: American College of Physicians, 1999.
42 Knottnerus JA (ed.) The evidence base of clinical diagnosis. London, BMJ Books, 2002.
43 Kassirer JP, Kopelman RI. Learning clinical reasoning. Baltimore, Williams & Wilkins Publ, 1991.
44 Haynes RB. Where's the meat in clinical medical journals? *ACP J* Club Nov–Dec 1993;**119**: A22–A23.
45 Henrion J, Schapira M, Luwaert R *et al.* Hypoxic hepatitis. Clinical and hemodynamic study in 142 consecutive cases. *Medicine* 2003;**82**: 392–406.
46 Pagnoux C, Mahr A, Cohen P, Guillevin L. Presentation and outcome of gastrointestinal involvement in systemic necrotizing vasculitides. Analysis of 62 patients with polyarteritis nodosa, microscopic polyangiitis, Wegener granulomatosis, Churg-Strauss syndrome or rheumatoid-associated vasculitis. *Medicine* 2005; **84**: 115–128.
47 Keljo DJ, Squires RH, Jr. Just in time, *NEJM* 1996;**334**: 46–48; letters: *NEJM* 1996;**334**: 1403–1405.
48 Clarke P, Glick S, Reilly BM. On the threshold – a diagnosis of exclusion. *N Engl J Me* 2005;**352**: 919–924.
49 http://www.cochrane.org/reviews/.
50 Rothwell PM. External validity of randomised controlled trials: 'to whom do the results of this trial apply?' *Lancet* 2005; **365**: 82–93.
51 Ridker PM, Cook NR, Lee I-M *et al.* A randomised trial of low-dose aspirin in the primary prevention of cardiovascular disease in women. *N Engl J Med* 2005; **352**: 1293–1204.
52 Pearson ER, Starkey BJ, Powell RJ *et al.* Mechanisms of disease. Genetic cause of hyperglycemia and response to treatment in diabetes. *Lancet* 2003;**362**: 1275–1281.
53 Chobanian AV, Bakris GL, Black HR. The seventh report of the Joint National Committee on prevention, detection, evaluation, and treatment of high blood pressure. The JNC 7 Report. *JAMA* 2003;**289**: 2560–2572.
54 Chassin MR. Appropriate use of carotid endarterectomy. *N Engl J Med* 1998;**339**: 1468–1471.
55 Spilker B. Guide to clinical trials. New York, Raven Press, 1991: 565–587.
56 Ioannidis JPA, Lau J. Completeness of safety reporting in randomised trials. An evaluation of 7 medical areas. *JAMA* 2001;**285**: 437–444.
57 Bodenheimer T. Uneasy alliance. Clinical investigators and the pharmaceutical industry. *N Engl J Med* 2000;**342**: 1539–1544.
58 Angell M, Is academic medicine for sale? *N Engl J Med* 2000; **342**: 1516–1518.
59 Garattini S, Bertelè V, Li Bassi L. How can research ethics committees protect patients better? *BMJ* 2003;**326**: 1199–1201.

60 Freemantle N, Calvert M, Wood J *et al.* Composite outcomes in randomised trials. Greater precision but with greater uncertainty? *JAMA* 2003;**289**: 2554–2559.
61 Easterbrook PJ, Berlin JA, Gopalan R *et al.* Publication bias in clinical research. *Lancet* 1991;**337**: 867–872.
62 Chan A-W, Altman DG. Identifying outcome reporting bias in randomised trials on PubMed: review of publications and survey of authors. *BMJ* 2005;**330**: 753–756.
63 Montori VM, Jaeschke R, Schunemann HJ *et al.* Users' guide to detecting misleading claims in clinical research reports. *BMJ* 2004;**329**: 1093–1096.
64 Bekelman JE, Mphil YL, Gross GP. Scope and impact of financial conflicts of interest in biomedical research. A systematic review. *JAMA* 2003;**289**: 454–465.
65 Als-Nielsen B, Chen W, Gluud C, Kjaergaard LL. Association of funding and conclusions in randomised drug trials. A reflection of treatment effect or adverse events? *JAMA* 2003;**290**: 921–928.

SESSION 8

Providing Scientific Evidence: RCTs and Beyond

Thorkild I.A. Sørensen, Antoine Hadengue, Francesco Salerno, Flemming Bendtsen, Jayant Talwalkar, Jenny Heathcote, Andres T. Blei and Juan Rodés

INTRODUCTION

In the previous Baveno workshops, a session was devoted to the methodological requirements for future RCTs in portal hypertension [1–5]. At Baveno IV, this session was replaced by one addressing various aspects of therapy in clinical practice that have not been or cannot be evaluated by randomised controlled trials (RCTs). Addressing these issues should contribute to Evidence-based Medicine (EBM) even though adequate information from RCTs is not possible to obtain or not yet available.

In portal hypertension as in any other clinical field, RCTs, wherever available, are the basis for establishing the evidence for choosing the best possible treatment of the clinical conditions that the portal hypertension may lead to – the principles of EBM [6]. However, for a variety of reasons, there are a broad panel of clinical therapeutic problems that cannot be solved by gathering evidence from the currently available RCTs, either because the relevant and adequate RCTs have not (yet) been conducted or because those conducted are inadequate for various reasons. For some of these problems, we could hope for adequate RCTs to be conducted that would contribute to the needed evidence, but for most of these problems it seems unfeasible to conduct such RCTs because the diseases are uncommon or the distinct features of common diseases are uncommon. In any case, we will need guidelines to optimise the current clinical decision-making in the absence of such evidence.

This task implies two important perspectives. One is that the guidelines emerging from addressing these problems are assumed to provide a better solution than would otherwise be the result if no such guidelines were adhered to. Thus, given that adequate evidence from RCTs is not available, then it is assumed that it is still possible to achieve a better outcome for the patients by applying such guidelines in creation of the basis for the clinical decision-making than to leave the decision-making to a more arbitrary basis. On the other hand, such guidelines will of course always suffer from an inherent doubt that better results might have been achieved by different decisions. This leads to the other perspective. Thus, the attempts to establish such guidelines should in no way be considered an argument or excuse for not pursuing any opportunities to conduct RCTs whenever and wherever feasible.

Need for international collaboration on clinical RCTs

To emphasise the latter perspective, the first guideline should be to conduct more, better and larger RCTs in the field of portal hypertension. It is clear from the systematic reviews conducted of RCTs in this field that they are greatly underpowered and often suffer from a variety of methodological weaknesses that can in principle be overcome in future RCTs [7]. Obviously, too many RCTs are conducted in local settings without the strength of available competence in conducting RCTs, that is, without access to the needed detailed knowledge and implemented technology of high-quality RCTs. It is likely that the competence may be easier to mobilise if the RCTs are set up as international collaborations. In other clinical fields, such as cardiology and oncology, we have seen that it is in fact feasible to conduct large-scale high-quality RCTs on a multinational basis, so why not also in the field of portal hypertension? Therefore, the first guideline is the following:

Need for international collaboration on clinical RCTs

- Almost all, if not all, RCTs in portal hypertension are underpowered and of low quality.
- This applies to uncommon but also common types of conditions associated with portal hypertension.
- In cardiology and oncology, very large international – multinational – high-quality RCTs are conducted, so it is feasible.
- We should do the same for solving our problems in management of portal hypertension.

Problems beyond the adequate RCTs

In this chapter, we suggest guidelines based on our attempts to answer the following questions related to clinical problems where adequate evidence from RCTs is not – or may not in a foreseeable future – become available.

- How do we interpret results of per protocol analysis when it yields results that differ from the intention-to-treat (ITT) results?
- How do we best assess the changes in treatment effects along the course of the progression of the disease?
- How do we best identify factors that may modify the treatment effect in a clinically significant way?
- How do we use the possible heterogeneity in meta-analysis of RCTs in research and clinical practice?
  - How do we handle the heterogeneity of RCTs in meta-analysis?
  - Is the solution for heterogeneity the use of stratified pooled data?
- How do we find the best possible approach to diagnosis and treatment in the type of single cases that we cannot get RCT evidence for?
  - To what extent can we rely on surrogate measures of the inaccessible evidence on hard clinical end-points?
  - Are there acceptable ways of accumulating the clinical experience from similar cases, which are so rare that RCTs will never be possible?
  - How do we deal with the fundamental problem of confounding by indication when trying to assess the effects of clinical actions in the observational setting?
- Do we have a problem in the portal hypertension field with effectiveness versus efficiency as defined by Archie Cochrane?
- What is the utility of the continuous monitoring of the clinical outcome of treatments in so-called clinical databases?
- How should we analyse the data on the multiple competing end points (e.g. bleeding and death) that prevails in studies of manifestations of portal hypertension?

How do we interpret results of per protocol (PP) analysis when it yields results that differ from the intention-to-treat (ITT) results?

In an ideal world, all subjects included into a clinical trial would comply with the allocated intervention and complete follow-up. In the real world, this never occurs, and the investigators are expected to anticipate how the resulting data should be analysed. The ITT principle, promoted both by the International Conference on harmonisation (ICH, www.ich.com) [8] and the Consolidated Standards of Reporting Trials (CONSORT) group [9] implies that 'primary analysis should include all randomised subjects'. With the only acceptable exception of eligibility violations identified prior to breaking the blind, ITT analysis means that all randomised subjects will be included into the full analysis set, irrespective of adherence to the protocol or completion of the trial.

In superiority trials (i.e. RCTs designed to show a difference between treatments), because a number of biases related to patient compliance are avoided by using ITT analysis, this strategy is viewed as conservative. Indeed, both compliance and follow-up can be linked to treatment efficacy and correlated to prognosis. Whatever treatment is applied, subjects who adhere usually have a better outcome than those who do not. Conversely, inclusion of non-compliers will usually decrease the observed treatment effect. ITT must therefore be chosen as the basis for primary analysis in such RCTs [9].

In non-inferiority trials (i.e. RCTs designed to show that one treatment is not inferior to another treatment, which may be called *equivalence trials* even though it is not feasible to show true equivalence), however, ITT strategies may miss the point. This may happen when uninformative noise, that is, patients who where randomised by error, did not get the allocated treatment, or failed to comply, brings differences between treatment arms towards zero. In this case ITT analysis will be non-conservative and lead to the erroneous conclusion that both arms are compatible with equivalent effects. In other cases, ITT analysis may falsely conclude for superiority, for example, in a trial comparing interventions A and B with similar efficacy, high adverse events rate in arm A can lead to drug discontinuation in that group. In that case, ITT analysis, although realistic by reflecting poor applicability of treatment A, may falsely conclude for the superiority of treatment B [10].

It has therefore been proposed that non-inferiority trials may benefit from both ITT and per-protocol (PP) analysis [11]. Obviously, the exclusion of an important fraction of patients from PP analysis may weaken the validity of the conclusions reached and the credit given to the study may decline. When ITT analysis yields a larger treatment effect than the PP analysis, one explanation may lie in the early discontinuation of the drug in one arm, inducing better apparent results in the other arm. When PP analysis yields a larger treatment effect than the ITT analysis, scrutiny of the patients excluded from analysis in both arms should help in analysing the discrepancy.

Definition of per-protocol analysis: Although ITT strategies are straightforward, the definition of 'per-protocol' analyses, meant to classify ambiguous patient situations, may vary from one study to another, and may have profound effects on the meaning of these studies. Any valid PP analysis implies that all criteria for excluding patients from the PP population are specified, all exclusions pronounced before breaking the blind, and the exact number of patients excluded in each arm according to each criteria are made available to the reader. Some criteria for PP analysis such as the exclusion of patients who failed to meet study entry criteria and the exclusion of patients who did not receive the allocated intervention are usually acceptable. However, since death or withdrawal may be related to side effects or inefficacy of the intervention, exclusion of patients who died or withdrew from the study before outcome assessment should be scrutinised with more care. Non-compliance is a crucial exclusion criterion, since compliance may be closely related to prognosis in many diseases. Indeed, compliance can be seen as a selective process by which compliant and non-compliant patients are expected to have different backgrounds and outcomes. Compliance may reflect side effects of the experimental treatment. In addition, the definition of compliance varies from all-or-none treatment adherence to any other compound or relaxed criteria. In the case of long-term mortality trials, including the actual treatment time as a variable into a Cox-proportional hazards model may be preferable to discarding significant information in subjects who discontinued the drug at some point [12–13]. Other exclusion criteria such as unspecified 'protocol violations' and 'missing data' that do not affect primary end point, should generally not be acceptable as valid for PP analysis.

In both *superiority and non-inferiority trials*, the key question to ask is 'How does the population that has been excluded from PP analysis drive the shift in the study results'? It will be important to scrutinise the number of patients excluded from each treatment arm, according to each single exclusion criteria. More specifically, was there an imbalance between groups in the number of randomised patients that did not receive allocated intervention, indicating that one intervention might not be applicable in a significant number of patients? Was there an imbalance between groups in the number of patients who discontinued the intervention, questioning the intervention's side effects in patients not analysed? Was the intervention's success associated with a better chance or quality of follow-up?

How do we interpret results of per protocol (PP) analysis when it yields results that differ from the intention-to-treat (ITT) results?

- In superiority trials, ITT strategies are preferred and PP analysis regarded only as supportive.
- In non-inferiority (or equivalence) trials, ITT and PP approaches (if appropriately predefined) may both contribute.
- When PP results differ from ITT results, the population excluded from PP analysis should be scrutinised. The applicability of the intervention may be questioned.

How do we best assess the changes in treatment effect along the course of the progression of the disease?

Defining outcome covariates in RCTs. Modelling the course of progression of a disease is a difficult task, especially during the course of portal hypertension, which may be due to different diseases. In RCTs, enrolling patients at different stages of the disease in question, delineating covariates associated with outcome is the easiest approach to this question. Some outcome-associated covariates, such as Child–Pugh's score, the MELD score or other composite scores may be known beforehand, and randomisation can be stratified accordingly, although this may not be necessary if the RCTs are large. Other outcome-associated covariates, however, will only be known after a predefined strategy has been applied to delineate baseline factors that are significantly associated with outcome in the particular study.

Baseline statistical comparisons of variables between study groups, although extensively used in most publications, do not stand as a valid method to evidence an interaction between treatment effect and outcome-associated covariates: depending on the strength of association between each covariate and outcome, some covariates with no statistically significant imbalance between groups may indeed be responsible for biased estimates of treatment efficacy [14–15].

Covariate adjustment. Accordingly, the proper way to address imbalance between groups and take into account baseline factors that may influence outcome is covariate adjustment. The ICH E9 international guidelines [8] state that it may be advisable to 'nominate the unadjusted analysis as the one for primary attention, the adjusted analysis being supportive'. We feel that whatever the results of baseline comparisons, both unadjusted results and results adjusted for strong outcome predictors should be given.

The best way to assess changes in treatment effects according to disease course is a test for interaction between treatment and covariates associated with outcome, which directly tests the hypothesis that treatment effects vary between subgroups. Using the whole data set to test for an interaction between treatment and covariates has the advantage of involving a single statistical test. It may often have the limitation of being underpowered if sample size was calculated for overall treatment effect rather than for testing the interaction. The same applies to the more complex type of analysis where the treatment effects during the follow-up after randomisation is assessed in relation to the progression of the disease. Interaction testing, however, is certainly preferable to subgroup testing, which exposes both to false negative results when underpowered analysis is performed in small subgroups, and to repeated post hoc testing [15–16]. Unless pre-defined with sufficient power and in general limited to the primary outcome, subgroup testing should be seen as exploratory method that can help design further studies, but should not modify the conclusions of RCTs [8].

How do we best assess the changes in treatment effect along the course of the progression of the disease?

- To assess how treatment effect may change with disease progression, use interaction tests between outcome predictors and the intervention(s).
- Both unadjusted results and results adjusted for strong outcome predictors should be provided, regardless of baseline comparisons.
- Any subgroup analyses should be predefined, have sufficient power and usually be limited to primary outcome. Otherwise, they are exploratory methods that can help design further studies but should not modify the conclusions of RCTs.

How do we best identify factors that may modify the treatment effect in a clinically significant way?

Adherence to evidence-based guidelines for clinical management is strongly encouraged [17–19]. Accordingly, the effects of individual treatments should be correctly predicted by the analysis of the results of appropriate RCTs. For example, when a cirrhotic patient bleeds from oesophageal varices, RCTs taught us that failure to control bleeding can depend on one or more of the following negative predictors: spurting varices at endoscopy, portal vein thrombosis, hepatic venous pressure gradient (HVPG) > 20 mmHg, development of bacterial infection, and high Child–Pugh score [20–23].

However, the reproducibility of the results of RCTs in the daily clinical practice is often unsatisfactory. Therefore, it is not infrequent that the outcome of an individual treatment is qualitatively or quantitatively different from what was expected from the results of RCTs. In addition, a new treatment is sometimes flawed by the occurrence of unpredictable side effects, because most RCTs explore adverse events with less systematic intensity than benefits [24]. This is exemplified by the recent experience with COX-2 inhibitors whose serious untoward vascular effects could have been evidenced only after a prolonged administration. Accordingly, it is crucial to develop strategies useful to identify the factors that significantly modify the outcome of individual treatments regarding both effectiveness and safety. The final effect of a treatment may deviate from what RCTs had reported because of two orders of factors: a defect of the quality (internal validity) or a defect of the external validity of the RCTs.

How to evaluate the quality (internal validity) of a trial

When the current effect of a treatment differs from the results of RCTs, this could depend on an overestimation (or less often an underestimation) of the treatment efficacy. In this case the poor reproducibility of the trial results is due to a low quality of the methodology used. The quality of RCTs can be assessed in its components according to the checklist of the CONSORT statement [9]. This checklist provides a clear picture of the progress of all participants in the RCT, from the time they are randomised until the end (Table 59). In particular, the following are relevant questions in evaluating the quality of RCTs:

1 How was the sample size calculated?
2 How were the patients randomly assigned to the different arms of treatment?
3 Was the treatment blinded? Blinded to the patients, to the investigators, or to both?
4 Was the analysis of the results made by intention-to-treat?
5 Were the statistical methods used to compare groups proper for both the primary and the secondary endpoints?

The probability that the results of the trial are appropriate is strictly related to the consistency of the sample size. RCTs with small sample sizes generate type I (by the multiple testing in several small RCTs compared to a single RCT of a size equal to the sum of the small RCTs) and type II errors and then they are of low quality [25]. Moreover, they have a low probability to identify side effects. Randomisation and blindness are two further prerequisites for avoiding bias. Randomisation favours the comparability between the different arms of the study. Sequence generation, allocation concealment, and implementation are three important aspects of the randomisation methodology to avoid selection bias. Adequate double blinding and follow-up of all patients are essential to avoid information bias. However, double blinding can be hardly obtained when a drug has a specific effect, such as bradycardia for propranolol, or when the trial includes surgical or invasive treatments, such as TIPS.

Finally, the interpretation of the results can vary according to the statistical methods. The use of an intention-to-treat analysis is usually

Table 59 Checklist according to the CONSORT statement [9].

Paper section and topic	Item	Description
Title and abstract	1	How participants were allocated to interventions (e.g. 'random allocation', 'randomised' or 'randomly assigned').
Introduction		
Background	2	Scientific background and explanation of rationale.
Methods		
Participants	3	Eligibility criteria for participants and the settings and locations where the data were collected.
Interventions	4	Precise details of the interventions intended for each group and how and when they were actually administered.
Objectives	5	Specific objectives and hypotheses.
Outcomes	6	Clearly defined primary and secondary outcome measures and, when applicable, any methods used to enhance the quality of measurements (e.g. multiple observations, training of assessors).
Sample size	7	How sample size was determined and, when applicable, explanation of any interim analyses and stopping rules.
Randomisation – sequence generation	8	Method used to generate the random allocation sequence, including details of any restriction (e.g. blocking, stratification).
Randomisation – allocation concealment	9	Method used to implement the random allocation sequence (e.g. numbered containers or central telephone), clarifying whether the sequence was concealed until interventions were assigned.
Randomisation – implementation	10	Who generated the allocation sequence, who enrolled participants, and who assigned participants to their groups.
Blinding (masking)	11	Whether or not participants, those administering the interventions, and those assessing the outcomes were blinded to group assignment. When relevant, how the success of blinding was evaluated.
Statistical methods	12	Statistical methods used to compare groups for primary outcome(s); methods for additional analyses, such as subgroup analyses and adjusted analyses.

Table 59 (Continued).

Paper section and topic	Item	Description
Results		
Participant flow	13	Flow of participants through each stage (a diagram is strongly recommended). Specifically, for each group report the numbers of participants randomly assigned, receiving intended treatment, completing the study protocol, and analysed for the primary outcome. Describe protocol deviations from study as planned, together with reasons.
Recruitment	14	Dates defining the periods of recruitment and follow-up.
Baseline data	15	Baseline demographic and clinical characteristics of each group.
Numbers analysed	16	Number of participants (denominator) in each group included in each analysis and whether the analysis was by 'intention-to-treat'. State the results in absolute numbers when feasible (e.g. 10/20, not 50%).
Outcomes and estimation	17	For each primary and secondary outcome, a summary of results for each group, and the estimated effect size and its precision (e.g. 95% confidence interval).
Ancillary analyses	18	Address multiplicity by reporting any other analyses performed, including subgroup analyses and adjusted analyses, indicating those pre-specified and those exploratory.
Adverse events	19	All important adverse events or side effects in each intervention group.
Discussion		
Interpretation	20	Interpretation of the results, taking in to account study hypotheses, sources of potential bias or imprecision and the dangers associated with multiplicity of analyses and outcomes.
Generalisability	21	Generalisability (external validity) of the trial findings.
Overall evidence	22	General interpretation of the results in the context of current evidence.

superior to a per protocol analysis in assessing the probability to obtain a result with a specific treatment (see above). When per-protocol analysis is made the number and the reasons of excluded cases must be clearly analysed.

How to evaluate the generalisability or external validity of a trial

The external validity of a trial is more difficult to assess. It involves the issue of the extent to which an individual patient could be part of the population of patients treated in the trial. To know this, one must take into account how the population of the trial was selected and what the main characteristics of such a population are.

Answers to the following questions can help this estimation:

1 How were the trial patients recruited and selected?
2 How was the diagnosis obtained?
3 Which were the demographic characteristics of the trial population?
4 Which were the inclusion and exclusion criteria?
5 Which were the schedule and dosage of the treatment?
6 How was the compliance of the patients?
7 How was the end point defined?
8 How long were the patients treated for?

The first questions directly refer to the issue of whether the population studied by the trial is representative of the general population affected by a specific disease. The setting where the patients are recruited can influence the average severity of the disease under study. Moreover, patients enrolled in a trial pass through a strict selection based on screening, inclusion criteria, agreement to participate, and randomisation. As a result the randomised patients represent a subset of the general population suffering from that disease.

The comparability of patients also depends on how the diagnosis was obtained. In several RCTs on portal hypertension HVPG was measured to estimate the severity of portal hypertension, whereas in clinical practice patients with portal hypertension are identified by clinical stigmata, such as varices or splenomegaly. This also may imply different severities of the cirrhosis.

The main clinical and demographic characteristics of patients enrolled in experimental treatments are reported by RCTs to demonstrate the similarity with the reference group taking placebo or standard therapy. The most important features concern age, sex, aetiology, scores which estimate the stage of the disease (i.e. Child–Turcotte–Pugh scores or MELD scores), laboratory tests and vital signs. Different ages or sex, as well as different stages of the disease, can affect the results of therapy [26–27]. Aetiology of liver disease is also important. Patients with alcoholic cirrhosis can become abstinent and thereby improve their prognosis [28]. Accordingly, it is difficult to extrapolate the results obtained in a population of cirrhotic patients with alcoholic aetiology to a patient with viral cirrhosis.

The inclusion/exclusion criteria are some of the most important variables, which define the population of RCTs. Most RCTs exclude patients with co-morbidities, such as diabetes, obesity, cardiac diseases or cancer. Most of these, however, are strong determinants of the outcome of individual patients. Moreover, co-morbidities require multidrug regimens, whereas RCTs often limit the use of medications. Drugs such as NSAIDs and ACE inhibitors adversely affect the renal function of patients with decompensated cirrhosis and this may interfere with the treatment effect, for example of diuretics.

The schedule of treatment is also important. Propranolol cannot be given at predefined dosages but should be titrated to obtain a 25% decrease of the heart rate, if possible. Accordingly, the final dose of propranolol can vary greatly depending on the heart rate response. Since starting terlipressin or somatostatin as early as possible is crucial for improving the chances to stop variceal bleeding, the effects of such treatments greatly depends on the timing variable.

The compliance of the patient markedly affects the treatment outcome: an irregular consumption of β-blockers could be more detrimental than no treatment. The compliance of patients is frequently greater in RCTs than in the current clinical practice. Trial patients are more motivated because they are aware of participating in an experimental study, they receive better counselling by doctors and nurses and they are more strictly monitored. Education is a further aspect that improves compliance. A bad adherence to a drug regimen, which also relies to drug safety, is the basis of a treatment failure.

The choice of the end points may vary greatly in RCTs and include survival, bleeding, quality of life, complications and symptoms. Sometimes surrogate measures of an outcome are used. This can generate errors of interpretations. From reduction of the HVPG obtained with β-blockers we cannot extrapolate the survival benefit that prophylaxis with β-blockers may generate.

Finally, many RCTs are conducted over weeks or months. The short-term nature of these studies precludes the ability to detect the benefit or harm associated with medications consumed over years for the treatment of chronic diseases.

How do we best identify factors that may modify the treatment effect in a clinically significant way?

- The physician must learn how to identify the factors that most often modify the clinical outcome at variance with the results of RCTs.
- The quality of the RCTs and their internal and external validities should be evaluated.
- The quality of a trial can be assessed according to the CONSORT checklist.
- The external validity can be assessed according to a list of variables which define how peculiar the trial population is with respect to differences in demography, co-morbidities, limitations due to inclusion/exclusion criteria, variability in the schedules and dosages of drugs, use of interfering drugs, low compliance, duration of treatment.

How do we use the possible heterogeneity in meta-analysis of RCTs in research and clinical practice?

This question has two aspects and it may be split into these two questions:

- How do we handle the heterogeneity of RCTs in meta-analysis?
- Is the solution for heterogeneity the use of stratified pooled data?

In the process of systematic reviews, information from all relevant studies are brought together and combined in an attempt to perform a meta-analysis. This process, without standardised criteria, will bring together studies with often large variation in terms of design (follow-up length, definitions of outcomes etc.), in types of patients studied (clinical characteristics) and eventually difference in the specific interventions applied in the studies.

These large differences in trial designs may eventually lead to conflicting results among the RCTs selected for the meta-analysis, with some showing a beneficial effect and others indicating a harmful effect of the actual intervention analysed. Statistical tests will then show heterogeneity, and conclusion based on meta-analysis may in these cases often seem meaningless, unless the cause of heterogeneity is clearly identified. Clinically important heterogeneity of treatment effects is often seen [29], when various groups of patients have very different risk of event. The results based on a broad range of evidence will in some cases be remote from the issue of how to treat the individual patient, although no one will argue against the fact that all treatments should be based on evidence, when it is available [30].

Stratified meta-analysis/subgroup meta-analysis

In case of heterogeneity, the problem of the gap between the evidence based on many patients and making decisions about treating individuals may be overcome by meta-analysis instead of analysing how treatment effects varies according to patients' characteristics within each trial [31]. Usually basic characteristics of patients recruited for the specific trials are given. This enables one to relate treatment effects in the different RCTs to the overall characteristics. We can for example, evaluate the treatment effects in RCTs dealing with primary prophylactic endoscopic treatment of oesophageal varices according to the number of patients with large varices or of Child–Pugh score C patients in each trial. This type of analysis is often called meta-regression, which however has several limitations and may potentially lead to misinterpretations in case of heterogeneity and diversity in treatment strategies, follow-up and others [32].

In order to look for beneficial effects in individual patients, subgroup analysis may be considered, although most RCTs are underpowered to show an effect in subgroup analysis. Subgroup analysis has several pitfalls increasing the risk of finding a false positive effect. Strategy for performing subgroup analysis should be specified in the protocol before initiating the study. Formal evaluation of interaction should be reported as the estimated difference in the intervention effect in each subgroup (with a confidence interval), not as p-values [33].

Meta-analysis is normally performed on the basis of fully reported articles published in scientific journals. Most often data are lacking for treatment effects according to certain characteristics or more complex variables. It is therefore not possible on the basis of the publications to perform stratified analysis on individual data.

Example of heterogeneity in portal hypertension

Endoscopic sclerotherapy reduces the risk of rebleeding and death in patients with previous variceal bleeding, although this treatment has now been replaced by endoscopic variceal ligation. The risk of rebleeding from oesophageal varices, without prophylactic therapy is high, and metaanalysis of the RCTs investigating the effect of sclerotherapy [34] showed no heterogeneity. This observation led to RCTs evaluating the effect of sclerotherapy as primary prophylaxis of variceal bleeding. The risk of a first bleed is dependent on many risk factors such as variceal size, presence of cherry red spots, severity of liver disease as evaluated by Child–Pugh score. Initial studies showed a beneficial effect on bleeding risk and some even on mortality. However, large multicentre RCTs that were performed later showed either no effect or even a harmful effect. Careful analyses of the studies have shown that RCTs with a high rate of bleeding in the control group tended to show a better effect in the sclerotherapy group. It was not possible from the available data to identify the reason for the large discrepancy of bleeding rates in the control groups, and it was therefore concluded that sclerotherapy could not be recommended as primary prophylaxis in variceal bleeding [35].

Recent studies comparing endoscopic ligation with β-blockade for primary prophylaxis indicate that endoscopic ligation reduces the bleeding risk especially in patients with a high risk of bleeding compared to treatment with a β-blocker [36]. This finding may explain the observation of heterogeneity in sclerotherapy studies, since sclerotherapy is not without complications, which for patients with a low risk of bleeding eventually may outweigh the potential beneficial effect on bleeding rate, while for patients with a high risk of bleeding the beneficial effect of sclerotherapy on bleeding rate is larger than the risk of complications, obviously with opposite effect on mortality.

Analysis of pooled data

Statistical analysis on pooled individual data is complicated and time consuming. The individual RCTs will often differ with respect to selection of patients, inclusion and exclusion criteria, treatment strategy, duration of treatment and follow-up. Pooling of the data is troublesome, and statistical analysis of the data difficult. To our knowledge systematic recommendations of how to perform this type of analysis do not exist [33]. Criteria for definition of situations, when stratified analysis of pooled data should be preferred for meta-analysis, are needed.

Pitfalls in stratified analysis of pooled data

The quality of the analysis of the pooled data is highly dependent on the design and execution of the individual RCTs being pooled. The design, conduct, and analysis of each trial should be clear and transparent and accurately described in the protocol and manuscript in order to evaluate whether it may be acceptable to pool the data and look for the following items among many other:

1 How and when were patients selected for the individual study (the effect of treatment may vary according to time interval between event and randomisation) [37].

2 Was the treatment in all studies compared to the same placebo or another uniform reference treatment?
3 Was the treatment appropriate in dose, frequency of treatment and others in all studies in order to make pooling of the data acceptable?
4 Are all data available from each trial in order to perform analysis according to an intention-to-treat strategy?
5 The definition of an end point should for each individual trial have been clearly stated and without major variations between the studies to be pooled.

It is therefore extremely important that the individual protocols be homogeneous according to patient selection, treatment strategy, analysis of data, which can only be overcome with consensus meetings defining these aspect, which then should be followed in order to be accepted as a manuscript in a scientific journal with peer review.

How do we use the possible heterogeneity in meta-analysis of RCTs in research and clinical practice?

How do we handle the heterogeneity of RCTs in meta-analysis?
• It can be used cautiously to suggest indications for a particular intervention.
• It requires that differences in trial methodology are not present and that the clinical source of heterogeneity has been identified

Is the solution for heterogeneity the use of stratified pooled data?
• Stratified analysis of pooled data can be done.
• Primary/secondary aims should be predefined.
• Plan for statistical analysis should be predefined (including multiple testing).
• Subsequent analysis can use the pooled data as long as the above protocol is followed.

How do we find the best possible approach to diagnosis and treatment in the type of single cases that we cannot get RCT evidence for?

This question may be made more specific by the following questions, which also will be addressed in this chapter:
• To what extent can we rely on surrogate measures of the inaccessible evidence on hard clinical end points?
• Are there acceptable ways of accumulating the clinical experience from similar cases, which are so rare that RCTs will never be possible?

• How do we deal with the fundamental problem of confounding by indication when trying to assess the effects of clinical actions in the observational setting?

Case report or case series formats have traditionally been used to identify novel approaches to diagnosis and therapy of rare conditions. Given the infrequency of these diseases, it has generally been accepted that RCTs will not be available to provide the highest level of scientific evidence for use in clinical practice. Nonetheless, a structured approach with collaboration from multiple institutions could facilitate standardised data collection for analysis and the development of guidelines for approaches to clinical management.

In terms of diagnosis, a preferred approach would be to predetermine what criteria are necessary for prospectively identifying affected individuals with disease. These criteria are usually identified from clinical epidemiological studies describing the demography, clinical presentation and laboratory features of the disease in question. Once diagnostic criteria have been established, a consensus agreement should be reached in terms of which data elements are required for diagnosis and longitudinal monitoring. The modified Delphi technique [38] has been successfully used in hepatology to derive explicit agreement on the clinical management of specific conditions. One notable example includes modifying the indication for home-based parenteral albumin in patients with symptomatic ascites [39]. Once a protocol is established, the study of alternate diagnostic methods can be incorporated within the core principles of management to determine their accuracy and effectiveness in clinical practice.

The administration of empiric medical therapy for patients with rare conditions remains an important part of clinical practice. Limitations in this approach, however, relate directly to the absence of scientific principles used to judge the level of internal validity. While a placebo effect may occur among single individuals without side effects or increased cost that may be appropriate, this may result in denying patients the opportunity to achieve further incremental benefit from an alternate therapy. Recently, the use of alternate (or quasi-experimental) study designs to examine the efficacy of medical treatments has emerged to improve the quality of scientific evidence linked with empiric therapy. Quasi-experimental designs are defined as experiments where balanced randomisation is not possible because of low sample size but where other features of internal validity (such as double blinding and concealed allocation) may be incorporated [40]. A well-described study design that may improve the validity and effectiveness of selected therapies for rare conditions is termed the N of 1 trial (see later).

To what extent can we rely on surrogate measures of the inaccessible evidence on hard clinical end points?

Objective endpoints such as death or liver transplantation are indisputable, unbiased events in observational and interventional studies. However, these end points may occur infrequently and will be difficult to use in specific clinical situations. This observation is based on several factors including hepatic disease severity of study participants, the need for large sample size requirements, increased trial duration and cost. The use of composite or multiple end points in a clinical trial, which can overcome limitations based on power and sample size requirements, may remain unhelpful if heterogeneity between the defined end points exists. Examples include variation of patient preference, the absence of significant and equivalent relative risk reduction, and the lack of biologic plausibility for all end points [41].

Recently, the use of surrogate markers of clinical end points to measure the efficacy of interventions has been the focus of intense study. In the field of portal hypertension, previous intervention RCTs were able to use hard end points to assess treatment efficacy given the increased rate of clinical outcomes such as death and rebleeding that occurred over short periods of time [42]. Examples of such RCTs include pharmacological prophylaxis against variceal haemorrhage [43], antibiotic prophylaxis for bacterial infection in cirrhosis [44], and transjugular intrahepatic portosystemic shunt (TIPS) compared to large-volume paracentesis for refractory ascites [45].

The validity of any surrogate marker will rely on evidence that links the measure to a definable clinical outcome. To date, the majority of surrogate markers in patients with cirrhosis and portal hypertension have been recognised to predict survival. Examples include the HVPG measurement for identifying bleeding risk and possibly survival [46], the Model of End-Stage Liver Disease (MELD) score for short-term survival [47], and the discriminant function for prognosis in alcoholic hepatitis [48]. Despite its widespread recognition, the Child–Turcotte–Pugh score remains too subjective and lacks the ability to predict survival on a continuous scale for use in future studies [49]. Other potential surrogate markers including serum ammonia and albumin levels are not useful despite their plausible link to pathophysiologic mechanisms of disease progression.

However, the ability to identify novel treatments for improving survival and related outcomes in cirrhosis and portal hypertension has become difficult over time. Continued improvements in the standard of medical care have reduced the incremental ability of new therapies to demonstrate greater efficacy in RCTs. In addition, longer study durations and increased cost will be required as the estimated survival of patients with compensated disease will further increase where effective treatment becomes available.

Therefore, the identification of a valid, reproducible, and responsive surrogate marker is needed to promote continued advances in the field. Ideally, the surrogate maker will have biologic plausibility in both static and longitudinal ways. A most recent example in patients with heart failure involves the clinical use of serum brain natriuretic peptide (BNP). Studies to date have linked the production and level of serum BNP with haemodynamic function in patients with heart failure and pulmonary hypertension. Evidence now supports the use of serum BNP as a highly accurate diagnostic test for patients with unexplained dyspnea from occult heart failure. Risk stratification is also associated with serum BNP as the magnitude of elevation appears to correspond with severity of ventricular dysfunction. Finally, the reduction in serum BNP level and correlation with functional improvement after therapeutic intervention may also provide a way to accurately measure outcome linked to prognosis [50].

A similar, non-invasive biomarker like serum BNP does not currently exist for widespread use in patients with cirrhosis and portal hypertension. Potential candidates for a similar biologic surrogate marker in portal hypertension may include: (1) serum markers of hepatic fibrosis and (2) soluble nitric oxide or similar biologic indicators of vascular endothelial injury.

Are there acceptable ways of accumulating clinical experience from similar cases, which are so rare that RCTs will never be possible?

As mentioned previously, the N of 1 study design may be of value in patients with rare manifestations of portal hypertension. The primary use for N of 1 RCTs is when uncertainty about a potential treatment's efficacy exists and where definitive intervention RCTs cannot be performed. N of 1 trials are designed to increase the scientific rigour of individual patient assessments and to provide a measure of effectiveness in clinical practice [51].

N of 1 trials are usually designed as randomised, controlled, multicrossover studies that examine an individual patient's response to medical therapy. Because clinical equipoise suggests that no accepted therapy is available for this situation, at least two or more therapies (including placebo) may be randomised individually or within paired treatment periods. Ideally, these treatments are provided in a double-blind fashion with concealed allocation. During the treatment periods, two or more assessments of disease status should be recorded for estimating treatment effect. The end point or outcome measure from N of 1 trials should be prespecified before a study is begun. Often, this will be related to finding a clinical or statistically significant response to a particular therapy. The results of a series of N of 1 trials may also identify that a drug therapy is ultimately not helpful despite prior assumptions that benefit would be experienced [52].

The advantages for using an N of 1 trial study design include: (1) providing information about new drug evaluations including optimal dose, duration and frequency and (2) defining preliminary estimates of treatment efficacy for power and sample size calculations in more definitive studies. Limitations associated with N of 1 trials include: (1) their specific use for assessments of symptomatic therapy in chronic disease, (2) their applicability only for therapies that allow for independent period measurements and (3) their time and labour intensive performance. In the literature to date, however, a number of conditions have been recognised as suitable for the successful application and completion of N of 1 trials [52].

However, the feasibility and internal validity of conducting N of 1 trials in patients with rare manifestations of cirrhosis and portal hypertension remains unknown. More recently, the conduct of randomised crossover RCTs in groups rather than individual patients may have supplanted the widespread application of N of 1 individual trials. Nonetheless, there will be a need to consider using these study designs in patients with rare manifestations of portal hypertension to improve the validity of utilised therapies.

How do we deal with the fundamental problem of confounding by indication when trying to assess the effects of clinical actions in the observational setting?

Prognostic factors influence the medical decisions to offer therapy to patients with chronic disease in observational settings. This creates a bias known as 'confounding by indication'. In these studies, the allocation to drug treatment is, by definition, not random. This means that the prognosis of patient groups is not comparable and thus inferences drawn about the relative effects of a particular treatment may be invalid [53]. In turn, confounding by indication has been identified as the most important limitation for determining the validity of treatment effect in observational studies [54].

Statistical methods for controlling the aggregate effect of confounding exist. When appropriately applied in a well-designed study, it may be possible that non-experimental studies assessing treatment effects should not be rejected unequivocally. However, the risk of failing to account for unknown risk factors given the absence of balanced randomisation always remains a threat. In the literature, the most common techniques to adjust for confounding are stratified analysis, multivariable logistic regression analysis, and use of the propensity score. A fourth technique called recursive partitioning has been used in the cardiovascular literature without extensive application in other fields and will not be discussed here.

In stratified analysis, the assessment of a risk factor's effect on outcome is done while holding other variables constant and thus minimising the effect of confounding. For example, cigarette smoking is associated with coronary artery disease (CAD). Sex may be a potential confounder in this association. If the association between smoking and CAD is measured for both men and women separately, the impact of sex as a confounder has been controlled. If smoking is no longer associated with CAD, then sex was confounding the relationship. This technique, however, is useful when only a few potential confounding variables (less than 3) are present. With more variables, the sample sizes for these calculations will be reduced with a loss of power in observed results [55].

The more common technique used in observational studies is multivariable logistic regression analysis. Similar to stratified analysis, this technique allows for many potential confounder variables to be assessed without loss of power. The weakness of this technique also includes the inability to control for variables that were not identified at baseline yet may be important confounders. Also, the estimates from models may be incorrect if too many variables are included when the number of events is low. Between 10 to 20 persons for each independent variable in a model is considered the 'rule-of-thumb' for preserving a model's reliability to explain or predict similar outcomes in different populations. With few events or outcomes, the precision of results will be low as represented by wide confidence intervals [55].

An emerging technique for controlling the effect of confounding is known as the propensity score [56]. This score is defined as the conditional probability of an individual patient receiving a particular exposure (or treatment) given a particular set of confounders. For the calculation of a propensity score (expressed as an estimated odds ratio), the confounder variables are retained in a logistic regression model to predict the exposure of interest without including the outcome. This collection of confounder variables is collapsed into a single variable, which represents the probability or propensity of being exposed. The appeal for using propensity scores arises in situations where studies with rare events and multiple confounders are being analysed. This single score allows one to potentially circumvent the notion of too many variables relative to the number of events with eventual loss of reliability. However, this hypothesis has not been tested extensively to date, especially in patients with cirrhosis and portal hypertension.

Both stratification and logistic regression analysis have been used in observational studies with patients affected by cirrhosis and portal hypertension. However, the degree to which these techniques have been appropriately used in this discipline remains unknown [57]. The proper application of these techniques should improve the ability to adjust for confounding by indication and to better assess the magnitude of treatment efficacy in non-intervention studies.

How do we find the best possible approach to diagnosis and treatment in the type of single cases that we cannot get RCT evidence for?

- Consensus-driven, clinical protocols are required to define the optimal methods for clinical management of rare manifestations of portal hypertension where RCTs cannot be performed.
- The treatment of rare manifestations of portal hypertension with evidence-based medicine awaits the identification of biologically plausible surrogate markers of clinical end points.
- Alternate study designs (database analysis, N of 1 trials) should be adapted to identify effective treatments for rare manifestations of portal hypertension.
- Observational studies of treatment effect require the application of statistical techniques to minimise confounding by indication.

Do we have a problem in the portal hypertension field with efficacy versus general and cost effectiveness?

Efficacy of interventions to either prevent initial variceal haemorrhage or prevent recurrent bleeding is assessed in the RCT format. However the effectiveness of any intervention needs also to be demonstrated outside the context of the RCT in the affected general population. Additionally, the outcome must not be too costly either to the individual or the payer – who may be one and the same individual. Thus, an intervention, which may show significant benefit in terms of efficacy, may not be effective because of undue side effects and/or because of undue financial cost.

Evaluation of general and cost effectiveness

The Markov model is the strategy most often employed to evaluate the effectiveness of an intervention. This model can be used to examine several strategies according to different grades of risk in different disease states and over time. However, the figures used in the model by necessity are taken from the published figures of RCT, and it is unusual for negative RCTs to be published. Thus, unavoidable bias can be introduced into the model. Additionally, as it may take several years for a trial to be completed and then published, the data used to subsequently determine effectiveness is often several years out of date.

Effectiveness of primary prevention for variceal bleeding (VB)

The study reported by Teran *et al.* [58] in 1997 assessed the cost effectiveness of β-blockers, sclerotherapy and surgery for primary prevention of variceal haemorrhage. They calculated the number of patients who needed to undergo the particular treatment for one (VB) to be prevented. This number was the smallest for surgery regardless of disease severity (Childs A, B and C) or degree of VB risk, but the cost in dollars to achieve this was high, even without including the costs of untoward side effects for all three strategies. When the dollar cost was combined with the number needed to treat to prevent one VB it was least in those treated with β-blockers that is, β-blockers appeared the most cost effective strategy of the three examined.

Again employing the Markov model, another approach was taken by Arguedas *et al.* [59]. These authors calculated the costs per years of life saved (CYLS) with four strategies (screening endoscopy and if varices are found either band or prescribe β-blockers or not screening at all and giving all patients with cirrhosis β-blockers or nothing). They calculated that whereas for patients with compensated cirrhosis (Child A score) screening and treatment of any large varices with β-blockers had the lowest CYLS, this was not the case for the decompensated cirrhosis – where screening and banding of any large varices was the most cost effective. All strategies except doing nothing were 'cost saving' in the decompensated cirrhotic. The authors did not address selective screening for varices according to platelet count [60], but selective screening was introduced into the model published by Spiegel *et al.* [61]. These authors determined that empiric β-blocker therapy cost $12,408/additional VB prevented whereas both universal screening and selective endoscopic screening (determined on factors such as platelet count of < 88,000/mL, PT < 70%, a portal vein diameter > 13 mm or splenomegaly) cost $175,833 and $178,400 respectively, per additional VB prevented. The 'do nothing' strategy is naturally the least expensive, but also the least effective. Sensitivity analyses were conducted to estimate the robustness of changes in base case estimates (e.g. the degree of reduction in incidence of VB over time), and this obviously depended on the effectiveness of the manoeuvre. Similarly, compliance with the manoeuvre markedly affects base case estimates – so the incremental cost effectiveness ratio (ICER) between strategies was \$50,000 when 80% were non-compliant and only \$4000 when 100% were non-compliant! This illustrates the importance of patient education. When the cost of endoscopy was changed from \$824 to \$281, the ICER of the empiric β-blocker strategy fell down to \$50,000. Similarly when the cost of β-blockers increased so the ICER for empiric β-blocker fell to \$50,000.

Effectiveness of secondary prevention strategies for prevention of variceal bleeding

The modern day equivalent of the surgical side-to-side shunt is TIPS. This procedure has been shown to very effectively reduce the risk of VB, but at great cost in terms of side effects, particularly portosystemic hepatic encephalopathy [62]. It also requires regular maintenance to avoid blockage; although the newer stents are less likely to clot off than the earlier versions, their price has also changed. A cost-utility analysis by Rubenstein *et al.* [63] indicated that TIPS had the highest costs in terms of dollars even though the benefit in terms of quality-adjusted life-years (QUALYs) gained was comparable to other manoeuvres, e.g. β-blockers, but not as beneficial in terms of QUALYs as endoscopic variceal ligation +/− β-blockers.

Issues to be addressed regarding effectiveness

Markov models are bound to make a number of assumptions, not all of which can be avoided, thus sensitivity analyses employing differing baseline case estimates are essential. Compliance, particularly with medical therapy has been evaluated, but compliance with follow-up strategies required for both TIPS and EVL needs to be included in models. Although they introduce further complexity into the model, changes in medical status over time need to be considered. This is particularly important in an ageing population. In the three assessments of primary prevention strategies discussed earlier the age at baseline of the cirrhotics was 40, 50 and 50 years. But in 2005 the average age of patients is probably greater, and many are already taking medications for other co-morbidities. Diabetes is very prevalent in patients with cirrhosis yet the effect of this co-morbidity has never been taken into account in any effectiveness analysis.

It is pertinent to include patient education into the formula as better understanding by the patient of the natural history of cirrhosis and its complications may influence the outcome of the strategies employed to reduce the consequences of portal hypertension.

Do we have a problem in the portal hypertension field with efficacy versus general and cost effectiveness?

- There are many problems in the terms of efficacy versus effectiveness in the management of portal hypertension.
- Effectiveness of any intervention needs also to be demonstrated outside the context of the RCT in the affected general population.
- Outcome must not be too costly either to the individual or the payer.
- It is imperative that editors consider publishing negative as well as positive RCTs of therapy so that the effectiveness of strategies can be more accurately evaluated.
- An assessment of availability and access to these strategies in terms of resources, facilities and competence is needed.
- Patient education should be included and may influence the outcome of the strategies employed to reduce the consequences of portal hypertension.

What is the utility of the continuous monitoring of the clinical outcome of treatments in so called clinical databases?

Single-institution trends on therapeutic outcomes in portal hypertension have been recently published [64], highlighting positive trends in survival over two decades. To our knowledge, there is no active inter-institutional database that monitors therapeutic outcomes in portal hypertension. Databases in multiple areas of medicine have been a constant source for analysis and publication. But, are the data reliable? In order to provide insight into the accuracy of such databases and registries, it is useful to review areas within the hepatological discipline where information is available. Liver Transplant-related databases, where both American and European registries have been operational for several decades, are a good example. Finally, specific proposals in the area of portal hypertension will be presented.

Background

Compulsory registries: the US transplant registry

In the United States, 10 transplant-related databases are operational. Participation in all, except one, is voluntary and may be related to specific problems within the spectrum of transplantation, focus on specific diseases or be age-related. Participation in one registry is compulsory, the Scientific Registry of Transplant Recipients (SRTR), mandated under provisions of the National Organ Transplantation Act. Approved transplant centres, in order to maintain their membership in UNOS (and be able to have their patients included in the computerised waiting list) have to provide data to the SRTR.

The SRTR contains information on 200,000 transplant recipients. It receives independent funding. Even with compulsory reporting, such as the

SRTR, concerns arise about the accuracy of the data collected. No systematic method to assure accuracy is in place. Recent evidence from SRTR suggests a relationship between poor form completion and lower graft and patient survival [65]. Adoption of Web-based data entry systems (of which multiple types are currently available) may be the key to accurate data recording. Such systems have built-in protections against the entry of inappropriate data [66].

Voluntary registries

Auditing of large databases appears *a priori* as a daunting task. The European Liver Transplant Registry (ELTR) embarked on such a project [67]. Active since 1968, ELTR has collected data on more than 45,000 liver transplants. Participation in ELTR is voluntary; nonetheless, more than 95% of the overall transplant activity in Europe is included in the ELTR registry (when compared to official data). Registry forms include 45 items, both pre- and post-transplant. An independent team visited 21/120 centres (17% of the group) with 10% of each centre's files chosen at random; 25 items were checked against the patient charts. The rate of completeness of forms was 95% and overall consistency was 98%. Still, inconsistencies were found in some specific items, including (surprisingly) cause of graft failure and patient outcome. The median cost per audited file was 44 EUR. Funding for the operation of ELTR originates from its partnership with European organ sharing organisations.

A database to monitor outcomes in portal hypertension

Arguments in favour

'Efficacy' of therapy, assessed in clinical RCTs, may not be equated with the 'effectiveness' of such treatments in clinical practice. A tool to monitor results across different institutions over time could be a valuable assessment of therapy in the 'real' world.

Unsuspected trends in outcome may arise from such data. The value of infection control in the management of variceal haemorrhage arose from analysis of data from different centres [44].

Selected problems in the area of portal hypertension, where data from clinical RCTs is scant, could be targeted (e.g. outcome of therapy of portal hypertension in patients awaiting liver transplantation).

Concerns

The GIGO effect: Analysis of clinical outcomes from a registry will be scientifically valid if they are based on accurate and complete data. Embarking on a project without all the necessary requirements in place risks generating incorrect, and at the end, misleading data.

Funding required for such a database includes several items. In 2000, it was estimated that development costs for a secure Web-based site for collaborative research was approximately US $20,000 [68]. Yearly maintenance of the web site was estimated to be $2,000. Auditing costs also need to be incorporated (see above).

Entry of data in voluntary databases requires the commitment of centres potentially burdened with many other obligations. It is unlikely that external funding could be generated for specific salary lines that support individuals responsible for data entry.

Procedure

Three elements need to be in place in order to launch such a project.

Scientific objective. A decision needs to be made on the scientific goals of such a database. Outcome measures to be explored need to be carefully discussed in order to balance out the inclination to include all possible variables.

Development of a secure Web site . Several software products are available for this purpose and should be tested by the investigators.

Funding. Agreement on the mechanisms to fund the database should be in place before starting the project.

What is the utility of the continuous monitoring of the clinical outcome of treatments in so called clinical databases?

- Development of a database to evaluate clinical outcomes in portal hypertension is a desirable goal.
- The scientific objective of such a database should be discussed by the conference.
- On one hand, general outcomes in the three main areas of primary prophylaxis of variceal haemorrhage, acute variceal bleeding and in the prevention of rebleeding can be followed. This general view may be complemented with specific populations within this spectrum.
- Agreement on the mechanisms to fund such an activity should be reached by the conference.
- Once the previous points have been agreed upon, it is recommended that a task force be set up to provide a proposal for the entire conference.

How should we analyse the data on the multiple competing end points (e.g. bleeding and death) that prevail in studies of manifestations of portal hypertension?

The Kaplan–Meier plot is often used to estimate the probability of survival free of other end points, for example, variceal bleeding. This produces non-interpretable results that may also be biased. The reason for the bias is that the Kaplan–Meier analysis censors patients when they get one of the competing end point. A fundamental principle in the Kaplan–Meier analysis, is that it is assumed that the probabilities over time of remaining free of the condition of interest, e.g. bleeding, would have been the same if the patients were not censored. When the patients are censored because of competing end points, for example, death, they cannot later get the end point of interest, and therefore they do not belong to the population of patients at risk after this time point. Since this is disregarded in the Kaplan–Meier analysis, the estimated probabilities have no meaning, and they are biased estimates of the true probabilities for those patients who remain under risk of the end point of interest. When the incidences of the competing end points are high compared to the incidence of the end point of interest, then seriously biased estimates may be obtained.

The estimation of the hazard function, as used in the Cox regression analysis, is unbiased by competing end point, and an unbiased illustration of, for example, treatment effect may be shown by the cumulative hazards. It is also possible to estimate the unbiased probability, analogous to the Kaplan–Meier estimates, but this is a more complicated procedure. The problem and the methods have been discussed and exemplified on the basis of a RCT of sclerotherapy for bleeding varices [69–70].

How should we analyse the data on the multiple competing end points (e.g. bleeding and death) that prevail in studies of manifestations of portal hypertension?

- The Kaplan–Meier plot is often used to estimate the probability of survival free of other end points than death, e.g. variceal bleeding, but this produces non-interpretable results that may also be biased.
- The cause is that analysis using censoring of patients assumes that those who die or reach other competing end points are still at risk for the primary end point, which is not true.
- For this type of analysis, cumulative hazard plots and Cox regression analysis are appropriate.

REFERENCES

1 de Franchis R, Pascal JP, Ancona E *et al.* Definitions, methodology and therapeutic strategies in portal hypertension. A consensus development workshop. *J Hepatol* 1992;**15**: 256–261.

2 de Franchis R. Developing consensus in portal hypertension. *J Hepatol* 1996;**25**: 390–394.

3 de Franchis R ed. Portal Hypertension II. Proceedings of the second Baveno international consensus workshop on definitions, methodology and therapeutic strategies. Oxford; Blackwell Science, 1996.

4 de Franchis R. Updating consensus in portal hypertension: report of the Baveno III consensus workshop on definitions, methodology and therapeutic strategies in portal hypertension. *J Hepatol* 2000;**33**: 846–852.

5 de Franchis R ed. Portal Hypertension III. Proceedings of the IIIrd Baveno international consensus workshop on definitions, methodology and therapeutic strategies. Blackwell Science, Oxford, UK, 2001.

6 [Luigi Pagliaro's chapter on EBM in these Proceedings. . .].

7 [Christian Gluud's chapter in these Proceedings based on the work carried out in the Cochrane Hepatobiliary Group].

8 Lewis JA. Statistical principles for clinical trials (ICH E9, www.ich.com): an introductory note on an international guideline. *Stat Med* 1999;**18**: 1903–1942.

9 Moher D, Schulz KF, Altman DG. The CONSORT statement: revised recommendations for improving the quality of reports of parallel-group randomised trials. *Lancet* 2001;**357**: 1191–1194.

10 Brittain E, Lin D. A comparison of intent-to-treat and per-protocol results in antibiotic non-inferiority trials. *Stat Med* 2005;**24**: 1–10.

11 Ebbutt AF, Frith L. Practical issues in equivalence trials. *Stat Med* 1998;**17**: 1691–1701.

12 Committee for Proprietary Medicinal Products. Points to consider on switching between superiority and non-inferiority. http://www.emea.eu.int/pdfs/human/ewp/048299en.pdf.

13 Tillmann HC, Sharpe N, Sponer G, Wehling M. Does intention-to-treat analysis answer all questions in long-term mortality trials? Considerations on the basis of the ANZ trial. *Int J Clin Pharmacol Ther* 2001;**39**: 205–212.

14 Assmann SF, Pocock SJ, Enos LE, Kasten LE. Subgroup analysis and other (mis)uses of baseline data in clinical trials. *Lancet* 2000;**355**: 1064–1069.

15 Pocock SJ, Assmann SE, Enos LE, Kasten LE. Subgroup analysis, covariate adjustment and baseline comparisons in clinical trial reporting: current practice and problems. *Stat Med* 2002; **21**: 2917–2930.

16 Brookes ST, Whitley E, Peters TJ, Mulheran PA, Egger M, Davey Smith G. Subgroup analyses in randomised controlled trials: quantifying the risks of false-positives and false-negatives. *Health Technol Assess* 2001; **5**: 1–56.

17 Institute of Medicine. Crossing the quality chasm: a new health system for the 21st century. Washington, D.C., National Academies Press, 2001.

18 The state of health care quality: 2003. Washington, D.C.: National Committee for Quality Assurance, 2003.

19 McGlynn EA, Asch SM, Adams J *et al.* The quality of health care delivered to adults in the United States. *N Engl J Med* 2003;**348**: 2635–2645.

20 D'amico G, de Franchis R. Upper digestive bleeding in cirrhosis. Post-therapeutic outcome and prognostic indicators. *Hepatology* 2003;**38**: 599–612.
21 Bernard B, Cadranel JF, Valla D, Escolano S, Jarlier V, Opolon P. Prognostic significance of bacterial infection in bleeding cirrhotic ptients: a prospective study. *Gatsroenterology* 1995;**108**: 1828–1834.
22 Ben Ari Z, Cardin F, McCormick AP, Wannamethee G, Burroughs AK. A predictive model for failure to control bleeding during acute variceal hemorrhage. *J Hepatol* 1999;**31**: 443–450.
23 Moitinho E, Escorsell A, Bandi JC *et al.* Prognostic value of early measurements of portal pressare in acute variceal bleeding. Gastroenterology 1999;**117**: 626–631.
24 Ioannidis JP, Lau J. Completeness of safety reporting in randomised trials: an evaluation of 7 medical areas. *JAMA* 2001;**285**: 437–443.
25 Kjaerdard LL, Villumsen J, Gluud C. Quality of randomised clinical trials affects estimates of intervention efficacy. VII Cochrane colloquium Rome 1999; 57.
26 Guyatt GH, Sackett DL, Cook DJ. Users' guides to the medical literature. II. How to use an article about therapy or prevention. B. What were the results and will they help me in caring for my patients? *JAMA* 1994;**271**: 59–63.
27 Gross CP, Mallory R, Heiat A, Krumholz HM. Reporting the recruitment process in clinical trials: who are these patients and how did they get there? *Ann Intern Med* 2002;**137**: 10–16.
28 Vorobioff J, Groszmann RJ, Picabea E *et al.* Prognostic value of hepatic venous pressure gradient measurements in alcoholic cirrhosis: a 10-year prospective study. *Gastroenterology* 1996;**111**: 701–709.
29 Thompson SG, Higgins JPT. Treating individuals 4. Can meta-analysis help target interventions at individuals most likely to benefit? *Lancet* 2005;**365**: 341–346.
30 Rothwell PM. Treating individuals 2. Subgroup analysis in randomised controlled trials: importance, indications and interpretation. *Lancet* 2005;**365**: 176–186.
31 Higins JPT, Whitehead A, Turner RM, Omar RZ, Thompson SG. Meta analysis of continuous outcome data from individual patients. *Stat Med* 2001;**20**: 2219–2241.
32 Sharp SJ, Thompson SG, Altman DG. The relationship between treatment benefit and underlying risk in meta-analysis. *BMJ* 1996;**313**: 735–738.
33 Altman DG, Schulz KF, Moher D *et al.* The revised CONSORT statement for reporting randomised trials: explanation and elaboration. *Ann Intern Med* 2001;**134**: 663–694.
34 Franchis Rd, Primignani M. Endoscopic treatments for portal hypertension. *Seminars in Liver Disease* 1999;**19**: 439–456.
35 Pagliaro L, D'Amico G, Sørensen TIA *et al.* Prevention of first bleeding in cirrhosis: a meta-analysis of randomised trials of nonsurgical treatment. *Ann Intern Med* 1992; **117**: 59–70.
36 Khuroo MS, Khuroo NS, Farahat KLC, Khuroo YS, Sofi AA, Dahab ST. Meta-analysis: endoscopic variceal ligation for primary prophylaxis of oesophageal variceal bleeding. *Aliment Pharmacol Ther* 2005;**21**: 347–361.
37 Burroughs A, Mezzanotte G, Philips A, McCormick PA, McIntyre N. Cirrhotics with variceal hemorrhage: The importance of time interval between admission and start of analysis for survival rates and rebleeding rates. *Hepatology* 1989;**9**: 801–807.

38 Meijer R, Ihnenfeldt D, Vermeulen M, De Haan R, Van Limbeek J. The use of a modified Delphi procedure for the determination of 26 prognostic factors in the sub-acute stage of stroke. *Int J Rehabil Res* 2003;**26**: 265–270.

39 Gentilini P, Bernardi M, Bolondi L *et al.* The rational use of albumin in patients with cirrhosis and ascites. A Delphi study for the attainment of a consensus on prescribing standards. *Dig Liver Dis* 2004;**36**: 539–546.

40 Guyatt GH, Heyting A, Jaeschke R, Keller J, Adachi JD, Roberts RS. N of 1 randomised trials for investigating new drugs. *Control Clin Trials* 1990;**11**: 88–100.

41 Montori VM, Permanyer-Miralda G, Ferreira-Gonzalez I *et al.* Validity of composite end points in clinical trials. *BMJ* 2005;**330**: 594–596.

42 Talwalkar JA, Kamath PS. An evidence-based medicine approach to β-blocker therapy in patients with cirrhosis. *Am J Med* 2004;**116**: 759–766.

43 D'Amico G, Pagliaro L, Bosch J. Pharmacological treatment of portal hypertension: an evidence-based approach. *Semin Liver Dis* 1999;**19**: 475–505.

44 Bernard B, Grange JD, Khac EN, Amiot X, Opolon P, Poynard T. Antibiotic prophylaxis for the prevention of bacterial infections in cirrhotic patients with gastrointestinal bleeding: a meta-analysis. *Hepatology* 1999;**29**: 1655–1661.

45 Gines P, Uriz J, Calahorra B *et al.* Transjugular intrahepatic portosystemic shunting versus paracentesis plus albumin for refractory ascites in cirrhosis. ss*Gastroenterology* 2002;**123**: 1839–1847.

46 Abraldes JG, Tarantino I, Turnes J, Garcia-Pagan JC, Rodes J, Bosch J. Haemodynamic response to pharmacological treatment of portal hypertension and long-term prognosis of cirrhosis. *Hepatology* 2003;**37**: 902–908.

47 Kamath PS, Wiesner RH, Malinchoc M *et al.* A model to predict survival in patients with end-stage liver disease. *Hepatology* 2001;**33**: 464–470.

48 Ramond MJ, Poynard T, Rueff B *et al.* A randomised trial of prednisolone in patients with severe alcoholic hepatitis. *N Engl J Med* 1992;**326**: 507–512.

49 Forman LM, Lucey MR. Predicting the prognosis of chronic liver disease: an evolution from child to MELD. *Hepatology* 2001;**33**: 473–475.

50 Cowie MR, Jourdain P, Maisel A *et al.* Clinical applications of B-type natriuretic peptide (BNP) testing. *Eur Heart J* 2003;**24**: 1710–1718.

51 Zucker DR, Schmid CH, McIntosh MW, D'Agostino RB, Selker HP, Lau J. Combining single patient (N-of-1) trials to estimate population treatment effects and to evaluate individual patient responses to treatment. *J Clin Epidemiol* 1997;**50**: 401–410.

52 Guyatt GH, Keller JL, Jaeschke R, Rosenbloom D, Adachi JD, Newhouse MT. The n-of-1 randomised controlled trial: clinical usefulness. Our three-year experience. *Ann Intern Med* 1990;**112**: 293–299.

53 Grobbee DE, Hoes AW. Confounding and indication for treatment in evaluation of drug treatment for hypertension. *BMJ* 1997;**315**: 1151–1154.

54 Johnston SC. Identifying confounding by indication through blinded prospective review. *Am J Epidemiol* 2001;**154**: 276–284.

55 Katz MH. Multivariable analysis: a primer for readers of medical research. *Ann Intern Med* 2003;**138**: 644–650.

56 Joffe MM, Rosenbaum PR. Invited commentary: propensity scores. *Am J Epidemiol* 1999;**150**: 327–333.

57 Moss M, Wellman DA, Cotsonis GA. An appraisal of multivariable logistic models in the pulmonary and critical care literature. *Chest* 2003;**123**: 923–928.

58 Teran JC, Imperiale TF, Mullen KD, Tavil AS, McCullough AJ. Primary prophylaxis of variceal bleeding in cirrhosis: a cost-effectiveness analysis. *Gastroenterology* 1997;**112**: 473–482.
59 Arguedas M, Heudebert GR, Eloubeidi MA, Abrams GA, Fallon MB. Cost-effectiveness of screening, surveillance, and primary prophylaxis strategies for esophageal varices. *Am J Gastroenterol* 2002;**97**(9): 2441–2452.
60 Schepis F, Camma C, Niceforo D *et al.* Which patients with cirrhosis should undergo endoscopic screening for esophageal varices detection? *Hepatology* 2001;**33**(2): 333–338.
61 Spiegel BMR, Targownik L, Dulai GS, Karsan HA, Gralnek IM. Endoscopic screening for esophageal varices in cirrhosis: is it ever cost effective? *Hepatology* 2003;**37**(2): 366–377.
62 Luca A, D'Amico G, La Galla R, Midri M, Morabito A, Pagliaro L. TIPS for prevention of recurrent bleeding in patients with cirrhosis: meta-analysis of randomised clinical trials. *Radiology* 1999;**212**(2): 411–421.
63 Rubenstein JH, Eisen GM, Inadomi JM. A cost-utility analysis of secondary prophylaxis for variceal hemorrhage. *Am J Gastroenterol* 2004;**99**(7): 1274–1288.
64 Carbonell N, Pauwels A, Serfaty L, Fourdan O, Levy VG, Poupon R. Improved survival after variceal bleeding in patients with cirrhosis over the past two decades. *Hepatology* 2004;**40**: 652–659.
65 Hanto DW. Reliability of voluntary and compulsory databases and registries in the United States. *Transplantation* 2003;**75**: 2162–2164.
66 Daily P, Kauffman HM. Quality control of the OPTN/UNOS transplant registry. *Transplantation* 2004;**77**: 1309.
67 Karam V, Gunson B, Roggen F *et al.* Quality control of the European Liver Transplant Registry: results of audit visits to the contributing centers. *Transplantation* 2003;**75**: 2167–2173.
68 Marshall WW, Halet RW. Use of a secure Internet web site for collaborative medical research. *JAMA* 2000;**284**: 1843–1849.
69 Thomsen BL, Møller S, Sørensen TIA, The Copenhagen Esophageal Varices Sclerotherapy Project. Optimized analysis of recurrent bleeding and death in patients with cirrhosis and oesophageal varices: Ap-plication of a multi-stage competing risks model. *J Hepatology* 1994;**21**: 367–375.
70 Thomsen BL, Sørensen TIA, The Copenhagen Esophageal Varices Sclerotherapy Project. Analysis of the treatment effect on recurrent bleeding and death in patients with cirrhosis and oesophageal varices: multi-stage competing-risks model compared to conventional methods. *J Hepatology* 1998;**28**: 107–114.

Baveno IV Consensus Statements: Providing Scientific Evidence: RCTs and Beyond

Thorkild I.A. Sørensen, Juan Rodés (Chairpersons), Flemming Bendtsen, Andres T. Blei, Antoine Hadengue, Jenny Heathcote, Francesco Salerno and Jayant Talwalkar

Possible use of per protocol analysis

- In superiority trials, ITT strategies are preferred and PP analysis regarded only as supportive.
- In non-inferiority trials, ITT and PP approaches (if appropriately predefined) may both contribute.
- When PP results differ from ITT results, the population excluded from PP analysis should be scrutinised. The applicability of the intervention may be questioned.

Assessing changes in therapeutic effects with progression of the disease

- To assess how treatment effect may change with disease progression, use interaction tests between outcome predictors and the intervention(s).
- Both unadjusted results and results adjusted for strong outcome predictors should be provided, regardless of baseline comparisons.
- Any subgroup analyses should be predefined, have sufficient power and usually be limited to primary outcome. Otherwise, they are exploratory methods that can help design further studies but should not modify the conclusions of RCTs.

Handling the heterogeneity of RCTs in metaanalysis

- Heterogeneity can be used cautiously to suggest indications for a particular intervention.
- This requires that:
  (a) Differences in trial methodology are not present.
  (b) Clinical source of heterogeneity is identified.
- Stratified analysis of pooled individual data can be done.
  (a) Primary/secondary aims should be defined.
  (b) Plan for statistical analysis should be predefined (including multiple testing).

(c) Subsequent analysis can use the same pooled data as long as the above protocol is followed.

Identification of factors that modify therapeutic effects in a clinically significant way

- Physicians must learn how to identify the factors that most often modify the clinical outcome at variance with the results of RCTs.
- The quality of RCTs (internal and external validity) should be evaluated.
- The internal validity can be assessed according to the CONSORT statement.
- The external validity can be assessed according to a list of variables which define the peculiarity of the trial population: differences in demography, co-morbidities, limitations due to inclusion/exclusion criteria, variability in the schedules and dosages of drugs, usage of interfering drugs, low compliance, duration of treatment.

Approach to the diagnosis and treatment of uncommon cases where evidence from RCT is not forthcoming

- Consensus-driven, clinical protocols are required to define the optimal methods for clinical management of uncommon conditions where RCTs cannot be performed.
- Treatment of uncommon manifestations of portal hypertension with evidence-based medicine awaits the identification of biologically plausible surrogate markers.
- Alternative study designs (clinical databases, N of 1 trials) should be adapted to identify effective treatments for uncommon manifestations of portal hypertension.
- Observational studies of treatment effect require statistical techniques to minimise confounding by indication.

Continuous monitoring of the clinical outcome of treatments in so-called clinical databases

- Development of a database to monitor outcomes is desirable.
- Goals should include monitoring outcome in:
  (a) Three major clinical areas in portal hypertension.
  (b) Specific sub-groups.
- Funding mechanisms should be identified.
  (a) Focus on complications of cirrhosis rather than portal hypertension.
  (b) Selected mix of institutions.

(c) Potential interest from both government and industry for funding such a database.

'Survival analysis' for competing end points other than death

- The Kaplan–Meier plot is often used to estimate the probability of survival free of other end points, for example, variceal bleeding. This produces non-interpretable results that may also be biased. The cause is that analysis using censoring of patients assumes that those who die or reach other competing end points are still at risk for the primary end point, which is not true.
- For this type of analysis, cumulative hazard plots and Cox regression analysis are better.

Need for international collaboration on clinical trials

- Almost all, if not all, RCTs in portal hypertension are underpowered.
- This applies to uncommon but also common types of conditions associated with portal hypertension.
- In cardiology and oncology, very large international – multinational – trials are conducted, so it is feasible!
- We should do the same for solving our problems in management of portal hypertension.

Index